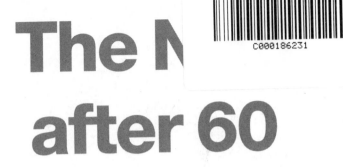

The N
after 60

For patients or profits?

The NHS after 60

For patients or profits?

John Lister

Middlesex
University
PRESS

First published in 2008 by Middlesex University Press

Copyright © John Lister

ISBN 978 1 904750 30 7

A CIP catalogue record for this book is available from
The British Library

Design by Helen Taylor

Printed in the UK by Ashford Colour Press

Middlesex University Press
North London Business Park
Oakleigh Road South
London N11 1QS

Tel: +44 (0)20 8411 4162
Fax: +44 (0)20 8411 4167

www.mupress.co.uk

Author's preface

This book aims both to celebrate the 60th anniversary of the NHS, and to reinforce the underlying values that it represented, which today are under sustained attack from the latter-day Labour Party in a way that few Labour activists would ever have imagined possible even ten years ago.

It takes a historical look at the NHS to show the process that has brought us to the present situation, and to help put the current stance of the major parties in context. Interestingly, both New Labour and the Conservatives under David Cameron are now trying to claim credit for the establishment of the NHS in 1948, and to peddle the line that its formation was the result of a "consensus" after the war.

Not only is this wholly untrue – there was no consensus: the Conservatives repeatedly and consistently voted against the NHS up to and including the final Commons division on the issue in February 1948, less than five months from the launch of the NHS on 5 July – but it obscures the unique and special qualities of the NHS which, thanks to Aneurin Bevan's bold vision and courage, became the most universal and comprehensive of all the public services.

Of course there is no consensus now either, no matter how much New Labour ministers may try to kid themselves. Their policy of carving off profitable slices of the NHS and sponsoring a new private sector remains highly controversial, not least among Labour's core supporters.

Bevan's huge contribution was in sweeping away the failed "market" of voluntary sector, private and municipal hospitals through a nationalisation which proved to be the decisive step in modernising services. The new, unified, tax-funded system was vital as a basis for the systematic training of doctors and nurses, for the development of modern medicine in larger hospitals, and for the closer integration of primary care, community and hospital services. It also made it possible to target resources on areas of greatest health need, regardless of market pressures to do otherwise.

Yet now, 60 years on, we see a New Labour government determined to roll back this historic modernisation, and explicitly hankering back to pre-1948 models (not least in the case of Foundation Hospitals). We see the NHS deliberately fragmented into a new, competitive market, in which a new, government-sponsored private sector is being nurtured at the expense of existing NHS services. We see this market increasingly shaped by the same priorities as the private sector, focusing disproportionate resources on (profitable) services for those with the most minor ailments at the expense of those with complex, chronic or urgent needs for treatment, and working to cash-driven targets that are reshaping today's NHS as "surplus-centred care" rather than patient-centred.

So while this book makes extensive use of historical facts and evidence, it is not primarily a book about the past, but one about the present and future of the NHS. That's why, despite the existence of a number of valuable books charting the origins and history of the NHS, I still felt the need to produce a new one.

This is my third, and by far my most extensive attempt to analyse the history and development of the National Health Service. Twenty years ago, at the peak of the Thatcher government, I was invited by Journeyman Press to write historical chapters and edit chapters from many distinguished contributors, for a volume to mark the 40th anniversary of the NHS. It was rather unwisely entitled *Cutting the Lifeline*, with an even less well-advised scary cover photomontage of Thatcher snipping the oxygen supply to a premature baby in an incubator. The book said many useful things, but the presentation was sufficient to deter many potential readers, while shockingly poor distribution ensured that many who might have been interested remained unaware of the book's existence.

Ten years ago, in collaboration with Professor Colin Francome and Kay Caldwell, I again contributed historical chapters to a volume, more positively presenting the NHS as *The Envy of the World*, and commemorating the 50th anniversary less than a year after Tony Blair's landslide victory. It was published by the NHS Support Federation in 1998.

Some of the information from each of these earlier volumes has been updated in this most recent attempt at an overview and analysis of the changes that have taken place in the NHS as it nears its diamond jubilee.

The NHS has done much more than age over the last ten years – it has been repeatedly reorganised and transformed. The NHS Plan in 2000, coupled with the sustained, year-on-year, above-inflation increases in spending, opened up a whole new direction of policy. That's why the bulk of this new volume, assessing 60 years of the NHS, has had to focus on events and policies of the last seven years, changes which have been inadequately publicised or discussed in the media. It argues that these policies have been implemented despite mounting evidence of public disquiet – and a total absence of evidence that New Labour's so-called "reforms" would assist efficiency, effectiveness or equity in access to services.

The book is not an impartial study, but one that comes from a distinctive point of view. It is detailed and referenced like an academic study, but it is also a campaigner's book. It does not simply rehearse the facts (like Geoffrey Rivett's *From Cradle to Grave,* 1998) or the debates among the policy makers (as Nick Timmins *The Five Giants,* 1995 or Rudolf Klein's *New Politics of the NHS,* 2006) but also goes down to local level to seek examples and experience on how the policies work through in practice.

It presents a consistent critique of the policies, based, especially over the last 25 years, on the experience of analysing, campaigning and arguing against them at the time. This campaigners' eye view also means that the book addresses different issues and discusses in a different way from Julian Tudor Hart's excellent and inspiring *The Political Economy of Health Care* (2006), and allows a fresh look at some of the issues that are also raised in Allyson Pollock's 2005 landmark volume *NHS plc.*

My starting point is that the NHS is under sustained threat, but that as a provider of publicly funded health care the private sector, despite its recent gains and its forward momentum under government patronage, is, as yet, still operating on a very small scale. It has limited ambitions to take over more mainstream NHS work. This means that we the public, as users of the service and as citizens concerned for the future of public services, still have a lot to defend in the NHS. That defence becomes more urgent as the impact of the private sector on existing NHS care continues to widen.

In every aspect of the book I have been able to draw inspiration, material support, and a fund of information from my work since 1984 with London Health Emergency and the many projects which have involved work alongside trade unions and campaigners and research at local, regional or national level. LHE is itself in its 25th year in 2008, and we have been able – despite occasional periods of adversity – to maintain it as a resource for campaigners and the media more than two decades after the demise of the GLC which originally funded it. This is thanks to the continued loyal support of individuals and affiliated trade unions and other organisations across the country. We have attempted to repay this support through a consistent defence of principles, backed up by solid research and information.

More recently, fresh impetus has been generated in health campaigning through the launch in 2005 of the Keep Our NHS Public campaign, inspired and urged on by Allyson Pollock, along with many from the NHS Consultants Association including Peter Fisher, Harry Keen, Jackie Davis, Wendy Savage, Julian Tudor Hart, and many more, and academics including Sally Ruane, as well as drawing in the NHS Support Federation and London Health Emergency.

Despite woefully limited resources, Keep Our NHS Public has established itself as a serious source of information and expertise, with a website boasting briefing papers, a searchable news roundup and much more, and it has given a lead on some legal challenges to the government's privatisation offensive and widened and strengthened the network of campaigners rejecting the market-style policies in the NHS.

It has been a pleasure and an inspiration working with these dedicated campaigners as we all battle to keep the flame alight for the universalist values embodied in Bevan's 1948 National Health Service, and ensure the NHS remains intact through a seventh decade and beyond.

This book is written above all for campaigners, by a campaigner: let's keep our NHS, and let's keep it public!

John Lister, PhD
Oxford, March 20 2008
j.lister@coventry.ac.uk

Acknowledgements
and dedication

While much of the last 20 years has been analysed from first-hand involvement and official documents, I have not attempted to write the early history from primary sources, and I readily acknowledge my reliance on established publications for many of the framework facts and historical detail of the early NHS, notably Nick Timmins (1995) Geoffrey Rivett (1998) and Rudolf Klein (2006).

More recent chapters have also been able to make use of revised versions of my own material, first published in my monthly column in the *Morning Star*.

I must also pay respects to the ongoing efforts of my old mate at London Health Emergency, Geoff Martin, who is still working with me, feeding the press and mass media with the hard facts, data and comment we need to publicise if we are to keep the NHS high on the news agenda week by week.

And I would like to mention a few of the many trade union activists who have most inspired and encouraged me over many years, not least from UNISON: Brian Lumsden, Kevin O'Brien, Nora Pearce, Helen Martin, Mick Griffiths and Adrian O'Malley, Mark Ladbrooke, Caroline Bedale, Frances Kelly, Alun Jennings, Chris Jones, Dennis English and others from Gwent healthcare, and too many more individuals and branches to name, plus a good number of UNISON officials, past and present, at regional and national level, whom I will not embarrass by naming in this list, but who have provided invaluable support and encouragement, through the good times and the bad.

From Amicus-Unite I would single out Ian Rez, Judy Atkinson and Gill George among many long-standing colleagues who have shared information and given solid support. Paul Evans from the NHS Support Federation and Alex Nunns from Keep Our NHS Public also deserve a special mention, but so do so many local campaigners who have kept the flag of protest flying and made it all worthwhile. If your name is not included, please share in this general acknowledgement of your contribution.

I must also note the support I have received from colleagues at Coventry University, both in the School of Art and Design and the Faculty of Health and Life Sciences where I have taught health policy at MSc level for many years.

On the nitty gritty of getting the book published and completed, I owe a massive thank you to Paul Jervis and Celia Cozens from Middlesex University Press for taking it on, and to Matt Skipper, the long-suffering copy-editor for his prodigious efforts in preparing the text for publication and patiently highlighting my errors and omissions. My brother Paul has, as ever, played a vital role in assisting with the production of the index.

Most of all I must thank my wife Sue for 37 years of unswerving support and allowing me the time to complete this book. I also owe her sister, Diane Plamping, a big thank you for persuading me to include a specific chapter on primary care.

And while I am proud and happy to acknowledge so many people as sources of information or inspiration, the final text is mine. So for any errors in fact or analysis, and for any unwitting omissions, I have nobody to blame but myself.

DEDICATION

I would like to dedicate this book to one NHS doctor who has shown me that it is possible to work a lifetime in the "Cinderella" specialty of geriatrics and still emerge as a caring, principled human being, justifiably proud to have witnessed and contributed to some significant, if unsung improvements in the quality of care. He is now my brother-in-law, Dr David Griffith, who retires this month.

Contents

v   Author's preface

ix   Acknowledgements and dedication

INTRODUCTION
1   From NHS to DIY? The decisive modernisation – and today

CHAPTER ONE
11   Bevan tackles the failure of the British health "market"

CHAPTER TWO
23   Consensus under strain: the first 30 years 1948–1979

CHAPTER THREE
49   The end of consensus: the road back to the market 1979–1988

CHAPTER FOUR
75   The first steps into the marketplace 1988–1997

CHAPTER FIVE
113   New Labour – new market? Picking up the pieces 1997–2000

CHAPTER SIX
135   The NHS Plan – Mr Milburn heads back to market 2000–2005

CHAPTER SEVEN
167   Hewitt and Blair crank up the pace 2005–2008

CHAPTER EIGHT
205   National Health Services? The changing model in Scotland, Wales and Northern Ireland

CHAPTER NINE
223   New dimensions in privatisation

CHAPTER TEN
267   The evolution of primary care

CHAPTER ELEVEN
291   The NHS in an international context

CHAPTER TWELVE
303   Into a seventh decade: what have we got left? Alternatives and conclusions

317   References

343   Index

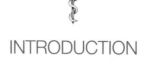

INTRODUCTION

From NHS to DIY? The decisive modernisation – and today

SIXTY YEARS AFTER IT WAS LAUNCHED to a tremendous wave of public enthusiasm and relief, Britain's National Health Service is still far and away the most popular of the public services – a jewel in the crown of welfarism, and very much the envy of billions of people around the world whose health services are less developed, less accessible, more expensive and more exclusive. The NHS has of course expanded massively, advanced technically and clinically, and changed in many respects – most of them for the better. But for much of its six decades, and most especially in the last 20 years, it has remained, as it began in 1948, the subject of furious debate over values, resources and policy.

Perhaps those differences are summed up by the New Year statement from the Prime Minister suggesting that the sixtieth anniversary of the NHS should be marked by adopting a typically New Labour "constitution" defining "rights and responsibilities" – and effectively enshrining and consolidating Tony Blair's controversial counter-reforms, undertaken since 2000. While the notion of a right to health care would be something that many socialists would in principle welcome – one that has been studiously avoided by successive governments since 1948 – any move that might make those rights conditional on lifestyle choices (such as losing weight or giving up smoking) would effectively be a means of restricting entitlement. Similarly, any move to push responsibility for a range of home-based procedures onto patients would raise serious safety issues, and could destroy what is left of the district nursing service – a service already damaged by years of localised NHS cuts, despite the government's stated policy of providing more personalised care in the home. A drive to force patients to manage their own blood pressure, pain control and a range of other procedures could open the door to an all-out assault on district and community nursing budgets. Like so many of New Labour's so-called 'reforms', this threatens to roll back the clock to the bad old days before the NHS, when DIY health care was all most people could access.

There are other contradictions, too. The promise from Gordon Brown and Health Secretary Alan Johnson of more systematic screening programmes to detect potentially life-threatening diseases flies in the face of reductions in local budgets for public health and preventative services over the last two years. And the pressure on GPs to offer primary care services over extended hours has been

1

botched by premature policy announcements – not least by Lord Darzi's ill-advised proposals for polyclinics in London and widespread private sector provision in primary care. These have predictably antagonised many GPs and their organisations, rather than winning their commitment to innovative proposals (Plumridge 2008).

Proposals to give individual patients the funds to buy in their own package of care raise even more questions – over the availability and quality of the care on offer, and the danger that such payments could be an undercover way of avoiding public spending by landing increased bills and responsibility onto individuals and their families. And there are underlying doubts over the transfer of long-term care from the NHS – where it remains free at point of use and collectively funded through taxation – to social services, where care and services have always been subject to means-tested charges (Plumridge 2008).

Most debate on the NHS in its first 60 years has, interestingly, not centred on the "Beveridge" proposal for a government (tax)-funded provision of health care to fill in the gaps left by free-market capitalism: that is now widely recognised (by all but a fringe right wing who favour reviving the private sector) as the most efficient and equitable means of sharing risk across the widest cross section of the population (Wanless 2003; Dixon and Mossialos 2002). There was a need for collective provision of services not only to meet visible health requirements, but also as a basis for British capitalism to secure a fresh social settlement between ruling and working classes in the aftermath of the Second World War. This need became a point of consensus between all three major political parties: Beveridge's report was commissioned by a Tory-led coalition, written by a Liberal and eventually implemented by a Labour government.[1]

Instead, differences have centred on the extent to which Aneurin Bevan's model of a National Health Service effectively superseded the market system, creating within a capitalist society a new type of service, one which has been uniquely based on need rather than on profit and ability to pay – and the extent to which this has been a positive and progressive step.

Critics from the left – not least in Bevan's own party – were concerned from the outset on the level of concessions which Bevan made to the medical profession (GPs and consultants) in order to secure the doctors' acceptance of the new system. His legislation broke with Labour Party policy and with demands that had been raised since 1930 by the left wingers of the Socialist Medical Association (Stark Murray 1971; Stewart 1999). The result has not only been the semi-detached contractor status of GPs and primary care, but the running sore of NHS "pay beds", part-time consultant contracts, and six decades of unresolved conflicts with the medical profession. And the SMA, later the Socialist Health Association, continued to criticise the NHS as little more than a "sickness service", lacking as it did from the outset the occupational health system which

---

1   For a fuller account of the political background to the Beveridge proposals to address the "Five Giants" of Want, Disease, Ignorance, Squalor and Idleness, see Timmins 1995.

socialists had pressed for, and any systematic investment in public health and preventative measures that might yield long-term results in improved health status for the population as a whole.

By contrast, the Conservative right wing has never been able to accept the impact of the changes that were ushered in on 5 July 1948. This includes those who – for whatever reason, be it the hopes of personal profit or advancement, or ideological conviction – have never been properly reconciled to the notion of any public or state responsibility to provide or fund health care. The Conservative Party has always retained this type of backwoods wing, which has always argued against the nationalisation of hospital services and for some form of system based on private sector provision, or health insurance involving greater reliance on individual contributions. Almost 20 years after the NHS was launched the Conservative Shadow Health Minister, Bernard Braine, told the *International Medical Tribune*:

> We could ensure that more is spent on medical care by introducing charges which could be covered in part... or wholly by health insurance... or we could encourage the growth of private medical schemes... we might even look at the possibility of levying a hotel charge for a hospital stay.
>
> (Braine 1967)

Another 20 years later, one of Margaret Thatcher's favourite right wingers, Norman Tebbit, explicitly raised the thorny issue of privatisation, asking, in the midst of one of the worst winter crises ever to hit the NHS:

> Is the present structure of a nationalised hospital service the best way of getting the best and the most patient care out of each pound we spend? Could more provisions be privatised?
>
> (*Guardian*, 16 January 1988)

Almost 20 more years later, it is the tax-funding of the NHS and the elimination of fees for service which rankle the right-wing members of the so-called "Doctors for Reform" group, who explicitly press ministers to roll the wheel of history back towards a new "mixed economy" of health care in which an expanded private sector and extensive use of co-payments and "top-up" payments would become the norm:

> Ever since 1948, when the NHS was first established, no party has had the courage to face up to this challenge. The idea that the system must be fully funded by the taxpayer and remain absolutely free to all patients at the point of use has been sacrosanct for more than half a century, one of the fixed, immovable objects in our constitution.
>
> In a way, the caution of all parties has been understandable, because the British public, not particularly given to devout demonstrations of faith, has treated the NHS as our national religion, not to be tampered with by anyone.
>
> Even Mrs Thatcher, famous for her enthusiasm for rolling back the frontiers of the state, did not dare to touch the NHS. As the present mess proves, however, we cannot go on like this.
>
> (Sikora 2006)

However, the Beveridge consensus and the huge political popularity of the NHS since 1948 have left little room in the UK for the far more extremist notions argued by doctors, academics and others on the American far right. With powerful backing from organisations such as the Heartland Institute, they continue to insist that health care should be viewed and treated like any other commodity or service for sale, and that it should be priced and sold with minimal regulation in a free, competitive market, regarding any form of public or social provision or government intervention to be 'socialism' or even 'fascism' (Aubrey 2001).

Denied any popular base for such fundamentalist views, the political right wing in Britain has instead sought every opportunity over the years to carp at and play upon the all-too-obvious shortcomings of the NHS – the bureaucracy, the waiting lists and inefficiencies which flow, to a large extent, from inadequate investment in premises, equipment and staff. These critics imply – without any real attempt to produce supporting evidence, and with a blind eye firmly closed to the staggering additional costs of apparently more advanced and responsive insurance-based systems in the USA and Germany – that greater privatisation and an insurance-based system would somehow solve all of these problems at little or no extra cost.

Sikora, for example, articulating the mantra of Doctors for Reform, claims – contrary to all the published figures – that health spending in the UK is almost equal to that in France and Germany (Sikora 2006): in fact the UK spending has just crept up to 8 per cent of GDP, while France and Germany have continued to spend well in excess of 10 per cent – and their health systems have consistently over-spent their budgets. And one key factor in that higher spending is that around the world insurance-based systems, especially those embodying a multiplicity of insurance funds, are more complex and costly to administer (Lister 2005a). Tax-funded systems are relatively low in overhead costs, equitable in that they draw contributions linked to the ability to pay, and share risk on the widest possible (and most equitable) basis (Talbot-Smith and Pollock 2006).

Taking an opposing view, sections of the left, often backed up by people who have been mobilised in defence of endangered local services, or who have personal or family recollections of the miseries of life before the NHS, have often taken refuge in a somewhat self-deceptive defence of the 1948 system. It is not uncommon to find such people harking back to an imagined "golden age" of NHS egalitarian values and planning, and as a result downplaying the weaknesses and problems which have always undermined the service, many of which remain unresolved 60 years later.

It is a marked feature of today's NHS, as it enters a seventh decade, that the predominant political force promoting market-style policies, competition and private sector provision of services is no longer the Conservative Party[2] but New

---

2   The Conservatives under David Cameron have astonishingly sought to lay claim to the mantle of the NHS, 60 years after Tory MPs in February 1948 loyally marched once more through the No lobby in the House of Commons, for a third and final time, in a last-ditch bid to halt the formation of the NHS a few months later.

Labour – the contemporary, neoliberal incarnation of the party which in 1948 boldly established the NHS as a break from a discredited and failing "market".

Only New Labour has been able to display a nostalgic affection for aspects of the failed system before the NHS, harking back affectionately to what ministers now portray as "localism" and a period of cooperatives and mutuals, and seeking means to stimulate the emergence of new "third sector" organisations reviving the spirit of "voluntary" work (McCartney 2002; Blears et al. 2002). Yet trade unions between the wars were among those pressing for a tax-funded health service, and Mohan (2003a, b) and Gorsky (2006) have ably exposed the mythology New Labour has created in its attempt to turn back the clock.

The 1948 NHS opened up a new relationship with hospital doctors and with GPs: it also created the conditions for the development of modern medicine and improved access to specialist care for the whole population, with more equal and rational allocation of resources than could ever have been achieved in a market system. But not by any means was all of this possible – or even imagined – at the point where the NHS itself was first launched. For this reason, while it is important to emphasise and celebrate the level of innovation and the turning point that it represented, it is not the intention of this study to portray the NHS of 1948 – or any subsequent year – as a perfect or finished model of a comprehensive and universal health care system.

The NHS emerged from a series of political compromises: it was established on the basis of a financially challenged, shambolic and unplanned mish-mash of public and private services, created in the aftermath of the economic devastation and social turmoil of the Second World War, in a country dependent on massive US loans to avert bankruptcy, and still to undergo another five-or-six years of rationing and shortages of basic goods. The NHS could never have begun perfect. But we should not underestimate the courage of those who took those first crucial steps along a previously uncharted route.

The new NHS cost £402 million in its first year – more than double its allocation of £180 million (Rivett 1998). Ophthalmic services, at £22 million, cost 22 times the projected budget. In a war-ravaged economy, still subject to widespread rationing, the demand for spectacles swiftly outstripped the capacity of the industry to supply them. Bevan had to face up to what then appeared to be unlimited, runaway increases in costs, and explain to his cabinet colleagues that much of this was working people properly accessing services they needed, but could never previously have afforded. On that basis he was proud to boast that – in pretty desperate economic conditions – in its first year the NHS issued 187 million free prescriptions. By contrast, the latter-day incarnation of Bevan's party in government is levying punitive prescription charges of £6.85 per item on low-paid workers in England (the Welsh Assembly, meanwhile, has scrapped prescription charges altogether, with Scotland and Northern Ireland seeking to follow suit).

The British economy's gross domestic product in 1949 was a relatively puny £12.4 billion: in 50 years it increased 63-fold to an estimated £787 billion in

1997–8. Amid this fabulous wealth, the share allocated to NHS spending rose, unevenly, from 3.5 per cent to just 5.6 per cent – leaving it well below the average for most comparable European or OECD countries. In real terms, adjusted to 1993–4 prices, NHS spending rose less than six-fold in 50 years, from £7.9 billion in 1949 to £40.2 billion in 1996–7 (Rivett 1998). There seems little doubt that if the tight-fisted attitude of the 1980s and 1990s had been adopted in 1948, the NHS would never have been established on sufficient scale to win its current pride of place in public affections, regarded as it is by many as the very heart of the welfare state.

Indeed the under-funding, both of capital and revenue, has been one constant through most of the 60 years of the NHS. And partly because of this, a variety of political, social and economic factors have combined to ensure that even though the NHS has expanded and improved, many of the early weaknesses have remained embedded in the growing structure.

But while the 1948 NHS was by no means perfect, it still represented a fundamental, radical and historic break, on a level that is not sufficiently appreciated today. It was a "modernisation" of a completely novel type, in that it superseded the failed "mixed economy" and "market" in health care that had evolved over two centuries of capitalism, and replaced it with a new, alternative system which effectively "decommodified" health care – in a way which never applied to the other industries nationalised after the war, such as railways, coal and steel – even though the framework of British capitalism was left intact, or even strengthened around it.

It is this dynamic, modernising role which means that the core principles of the NHS in 1948 can still offer an attractive and popular rallying point today for those resisting a slide back towards a market-style system, self-help, and greater reliance upon private sector providers. In this sense, the conclusion of this book, and the view held by many campaigners challenging the current direction of government policy, is that the progressive direction for genuine reform would be "back to the future" – back to the first principles which allowed the NHS to break from the chaos and inequality of the market, and back to the sense of public service which has continued to attract the best professionals and most dedicated staff to work in health care.

There is no significant popular public lobby in favour of more private sector involvement or in support of market-style policy reforms: none of New Labour's most loyal supporters in the trade unions endorses these policies. Indeed, the only organised weight of opinion backing such reforms is the private sector which stands to gain from changes which enhance the role of private corporations, the involvement of more private medical providers, the employment of growing numbers of management consultants, and the use of private finance to resource new hospitals, clinics and health centres. New Labour has to decide whether to remodel the NHS to maximise the opportunities for these influential organisations to accumulate profits at the expense of public services, or whether to focus on the needs and views of patients, virtually none of whom have asked for or support the current line of policy.

Most of the following chapters follow a broadly chronological sequence, charting the development of the NHS from its formation, through the years of apparent political consensus, and into the period from 1979 in which that consensus was quite deliberately shattered by the Thatcher government. Of course, we now know that the radicalism of that government in its approach to the NHS was always balanced by Thatcher's strong sense of the political damage that would be suffered by a party that was perceived to be undermining or privatising such a vital, popular and universal public service. Nonetheless, as chapters three and four outline, Thatcher's privatisation of non-clinical support services, restructuring of NHS management, and the "internal market" reforms later implemented under John Major did begin a much more fundamental process which has led in more recent years to an explicit embrace of market-style policies.

Just as the Tory government's policy breaks logically into two distinct phases, prior to and following the introduction of the internal market, New Labour policy has also evolved and changed in three quite distinct phases since 1997. The first saw limited attempts to restrain and replace the internal market, while retaining the "purchaser–provider split". The second phase saw the publication of the NHS Plan and the decision by Blair and Brown to promote a qualitative increase in the funding of the NHS. And the third phase, which began around 2005, marked a rapid acceleration and broadening of the drive towards the privatisation of clinical services and increased reliance upon private sector provision of services, service models and consultancy. It is an indication of how far and how fast New Labour has driven the NHS along this road to a market-style system that the three chapters (five, six and seven) dealing with developments in the eleven years since Tony Blair took office are far longer than the preceding chapters dealing with the first 49 years of the NHS.

The constraints imposed by a largely chronological account make it impossible to do full justice to some of the central themes and issues which have emerged, especially over the last decade. For this reason, a number of thematic chapters explore these in far more detail, beginning, in Chapter eight, with a comparative study of the NHS in post-devolution Wales, Scotland and now Northern Ireland. This helps to highlight the extent to which the more extreme market-style policies and the drive to privatisation have relied heavily on the lack of democratic control over health services in England, compared with the more overt systems of accountability to the Welsh Assembly, the Scottish Parliament and now the Northern Ireland Assembly in Stormont. All of these devolved assemblies have, under nationalist or even Unionist leadership, adopted more traditionally social democratic policies than New Labour in Westminster.

Chapter nine explores "new dimensions in privatisation", New Labour's complex and rapidly developing relationship with the private sector since 1997, and more especially since 2000, with an extended section analysing the Private Finance Initiative and its implications for Trusts and for local health services.

Chapter ten charts the evolution of primary care over 100 years, and questions the wisdom of government policies which appear to be undermining the qualitative elements of primary care and encouraging an ever-greater private sector involvement.

Chapter eleven takes a step back to explore the historical and international context in which the NHS was established. It also discusses the varying political factors which prevented a handful of countries such as the USA along with many colonial countries from joining what was clearly a global movement towards collective and social provision of health care services and sharing of risk in the period after the Second World War.

The final chapter, a discussion of 'alternatives and conclusions', seeks to present an objective balance sheet of the undoubted gains and benefits which have flowed from the establishment and continued expansion of the NHS. This book has only been written because the author is convinced that, whatever the weaknesses and negative recent developments, there is a tremendous amount that health workers and the British people should still feel proud of in the NHS – we still have a lot to lose if current policies are not reversed.

With this in mind, the final section argues that – in a paraphrase of the anti-globalisation protesters and the European and World Social Forum movements – 'Another NHS is Possible'. This alternative would consciously go back to the future, to build on the strengths of the 1948 model, and integrate this with the scientific and technical advances which have opened up new lines of treatment and reduced lengths of stay in hospital; the improvements that have been made in care of older people and care for mental health; and the growing wider awareness of the need to shape health care and health provision to tackle inequalities, discrimination and social disadvantage.

As a final note to this introduction, it is appropriate to recognise some limitations in this study. While many of the examples and the breadth of information flow from the author's active role as a campaigner working with health unions and local community activists over the last 24 years, this also implies weaknesses and areas of unequal and inadequate knowledge. As a result, even at its present length, this book does not pretend to be comprehensive, and has not really tried to be so. Some important areas of health and social care have been left out of the running analysis – most notably learning disabilities. In 1948, this was regarded as firmly a health issue to be dealt with by nurses and doctors in large institutionalised hospitals, but it has been progressively redefined as increasingly a social care issue to be dealt with through social services in community settings. A history of the evolution of this area of care would merit a book-length study on its own, and this author has never been called upon to carry out any systematic analysis of these policies.

Another area of health care which has been inadequately discussed in these pages is dentistry – perhaps one of the greatest failures of the NHS. A large proportion of dental care is now provided outside of the NHS altogether; and even where NHS dentists are still available, the charges have been raised to punitive and unaffordable levels for many on low and even medium wages. Here too, the author's lack of detailed policy research work has impeded any more extended coverage, although the rise and fall of NHS dentistry clearly cries out for investigation as a case study.

Despite these omissions and others, this account of the evolution of the National Health Service over six decades makes no apology for focusing the majority of its attention on the most recent period, and the unprecedented scale and pace of the changes that are taking place even as the book goes to press. For those who value the NHS and wish to celebrate its many strengths there is a real dilemma – whether to stand idly by and watch some of the core strengths of the NHS be undermined by policies promoting a private sector that is exclusive, restricted in scope and driven by profit; or to join those at local and national level, such as Keep Our NHS Public and London Health Emergency, who continue to challenge these policies and uphold the basic values of the NHS.

At root, therefore, the question is: in whose interests should the NHS operate? Who should most benefit from the huge allocation of tax funding which no major party can now propose to reduce? Is this service to be run for patients, or for profits? If the answer is patients, then the great modernising reform of 1948 which scrapped a failed market must become the model for policies in a seventh decade of our most popular and universal public service.

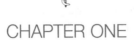

CHAPTER ONE

Bevan tackles the failure of the British health "market"

ALTHOUGH HE WAS PART OF A LABOUR GOVERNMENT which resorted to nationalisation as a means to rescue a variety of flagging and bankrupt industries, Bevan did not invent the idea of government intervention in health care. For more than a century before the NHS, the British experience had increasingly revealed the limitations of private and charitable systems for delivering health services to those who need them most.

Poverty, poor housing and malnutrition generated both ill health and a layer of the population unable to pay even modest fees for health care. The public sector was obliged to fill the resultant growing gap, most notably in the areas of infectious diseases and mental health – which posed a potential public risk, but were beyond the means of charitable efforts. In the final decade of the nineteenth century bed numbers in public infectious hospitals and workhouse institutions increased 85 per cent to reach 154,000 in 1901, almost four times the number (43,000) available in voluntary sector hospitals (Timmins 1995).

From 1906 onwards the governing Liberal Party, facing a growing political challenge from trade unions and the newly formed Labour Party, came under increased pressure to deliver a wider access to health care for workers. The result was Lloyd George's 1911 National Health Insurance Act, which from 1913 instituted compulsory medical insurance for low-paid workers and sections of the middle class.

The scheme covered just one third of the population, and while it provided free care from GPs, free prescriptions, free treatment for TB and sickness benefits, it did not cover children, child birth, or hospital treatment. Nor did it cover wives who did not work, the self-employed, many older people, or higher-paid workers (Abel-Smith 1978). There was a separate system offering free health care for school children, and the poor could only access free care if they consulted a local "poor law doctor".

Inverse Care Law

While the new Act offered a significant increase in fees for GPs, who picked up double what they had previously been paid by trade unions and mutual benefit societies, and were often able to expand their list of patients, there was still more money to be made from private fee-paying patients. Many GPs ran separate

11

waiting rooms for the Health Insurance patients to segregate them from private patients, while others would see private patients only in their own homes. The attraction of the higher incomes from attending to wealthier patients led to huge inequalities in the distribution of GPs – with twice as many GPs per head of population in London compared with South Wales and four times more in Bournemouth than the industrial midlands (Abel-Smith 1978); by 1945 Kensington had seven times more doctors per head than South Shields (Eckstein 1970).

The same pressures also led to massive inequalities in access to hospital services. In the more prestigious voluntary sector hospitals, consultants had honorary, unpaid appointments, and relied for their income on charging private patients, allowing them to treat the poorest free of charge. However as Timmins (1995) points out, this meant that specialist care was available only in areas where there was a sufficient concentration of wealthy patients to pay fees for treatment, while the most deprived areas, with the greatest level of health need, found themselves dependent upon less attractive municipal hospitals.

In both these cases the origins of Julian Tudor Hart's often-quoted "Inverse Care Law" – "that the availability of good medical care tends to vary inversely with the need of the population served" – can be seen in the failed "market":

> In areas with more sickness and death, general practitioners have more work, larger lists, less hospital support, and inherit more clinically ineffective traditions of consultation than in the healthiest areas: and hospital doctors shoulder heavier caseloads with less staff and equipment, more obsolete buildings, and suffer recurrent crises in the availability of beds and replacement staff. These trends can be summed up as the Inverse Care Law: that the availability of good medical care tends to vary inversely with the need of the population served. …

> If our health services had evolved as a free market, or even on a fee-for-item-of-service basis prepaid by private insurance, the law would have operated much more completely than it does: our situation might approximate to that in the United States, with the added disadvantages of smaller national wealth.

> The force that creates and maintains the Inverse Care Law is the operation of the market…. The more health services are removed from the force of the market, the more successful we can be in redistributing care away from its 'natural' distribution in a market economy…

> (Hart 1971)

Tudor Hart, perhaps annoyed by the way in which New Labour ministers and private sector corporations have attempted to exploit the concept as a rationale for privatisation of care in "under-doctored areas"[3] has in recent years stepped back from the Inverse Care Law, describing it recently as a "banal truism" (Hart

---

3 "The Secretary of State for Health, Patricia Hewitt, has said that her goal in encouraging new providers to take on primary care in England is to break the 'Inverse Care Law', which holds that the greater an area's deprivation and need, the poorer the medical services it will have. But Julian Tudor Hart, a research fellow at Swansea University Clinical School, who first

2006: 67). However, the concept has been explored by others in various contexts both at home and on a global level, and found to be a useful, consistent and materialist summary of market failure. On a world scale, too, for example, those who suffer the greatest burden of disease are the poor; and not only are they least in a position to pay a market price for their own health care: their poverty, often reinforced by the social isolation of poor rural populations and social exclusion of the masses in slums and shanty-towns, also results in a lack of political power and influence to press for alternative, progressive systems that could deliver universal health care. On a world scale, the private sector (most notably the for-profit private sector) in health care allocates its resources not according to levels of need for health care, but instead singles out the least complex and risky specialist services and, often, the geographical areas most likely to attract a sufficiently wealthy or well-insured clientele (Lister 2005a).

Inequalities

The "mixed economy" of the health care market continued to display growing gaps and inadequacies in Britain in the early twentieth century. The lack of any proper, systematic coverage of childbirth and young children brought a dreadful and rising toll of avoidable deaths and illness in the 1930s, with increased preventable deaths in childbirth and 2,000 children a year dying of whooping cough.

In 1935, 42 infants per 1,000 died in the relatively prosperous South East, compared with 63 in Glamorgan, 77 in Scotland, 92 in Sunderland and 114 in Jarrow. By 1937, an examination of over 1,600 children in County Durham found less than 12 per cent were free from rickets. TB was killing 30–40,000 young adults each year, with death rates twice as high among the working class (Iliffe 1983).

Many of those most in need found themselves outside of the health care system and unable to access the care they required, but these inequalities also applied to the providers of health care, which were inadequately and unequally funded to an unsupportable degree. It became increasingly obvious that the problems were on such a scale that only government action could hope to plug the gaps.

The hospital system was floundering, being chaotic and hugely under-resourced. As early as 1920, a report from a committee headed by Lord Dawson, commissioned by the newly established Ministry of Health, argued for a nationalised health service. Dawson suggested a system in which primary care should be delivered from centres rather than by single-handed GPs, and should be linked to district-level hospitals and regional centres with university teaching hospitals (Rivett 1998).

---

described the Inverse Care Law in 1971, said Ms Hewitt misunderstood his theory. 'Politicians love one liners, but they've missed the second line: that this is a market effect, and any return to the market will make it worse.'" (Dyer 2006)

In 1926, a Royal Commission on the National Health Insurance system also concluded that health services should be directly financed from public funds. By 1930 even the British Medical Association had joined the call for wider provision and called for national health insurance provision. And by the mid-1930s the state hospital sector, which had continued to grow much faster than the voluntary sector, accounted for around 80 per cent of the nation's total hospital beds (Taylor 1984).

From 1937 onwards, with the looming threat of war, gaps were identified in the hospital system which again only the public sector could fill. An Emergency Medical Service (EMS) was established, organised on regional lines to facilitate better planning (Rivett 1998). By October 1939 the government had funded almost 1,000 new operating theatres and tens of thousands of additional beds in prefab "annexes" – some of which lasted until the dawn of the new millennium.

The list of those eligible for free treatment was extended to give 43 per cent of the adult population cover from a "panel" doctor by 1938 – leaving only the elderly and some other groups outside the new system (Timmins 1995: 103, 107). The first elements of a national blood transfusion service were created in 1939, run by the Medical Research Council, while a more developed service took shape from 1946, opening up the possibility of more advances in surgery and other forms of treatment (Rivett 1998).

Voluntary hospitals

By this point there were 1,334 voluntary hospitals, ranging from 500-or-more beds in the big teaching hospitals to a mere handful in many cottage hospitals (with an average size of 68 beds). The Goodenough Report in 1942 argued that a medical school admitting 100 students a year needed access to 950–1,000 acute beds – far more than the number available in most of the existing teaching hospitals (Rivett 1998). Any expansion would require government intervention and public funds.

The teaching hospitals also demonstrated the huge inequalities in access to specialist care: 12 of the 23 teaching hospitals, and all nine of the postgraduate teaching hospitals, were in London. So too were many of the most advanced municipal hospitals (Rivett 1998). To make matters worse, medical education was held back by the fact that most specialists had to make their living from private practice, leaving little time for either teaching or research: it was not until salaried staff were employed by academic clinical units that this limitation could be overcome (Rivett 1998).

But the funding base of the voluntary hospitals had changed dramatically since the turn of the century: just 33 per cent of their income arose from gifts and investments in 1938, compared with 88 per cent in 1891, while almost 60 per cent of income now came from payments from patients, whether paid "out of pocket" or through some form of insurance: in other words the voluntary hospitals had become private hospitals in all but name. And by the end of the 1930s many were in deep financial problems and seeking support from the Ministry of Health (Timmins 1995; Rivett 1986).

The financial crises of the voluntary hospitals had deepened still further by the end of the war: the newly appointed Minister of Health Aneurin Bevan was advised that any attempt to rescue them would involve heavy state subsidies equivalent to 80–90 per cent of the hospitals' income. Bevan concluded that this, together with the problem of controlling the ramshackle hospital system and creating a basis to plan services in a new national system, tipped the balance in the argument towards the nationalisation of both the voluntary and municipal hospitals as part of a National Health Service – bringing the "extinction" of the voluntary hospital sector (Timmins 1995: 116).

While the Conservatives focused much of their campaign against the National Health Service Bill on defending the voluntary hospitals, Bevan was not among those who lamented their demise. He made clear his disapproval of their fund-raising flag-days, begging bowls at the end of each ward and reliance upon the benevolence of a self-selecting group of wealthy and aristocratic patrons:

> I believe it is repugnant to a civilised community for hospitals to have to rely upon private charity. I believe we ought to have left hospital flag days behind. I have always felt a shudder of repulsion when I have seen nurses and sisters who ought to be at their work, or students who ought to be at their work, going about the streets collecting money for the hospitals.
>
> (*Hansard* 1946)

According to the amendment tabled by the Conservative opposition, the new NHS:

> gravely menaces all charitable foundations by diverting to purposes other than those intended by the donors the trust funds of the voluntary hospitals.

In fact the nationalisation was to lift the burden of debt from the teaching and voluntary hospitals, but leave their trust funds intact. Bevan hit back, arguing strongly that:

> The only voluntary part of hospital service destroyed by the Bill is the necessity to sell flags and to collect money. Honourable Members opposite, as they represent the party of property, always imagine that the only voluntary act which has any sanctity behind it is the writing of a cheque.
>
> (*Hansard* 1946)

Municipal hospitals

The municipal hospitals, on the other hand, had their origins in poor-law provision for the poor and chronic sick, and some dated back to the early 1800s. Some developed more intensive treatment facilities or "infirmary" sections that employed medical staff and provided facilities for diagnostic tests.

In 1929 the Local Government Act placed 150 counties and county boroughs in charge, replacing the previous boards of guardians: funding was to come 60 per cent from local rates and 40 per cent from central government. The municipal hospitals remained relatively large units, mainly caring for the elderly and chronic sick, and others purely focused on mental illness.

By 1930 only three local authorities were running general hospitals. However, in parts of London and other centres some local authorities were beginning to take advantage of their new powers to invest and expand the hospitals as modern acute hospitals: some were purpose built as such in the 1930s and were able to recruit high-quality specialist medical staff. Access to beds was means-tested, and subject to charges for those deemed able to pay – although relatively small amounts were raised through patient fees (Timmins 1995).

In many areas, however, the municipal hospitals tended to be the "dumping ground" for patients deemed too difficult or expensive for the voluntary hospitals to accept – such as terminal cancer patients, and those with infectious diseases, for which local authorities had primary responsibility: almost 33,000 municipal hospital beds were in TB sanatoria, with 23,000 deaths from TB and 52,000 new cases in 1947 (Rivett 1998).

As with the voluntary hospitals, many of the municipal hospital buildings were extremely old, unsuitable, and poorly maintained. By 1945 two-thirds of all hospital buildings were over 50 years old and over 20 per cent dated back to before 1861. Many had steam heating systems installed around 1900, with boilers having a life expectancy of 50 years (Rivett 1998: 5).

Not only was the capital stock aged and in need of renewal, there was no coherent system linking the voluntary and municipal hospitals, or allocating resources according to need. In many areas municipal hospitals ran without specialist medical staff, and surgery was a sideline pursued (and jealously defended) by GPs, often self-taught. There was just one gynaecologist and no radiologist in Lincolnshire, for example. In Rotherham, Rivett reports:

> GPs objected to the appointment of full-time surgeons, but examination of their results showed that four prostatectomies had been carried out the previous year, only two of the patients leaving hospital alive.
>
> (Rivett 1998: 27)

Several hundred local authorities ran a variety of services with varying levels of quality and investment: councils were responsible for the medical service in schools, some home nursing, and ante- and post-natal care, while most births were under the care of midwives at home (Timmins 1995: 107).

The various elements of the health care market were therefore conflicting and competing unproductively against each other, leaving huge gaps in care affecting vulnerable sections of the population, while there was a total absence of overall responsibility or planning – a situation which only government intervention and the creation of a new system could remedy.

It is also interesting to note that mental health services have also always depended primarily upon public sector support. The main provision from the beginning of the nineteenth century was the network of large-scale county asylums: provision for mental health was made a mandatory duty of county councils from 1845, and by 1930 there were 98 asylums – some very large, with over 2,000 patients – accommodating a total of around 120,000 patients in England and Wales (Ham 1999, citing Jones 1972).

The nationalisation of the municipal hospitals brought mental health services into the new NHS, but the integration was far from instant or willing, and these services have remained at the neglected fringe of public sector health care through successive governments, restructurings and reforms to the present day.

Health and local government

The Bevan scheme for the new NHS was strongly driven by the desire to avoid any formula that gave control over health services (and especially GP services) to local government. There was a political argument against giving such powers to local government, but also a strong pragmatic argument: after negative experiences in the early decades of the twentieth century of working under the less-than-friendly direction of Medical Officers of Health, GPs in particular were strongly opposed to any formula which would place them as salaried employees of local government or "civil servants" (Timmins 1995).

Bevan's approach was a breach of Labour Party policy, which had argued for greater municipalisation but not for nationalisation. The Socialist Medical Association (SMA) had for years set the line of Labour policy, calling for GPs to be salaried employees working from health centres; and there had been a general expectation among all parties that any national health system would – like the municipal hospitals – be controlled by local councils.

Criticism from within Bevan's own government colleagues and Party centred on two issues: the vexed question of who was to control the new system, and how, if at all, it would be locally accountable; and the left-wing allegations by the SMA that Bevan's concessions to the medical profession had also diluted and discarded much existing Labour Party policy on private practice.

Herbert Morrison, a former leader of the London County Council, led the calls for the new service to be run by local government, opposing the system of appointed hospital boards which Bevan proposed should be accountable directly to him, and through him to Parliament (Timmins 1995).

In what proved a tellingly accurate forecast of the ossification of the new network of quangos, Morrison warned that:

> Subject to the Minister's directions on all questions of policy, finance, establishments and so on… they will be mere creatures of the Ministry of Health with little vitality of their own.

> (Timmins 1995: 117)

Bevan responded with some justification that leaving the new service in the hands of local authorities would lead to serious inequalities, and then added the killer argument that if the Minister of Health had to remain answerable for the policies implemented at local level, then he had to have some control over who was appointed to the boards taking these decisions.

Bevan eventually won the backing of the cabinet for his position, which – despite repeated and strident calls over the years for elected health authorities from the Socialist Health Association and others on the left in the unions and Labour Party – has shaped the internal structures of the NHS to the present day.

The deal with the doctors

However, other critics on the left of the party were less than happy with Bevan's series of concessions both to consultants and GPs, which were clearly incorporated as a means to secure their support and participation in the new NHS.

The consultants were the first to agree to Bevan's plans, encouraged by the development for the first time of a national career structure and salary scale. These would open up the possibility of recruiting consultants to some of the less attractive provincial hospitals. Bevan moreover agreed to allow them to maintain a limited level of private practice and for the incorporation of private beds in NHS hospitals. A crowning final touch was the allocation of an additional annual fund, to be distributed as substantial "merit payments" to consultants, by a secretive panel of medics.

The market system had left hospitals terribly stunted in development: by 1946 just half of the country's 3,000 acute hospitals had 50 beds or more,[4] and only 350 had over 200. The NHS would have to expand the availability of specialist services, and to ensure that the consultants were as fully engaged as possible with the new service (Timmins 1995).

Bevan made no secret of the concessions he made both to the consultants and then repeatedly to the GPs. In a further parliamentary debate on 9 February 1948 to endorse the Act – in which once again the Tory Party voted against it – he spelled out the situation:

> These negotiations have been a long series of concessions from us, and not one from the medical profession – not a single one. Indeed, one member of the Negotiating Committee boasted that during these negotiations they had not yielded a single inch.
>
> Consider what we have done. Consider the long record of concessions we have made. First of all, in the hospital services we have accorded paid bed blocks to specialists, where they are able to charge private fees. We have accorded, in addition to those fees for those beds which will have a ceiling, a limited number of beds in the hospitals where there is no ceiling at all.
>
> I agree at once that these are very serious things, and that, unless properly controlled, we can have a two-tier system in which it will be thought that members of the general public will be having worse treatment than those who are able to pay. That is a very grave danger, and it is a very serious and substantial concession made to the medical profession.
>
> We have also conceded that general practitioners and specialists can have private patients. That was repugnant to many of my honourable Friends. They hated it, because they said at once that we can have, if we are not careful, a revival of the

---

4   Interestingly, private hospitals have persisted with the model of very small hospitals, focused upon low-risk elective treatment, requiring minimal provision of intensive care or out-of-hours medical cover. The average size of the largest chain of private hospitals in England is just 50 beds: all of the core work of modern medicine is delivered elsewhere, by large-scale NHS hospitals delivering a comprehensive mix of emergency and elective treatment.

old Poor Law system, under which the man who does not pay does not get the same treatment as the man who does.

This kind of propaganda contains the possibility of developing that atmosphere. I would warn honourable Members opposite that it is not only the British working class, the lower income groups, which stands to benefit by a free health service.

Consider very seriously the tradition of the professional classes. Consider the social class which is called the 'middle class'. Their entrance into the scheme, and their having a free doctor and a free hospital service, is emancipation for many of them. There is nothing that destroys the family budget of the professional worker more than heavy hospital bills and doctors' bills. There is no doubt about that at all, and if honourable Members do not know it, they are really living in another world.

I know of middle class families who are mortgaging their future and their children's future because of heavy surgeons' bills and doctors' bills. Therefore it is absolutely vital, not only for the physical good health of the community, but in the interests of all social groups, that they should all be put in the system on 5 July and that there should not be some in and some out of the scheme.

(*Hansard* 1948)

General practice

The main opposition to Bevan's proposals was led by the general practitioners, then the driving force of the BMA and, as Timmins (1995) points out, very much dominated by the more prosperous and conservative layer of GPs who were able to make enough money to spare the time to attend BMA meetings and conferences. They interpreted Bevan's plan for them to be paid a basic salary topped up with capitation fees for the patients on their list as a move to make them into "civil servants", threatening their clinical and professional independence. They were less unhappy with his offer of a generous £66 million handout as compensation for ending the buying and selling of practices when GPs retired.

There had indeed been long-standing calls for general practice to be made a full-time salaried service. However, Bevan's proposals, which would leave GPs as semi-detached independent "contractors", were very similar to plans which had been drawn up and adopted by the BMA itself three years earlier (Timmins 1995; Rivett 1998).

Nevertheless there were prolonged and often acrimonious negotiations. One prominent BMA member, Dr Alfred Cox (who was later to be persuaded of the Bevan proposals) branded the health minister as some form of "national socialist" in the *British Medical Journal*:

I have examined the Bill and it looks to me uncommonly like the first step, and a big one, towards National Socialism as practised in Germany. The medical service there was early put under the dictatorship of a 'Medical Fuehrer'. This Bill will establish the Minister of Health in that capacity.

(cited in Timmins 1995: 119)

The BMA had long favoured an extension of National Health Insurance to cover 90 per cent of the population, leaving the more prosperous 10 per cent as the basis for continued private practice: but amid the debates over the shape of a new National Health Service it changed its line in July 1942, and pressed for the whole population to be covered. As Timmins points out, the implication of this was that doctors would for the first time ever become entirely dependent upon public funds – private practice would wither away, leaving GPs effectively facing the dreaded status of "civil servants" (Timmins 1995: 111).

The final concessions which tipped the balance of GP opinion in the final weeks before the launch of the NHS in 1948 involved Bevan's amendment to the legislation to forbid the introduction of a full-time salaried GP service without a further specific Act of Parliament, and the promise that if GPs felt their independence was compromised by the £300 per year flat-fee retainer that was part of their package as independent contractors to the NHS, they could hand the money back (Timmins 1995).

As his speech above demonstrates, Bevan knew that in the concessions that he made to create a basis for the medical profession to come in to the new NHS, he was reinserting elements of the market system: and he recognised that if the concessions were allowed to get out of hand the new structure could be derailed – into a two-tier service and a reconstitution of private practice. As NHS historian Charles Webster has pointed out, Bevan knew that if he failed to win and keep the consultants, the result would be "a rash of private nursing homes all over the country", while the GPs, too could be lured back towards private practice (Webster 1991: 73). However, Bevan also knew that he could count on the overwhelming popularity of the new NHS and the eagerness of much of the population to gain access to health care services that had for generations been beyond their reach. This created a favourable political balance of forces.

Even though almost 26,000 BMA members voted in a May 1948 ballot to oppose the Act, many of them were already signing up to work for the NHS by the end of that month. In July, the NHS was launched with 75 per cent of the population already on the list. By September this had reached 93 per cent (almost 40 million people), and soon after the figure hit 97 per cent. In its first two months 18,000 GPs signed up, out of a possible 19,600 in the whole of Great Britain. By October Bevan told a meeting of the Executive Councils Association that over 80 per cent of dentists (8,000 from a maximum 10,000) had signed up, and that a million people had received dental treatment in the first two months of the NHS. The new service immediately came under a huge strain as it grappled with a vast backlog of unmet need for medical attention.

For millions of women, for children, for the unemployed and the elderly and disabled – the forgotten people of previous schemes – the new system, which required no means test, no weekly stamp, no qualifying period and no prior enrolment on a 'panel', offered for the first time a remedy for ailments and discomfort.

No capital for investment

However, there was one immediate downside even as the new NHS was launched: in the dire economic conditions it was clear that there would not be the funds available to commence the promised wave of building new health centres to bring together GP practices and improve the range of services. One or two show-piece health centres were eventually built, but this shortage of capital investment also coloured the development of secondary care: no new hospitals were built until the 1960s. The new NHS was obliged to make do and mend, delivering health care in aged and dilapidated buildings for at least another two decades.

But while the nationalisation of what had evolved as a completely unplanned variety of thousands of voluntary and municipal hospitals established a potential to plan and organise a service, that potential depended above all on the ability to renew and upgrade the capital stock – and no resources for this existed. For over 20 years most of the NHS hospital premises remained where they had been on 5 July 1948 – an allocation which as discussed above flowed from the Inverse Care Law rather than any rational response to patterns of patient need for care. Large areas of deprivation and newly emerging centres of population lacked adequate primary care and hospital services, and big fights had to be waged for hospitals to be built in some of the "new towns" that sprang up in the Home Counties and in new dormitory towns around the country.

Unfair shares

The new NHS was no longer a market – but nor was there a sufficient allocation of available resources and supplies to allow it to be a planned system intervening at local, regional or national level to switch or increase resources to match needs.

So great had been the gaps in the previous market system that nobody had any clear idea what the costs would be of running a universal and comprehensive system. The first year's budgets, based on projections from spending patterns in the previous year, were overspent well before the end of the year. But these spending patterns, too, replicated the problems of the Inverse Care Law.

There were no democratic levers to help rectify the inequalities. Changes had to flow through the government at national level: there was little or no mechanism to alter the balance of provision or resources in a locality. The 1948 NHS was structured around 14 new Regional Hospital Boards overseeing a network of more local Hospital Management Committees, while the Teaching Hospitals, run by their own boards, would answer directly to the Ministry – a model later used by Conservative Health Secretary Kenneth Clarke as the basis for NHS Trusts in the 1990s. Bevan was at pains to argue that there should be only a "light touch" from the centre and at regional level, leaving maximum discretion to the most local bodies – which many were happy to see as a mandate for little or no change on the status quo (Rivett 1998).

Bevan had avoided falling into the trap of handing power to local and county councils – but at the expense of establishing a new network of unelected quangos which would deny local people any significant voice in the planning and allocation of services. The scale of the inequalities in the distribution of services and allocation of resources was to some extent obscured at first by the publication only of aggregated data from the whole of the new NHS, with no local figures to reveal who got what. And for many of the poorest, and for women and older people excluded for years from the possibility of accessing health care, the availability of any services at all – even if they were unequally distributed – seemed like a historic relief.

To plan – or not to plan?

There was another way in which Bevan's 1948 NHS broke from the previous, failed, market system. As Timmins (1995) argues, Bevan's reforms followed the broad outlines of proposals put forward back in 1939 by the Ministry of Health's Chief Medical Officer Sir Arthur McNalty. He had far-sightedly pointed out that the establishment of a national hospital service was a "revolutionary change" – and one that would imply a sizeable change of role for the Ministry, from a largely passive regulator and supervisor of services into a more decisive executive body:

> Hitherto, we have always worked on the assumption that the Ministry of Health was an advisory, supervisory and subsidising department, but had no direct executive functions.

> (cited in Timmins 1995: 109)

This dynamic towards greater central control was restricted from the outset by material shortages – of money, equipment, supplies. But the recognition of the need for firm government intervention to drive forward the development of a national service runs in sharp contrast to more recent structural "reforms" to the NHS since 2000. These reforms, following the "NHS Plan", have aimed at separating the "commissioning" role from the provision of health services at local and national level. This is intended to create a new competitive "market" in which a variety of public, private and "third sector" providers compete for contracts. In other words the most recent pattern of "modernisation" effectively looks back to the pre-1948 situation in Britain – and threatens to roll back the great modernisation which Bevan managed to achieve.

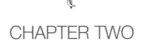

CHAPTER TWO

Consensus under strain:
the first 30 years 1948–1979

WHATEVER ITS FAULTS, THE NEW NHS PROVED IMMEDIATELY and lastingly popular, for good reasons. It represented a historic stride forward, a bold experiment which was at once the "envy of the world". As Rudolf Klein points out in opening *The new politics of the NHS*:

> It was the first health system in any Western society to offer free medical care to the entire population. It was, furthermore, the first comprehensive system to be based not on the insurance principle, with entitlement following contributions, but on the national provision of services available to everyone. It thus offered free and universal entitlement to State-provided medical care. At the time of its creation it was a unique example of the collectivist provision of health care in a market society.
>
> (Klein 2006: 1)

Health care in Britain was no longer operating as a conventional "market", and much of the private component of the pre-war "mixed economy" had been eclipsed, or vanished altogether beneath the flood-tide of enthusiasm for the new NHS. The NHS between 1948 and the 1980s has been recently described by Hart (2006) as a "gift economy". Hart outlines nine unique characteristics of the NHS, three of which (points 2, 4 and 5) are especially relevant here:

> It was a gift economy including everyone, funded from general taxation (of which the largest component was income tax), neither a contributory insurance scheme nor a commodity economy funded by consumers in an open market.
>
> ...
>
> Its products were potentially measurable as health gain for the whole population, not as processes acquired by individual consumers.
>
> Its staff and component units were not expected to compete for market share, but to cooperate to maximize useful service. Commercial secrecy had no function and became unthinkable.
>
> (Hart 2006: 9)

This concept of cooperation was perhaps the sharpest contrast with the chaotic period prior to 1948: to take one obvious example, in local areas, Hospital Management Committees were able for the first time to link up the work of the various local hospitals which had previously worked separately, forming district networks opening up the possibility of expanding specialist services and delivering care beyond the scope of any of the smaller hospitals before 1948.

The reduction in the burden of infectious diseases such as TB from 1950 onwards also enabled many of the beds that had been devoted to this area of care to be reallocated (Ham 1999). The larger management units were able to recruit new specialists, and numbers of hospital consultants began to grow, along with new methods and a new national framework for training consultants and hospital doctors.

Held back by the past

However, the NHS itself was still operating within a capitalist economy which was very much part of a market system at home and abroad. It was not so much the innovative elements of the NHS which held back the development of the system, but the extent to which in many areas it was still hedged about, inside and out, by hangovers of days gone by, the old boards of establishment worthies, backwards-looking medical men, and of course the capitalist market system.

As an island of socialist values, with no established alternative network of supplies, the NHS needed to be sustained by constant deliveries from the capitalist "mainland". This was to the profound irritation of socialists in and outside the NHS workforce, who lamented the contradiction of cash constraints in the NHS itself while lavish, guaranteed profits were increasingly to be notched up by its main suppliers.

Other problems flowed from the many compromises that had been made by Bevan as he sought to push through his ambitious reform by disarming as well as defeating his opponents. From day one, because of the character of the hospitals and facilities it had taken over, and because there was no additional capital investment, the NHS was centralized but unplanned and under-resourced. Sir George Godber commented that the new NHS was stuck with hospitals that were mostly old, defective in structure and in the wrong locations, and required not only:

> to waste effort maintaining service with inefficient plant, but also… to spend what little capital there was making these bad old units usable for modern treatment.
>
> (cited in Webster 2002: 40)

The NHS also lacked either central control or any form of democratic accountability to local communities, to patients or to health workers. Even the managerial apparatus and expertise was lacking for this centralized system that was still in essence "an experiment in administration" (Webster 1988: 121). The new system combined an element of decentralization "to preserve a sense of local responsibility" but in a manner carefully designed to avoid any direct accountability to local government or an elected authority. The governing boards had been opened up to allow participation by senior doctors, but all other health workers were very firmly excluded from the beginning.

Other important elements were also lacking from the outset. There was no provision for the occupational health schemes so long advocated by the Socialist Medical Association as a key component of a system of prevention and health promotion (Thunhurst 1982). And for years there were virtually none of the new-style health centres for which the SMA had lobbied so hard and so long. Nor was there any plan to improve health or promote health education.

Outsiders: primary care and community services

The provision of primary care remained hugely unequal, and despite the establishment of a Medical Practices Committee which attempted to prevent still more doctors setting up practice in well-provided (generally prosperous) areas, there was no mechanism to fill the vacancies in under-doctored parts of the inner cities and rural areas (Ham 1999; Rivett 1998). The overt hostility of most GPs in the run-up to the launch of the NHS left them increasingly marginalised in what developed as an increasingly hospital-dominated, consultant-led service, with priorities emphasising intervention rather than prevention, and acute care over services for the chronic sick.

But among the hospital doctors, too, there was evidence of a continued hierarchy, in which the less glamorous fields of mental health, mental handicap (learning difficulties) and care of the elderly were marginalised. Most community services – maternal and child welfare, health visiting, home nursing, vaccination and immunisation, and even ambulance services – were still run by local authorities, and were in this way cut even further adrift from the hospitals they ought to have complemented. This early obstacle to an integrated health care system has been explained away as a necessary compromise to avoid creating too large and unmanageable a service in one go: but there was a heavy price to pay.

The "second class" status it gave community services in the wider forum of health service planning has never been overcome. Even after these services were brought into the NHS they remained at the back of the queue for resources, while to this day every period of financial stringency has led first of all to cutbacks in the relatively low-profile and under-valued community services (Lister 2007a, 2007g).

Among NHS staff the elitism and male domination of the medical profession created a sharp differentiation between the vast army of low-paid workers (mainly women) who provided the day-to-day nursing and support services to patients, and the doctors and management, most of them white men. For many years this combination led to preventative and health promotion measures affecting women receiving especially low priority (Thunhurst 1982; Doyal 1985).

---

5   For a detailed study of twenty-first century cutbacks in Suffolk and East Anglia, for example, see Mandlestam (2007).

A network of quangos

The management challenge in establishing the NHS was considerable, but the structure of the service was also ramshackle from day one. In England and Wales, 15 new Regional Health Boards were established, each centred on a university with a medical school; but the teaching hospitals themselves were separately administered by boards of governors, and only answerable to the Ministry of Health. London, with its concentration of teaching hospitals, was deliberately carved up between four different Regional Boards, reaching deep into the home counties and out to the coast. Other hospitals or groups of hospitals were run by 388 Hospital Management Committees, leaving the hospital network itself in theory linked up across voluntary and municipal hospitals, but in practice still often divided into rival interest groups. Extra divisions and complications arose because the psychiatric hospitals, which had been run by local authorities, insisted on preserving their independence and were grouped into separate HMCs.

There were also real limitations on these new boards and committees which Bevan appointed to run the NHS. He had himself scathingly exposed the myth of "local responsibility" in the old voluntary hospitals, whose boards of governors he denounced as "a patchwork quilt of local paternalism", elected by nobody and accountable only to themselves: this style of organization, declared Bevan, is "the enemy of intelligent planning". He was equally contemptuous of the emotional commitment of the voluntary hospital boards, arguing that "warm gushes of self-indulgent emotion are an unreliable source of driving power in the field of health organization" (Bevan 1952). Yet when he came to appoint his new bodies, many of these same paternalists were simply drafted in, perhaps switching hats but still retaining a degree of unaccountable control over local hospital and health services.

Primary care – including the GPs who had taken the lead in opposing the new NHS and demanding independence from it, but also dentists, pharmacists and opticians – was run separately as the Family Practitioner Service, directed by their own Executive Councils. Executive Councils had the task of trying to coordinate the efforts of 18,000 determinedly individualistic GPs, almost all of them men – half of them working in single-handed practices, many from their own homes (Rivett 1998). Primary care facilities were no more modern than the hospitals. Eighty per cent of GP surgeries in working class areas – and half of those in the more prosperous areas – were 50 years old or more.

Each section of the NHS was responsible to the Ministry of Health, but none of the controlling bodies was responsible to its local electorate or to consumers of the service. Most health workers, too, were excluded from any part of the decision-making process, with only the handful of doctors appointed to boards or committees able to bring any frontline experience to bear.

Since then, every reform of the NHS has left this structure of appointment (and the resultant potential for patronage) intact. Indeed it was reinforced by the Conservative government's 1990 reforms, which drastically reduced the size of health authorities and in the process removed the four local authority representatives. These were generally councillors, and the "trade union member" – in other words all those closest of any of the HA members to having been elected to represent local people. In 2003 New Labour went further down the line of reduced accountability when it finally axed the Community Health Councils, which in many areas had since 1974 been the statutory body representing the consumer, and the nearest thing to a democratic voice for local people on NHS issues.

The pattern has continued into a new century, although New Labour has in general been somewhat more reluctant than their Tory predecessors to stuff the latest quangos (Trust boards, Primary Care Trusts and Strategic Health Authorities, each of which now pay substantial fees to their appointed part-time chairs and "non-executive" members) with their own party faithful and hangers-on. The most recent reorganization of the NHS saw a merger of Strategic Health Authorities to leave just ten covering England, none of them in any way elected or accountable to the millions of people living in their catchment areas. London's SHA, for example, now known as 'NHS London', controls a budget of more than £11 billion in 2007–8, has extensive powers, and spans a population of 7.2 million people – almost the population of Wales and Scotland combined; but while these countries within the UK enjoy devolved power to decide their own health policies through an elected Assembly and the Scottish Parliament, Londoners have no such influence over their own health care.

Hospitals

The HMCs took over 1,143 voluntary hospitals comprising 90,000 beds (average size 79 beds), and 1,545 municipal hospitals with about 390,000 beds (190,000 of which were beds for mental illness and mental handicap), many of them in extremely large, institutional, often Victorian buildings. Almost half the local authority and voluntary hospitals were over 50 years old, and 20 per cent were built before 1861. As well as being old, many of the buildings were in a shocking state of neglect, and most of the hospitals were very small, limiting their ability to provide modern treatment, afford modern equipment, or to incorporate a wider range of specialist services (Rivett 1998).

Even if there had been a plan for development and modernisation – which there wasn't – there were no extra resources available to fill the gaps by building new hospitals. Building materials were initially still in short supply, but so was capital – with a national allocation of just £10 million a year – and it was not until the mid-1950s that serious attention was devoted to the need for new hospitals, and not until the 1960s that serious cash was invested to make these schemes work. The 1950s were to see the slowest growth in hospital building for over 100 years, with the first new district general hospital the Queen Elizabeth II, opened by the Queen in Welwyn Garden City… in July 1963, 15 years after the launch of the NHS (Webster 2002: 41).

Cash pressures were there from the very outset, despite the fact that before the war health services had received an exceedingly low level of investment as a share of national wealth, with health and welfare budgets combined adding up to just 1.8 per cent of GNP in the 1930s – the sort of levels of the poorest developing countries in recent years (Gough cited in Webster 1988: 12; Lister 2005a). In 1946 the NHS was expected to cost £110 million a year. By the end of 1947 this estimate had been increased to £179 million. Later the Guillebaud Committee – set up by a sceptical Tory government in 1953 to investigate the cost effectiveness of the NHS – was to report that the actual cost for the first (part) year was £328 million – nearly three times the 1946 estimate. The first full year (1949–50) cost £372 million (Rivett 1998).

Far from "infinite" demand

Beveridge's naive expectation, echoing the long-held belief of some socialist campaigners, had been that costs and demand would reduce once the backlog of unmet need had been cleared (Rivett 1998). This hope was soon to be dashed. Capitalist society, with its pressures on the poorest, could be counted on to generate a constant stream of people needing medical help, even while rising levels of prosperity helped to eradicate some of the previous scourges of infectious disease. Bevan, however, was not surprised, and always recognised that resources would be under pressure:

> We will never have all we need. Expectations will always exceed capacity. This service must always be changing, growing and improving, it must always appear inadequate.

> (cited in Foot 1982: 209–10)

Bevan is clearly arguing here that there is a constant tendency for demand to outstrip very limited levels of supply that were available in the straitened times of 1948. He also expressed understandable concerns as Minister of Health that perhaps the initial surge of demand would get out of hand, when he told Parliament:

> I shudder to think of the ceaseless cascade of medicine which is pouring down British throats at the present time.

> (Campbell 1987: 183)

But it would be quite wrong to read either of these often-quoted statements as an acceptance of – let alone an argument for – the rationing of health services, whether through the imposition of charges for treatment or alternative methods of restricting access to care. His opposition to the imposition of charges was not a categoric point of principle: his drafting of the NHS Act had indeed left a loophole for charges for certain services to be imposed at the discretion of the government:

> The services so provided shall be free of charge, except where any provision of this Act expressly provides for the making and recovery of charges.

However, Bevan was never himself an advocate of charges: indeed he was soon to run into conflict on this point with government colleagues, when the pressures of a mounting international economic crisis forced a devaluation of the pound in 1949, and with it a panic-stricken debate in the Cabinet on cost-cutting proposals. Bevan under pressure agreed to amend the Act to give the government power to impose prescription charges – but managed to prevent those powers being used while Labour was in office.

The pressure on the NHS budget intensified with the outbreak of the Korean War in 1950 and the Labour government's decision to embark on a massive £4.7 billion three-year rearmament programme. Bevan himself was moved from Health and Housing to become Minister of Labour, but strongly resisted proposals in 1951 by the new Chancellor, Hugh Gaitskell, to impose charges on false teeth and spectacles – in order to cut just £13 million from the NHS budget that year and £30 million the following year. Defeated in cabinet, Bevan resigned, arguing angrily in the Commons – as he had with his ministerial colleagues – that the penny-pinching savings would make no significant difference to a £4 billion national budget, but represented a damaging precedent for the new NHS.

Nobody had known what scale of demand to expect, and the new NHS groaned under the strain of coping with patients emerging from years of silent suffering to seek the care they had longed for and were now entitled to receive. With the novelty of a service for the first time available free of charge, no doubt there were a few patients who, with the connivance of their GPs, secured more than they immediately needed in supplies of aspirin, laxatives, or even a previously unthinkable second pair of spectacles (Rivett 1998). Despite these occasional lapses, however, the launch of the NHS was a firm answer to those who embrace the concept of "moral hazard", and those who claim that demand for health care is "a bottomless pit" (challenged by Light 1997 and Frankel et al. 2000), or an "infinite" demand which can never be met, making rationing of care inevitable[6] (Klein 2006: 54, 60, 202; Ham 1997; Ham and Honigsbaum 1998; Smith R 1996a, b; Lenaghan 1997).

The NHS experience showed that even with a service abruptly opened up to all and levying no charges, demand was far short of "infinite", and the cost of the service did not rocket out of control. Bevan pointed out from very early on that while the rush for spectacles and dental treatment had "exceeded all expectations", one good reason for this had been the level of unmet need in the period prior to the NHS:

---

6   "Moral hazard", although referred to as an established fact by some health economists (Dunlop and Martins 1996) might more realistically be seen as a largely imaginary creation of health economists, under which patients may in theory be tempted to avail themselves of additional unnecessary treatment if it were available to them free of charge. However, as Deber (2000) points out, even where health care is available free, demand for it is far from infinite: people demanding it are restricted to those suffering the appropriate condition: "I doubt if many readers... would gladly accept free chemotherapy or free open-heart surgery, unless they 'needed' it."

But there is also, without doubt, a sheer increase due to people getting things they need but could not afford before, and this the scheme intended.

(cited in Klein 2006: 25)

The NHS caseload grew, but not astronomically: numbers of inpatients rose by over 20% in the first five years, outpatient attendances were up 10%, while spending in real terms rose 16%, much of it required for increased numbers of nurses (up 16%) and a 20% increase in medical and dental staff (Rivett 1998).

A continuing shortage of nurses meant that beds had to be left empty, and as a result waiting lists were created at once. Waiting lists for the first five years, which included mental health and mental handicap patients, hovered at around the 500,000 mark, although the quality of the data and monitoring of this statistic was often poor. As Julian Tudor Hart argues:

There were, and still are, all sorts of reasons why people who needed medical care in 1948 did not choose to receive it. Only one of those reasons changed in 1948, when doctors' fees were abolished. Of course there was a huge rise in demand, because costs of care had deterred many people from seeking treatment, most notably working class mothers who had borne and reared many children, and could only now afford to be ill or to contemplate surgery.

For the first 20 years of the NHS, there were huge waiting lists for gynaecological repairs, cholosystectomies for gallstones, hernia repairs and cataract surgery. …There was a huge rise in demand in GP workload and hospital referrals, resulting in long waiting lists for admission; but this was anticipated, calculable, and in the course of time it was coped with, despite always-inadequate funding and resources. Nowhere did demand approach infinity, whatever that means.[7]

(Hart 2006: 27)

Indeed, the Guillebaud Report in 1956 showed that though the headline spending figure was increasing year by year, in real terms spending on the NHS had risen less than inflation. The new service, concluded the Tory-appointed committee, was good value for money: indeed was under-funded and needed

---

7   Germany is a good example to refute the mythology of "infinite demand" – as well as showing that the separation of purchaser from provider in a health care market, which has prevailed since the system was first established in 1883, is no guarantee of efficiency or cost containment. The system is commonly described as "top-heavy", wasteful and carrying excess capacity (Garcia 2001). Costing around 11 per cent of GDP, the €270-billion-a-year German health care system is the most costly in Europe, despite more than two decades of attempts at cost-containment (MSI Healthcare 2000). But with Germany's waiting lists completely eliminated, and amid revelations that 20 per cent of German hospital beds were empty, hospitals seeking to ride out the squeeze on prices from the sickness funds and utilise their spare capacity began searching for private patients from Europe and beyond. A new private company GerMedic visited Ireland, Denmark and Sweden offering "package deal" operations in a network of 80 hospitals and clinics. The German example suggests that far from being "infinite", a comprehensive health care system can be provided at a cost somewhere between the 8 per cent of GDP currently being spent in Britain and the 11 per cent figure which has produced a surplus of beds and facilities and a shortage of patients in Germany.

more spent on it (Hart 2006; Webster 2002; Ham 1999; Rivett 1998; Timmins 1995). Guillebaud not only rejected the case for any additional charges for NHS treatment but also argued for some existing charges to be dropped. Far from raging out of control, NHS spending was actually less in real terms in the mid-1950s than it had been in 1948. This came after the Tory government, resenting every penny spent on collective provision, had begun from 1952 to squeeze back down the share of GNP allocated to the NHS, which peaked at 3.7 per cent in 1950–1, falling to 3.5 per cent and then lower throughout the 1950s. Throughout the 1950s Conservative governments struggled to contain NHS spending below £400 million: between 1950 and 1958 the NHS current budget increased in real terms by just 12.8 per cent (Klein 2006: 49).

The Guillebaud Report helped to make it more or less impossible for politicians to speak out in open opposition to the principle of collectively funded health care. Right wingers in the Tory cabinet were forced to retreat from proposals to cut NHS spending through imposing charges for overnight stays in hospital, abolishing dental or ophthalmic services, or limiting the list of drugs available on prescription: but these ideas simply went "underground". They continued to be bandied about in confidential discussions, periodically to resurface every few years in fresh calls for extended charges, means testing, a separate "health" stamp, and the expansion of private health schemes (Webster 1988; Webster 2002).

With the NHS occupying a focal point in the developing welfare state, and with its budget – driven by demographic pressures (a 10 per cent increase in population in its first 20 years) as well as by the costs of new technology – inexorably rising with the growth in the economy, it was perhaps inevitable that those who had only reluctantly accepted the principle of state-funded health care would repeatedly look for ways of holding down the cost, or ways of wriggling out of the commitment altogether.

From its very first year onwards, NHS spending had been squeezed by the impact of the British economic crisis, and throughout its first 50 years this was to bring a succession of conflicts, compromises and cutbacks. Nevertheless, although saddled with charges for prescriptions, dental treatment and spectacles, the NHS remained largely free at point of use. However the service remained starved of capital for investment in either hospitals or primary care – and far more accessible in some areas than others.

The real role of user fees

In the autumn of 1951 the weakened and battered Labour government went to the polls and was defeated by Churchill's Tories. The following year the new government widened charges for dental treatment and – no doubt happily utilising the legal powers introduced by its predecessors – imposed a one shilling (5p) prescription charge, designed to raise £20 million a year from the sick. Five years later it was to be increased to a shilling per item, and in 1961 the prescription charge was doubled to two shillings. The principle of an NHS free at point of use, funded from taxation, may have won the hearts of the general public, but it had not persuaded the diehard political defenders of free market capitalism.

The prescription charge issue retained an emotional significance. In 1964 the incoming Labour government won popular support by implementing its promise to scrap the charge. But as the economic situation once more lurched into crisis in 1968, it was reintroduced – this time as an attempt by Minister of Health Kenneth Robinson to avoid inflicting any cuts on the main body of hospital and primary care services. However, Robinson did seek to minimise the blow by introducing extensive exemptions which at that stage left 60 per cent of prescriptions dispensed free of charge (Klein 2006): this proportion has risen over the years.

Indeed while they are normally introduced as concessions to financial stringency and economic austerity, prescription charges and other user fees generate little if any significant additional revenue: they are above all a means of restricting demand. In Britain the persistence of widespread exemptions from prescription charges (children, pensioners, students, the unemployed, pregnant women) means that the vast majority are dispensed without charge, leaving the greatest burden on low-paid workers for whom the fee of £6.85 per item in 2007 is often too high for them to afford more than one item, regardless of their health needs. The totals raised through prescription charges (£427 million in 2005–6 (DoH 2007a)) remain derisory in comparison to the drugs budget (£7,240 million) and the total NHS budget (£74,000 million). They are high enough to deter low-paid workers with serious health needs, but not significant as a contribution to the running costs of the wider NHS. In Wales the National Assembly has in 2007 finally scrapped the prescription charge – at a relatively marginal cost.

The issue is not one restricted to the UK: the main claim that user fees help improve "efficiency" revolves around their effectiveness in discouraging "unnecessary" demand, or in some cases in generating additional revenue for funding health care when alternative funds are not available. However, such a policy is more accurately seen as "public sector cost containment" (Robinson 2002).

Surveys conducted in 1998 and 1999 including Russia, Central Eastern Europe and former Soviet Union republics of Central Asia, show that user fees are widely used by most countries in the form of co-payments for pharmaceuticals – covering as much as 35 per cent of the drug cost in Hungary – while nine EU countries imposed charges for general practitioner consultations, and most EU countries imposed co-payments for specialist consultations. Sweden levied extensive user charges, including for children's outpatient services. However, only Greece, Italy and Portugal relied upon user charges to raise more than 20 per cent of health care funding (Robinson 2002: 174).

The evidence of limited research shows that while total revenue from user charges rarely exceeds 5 per cent of total health revenue in wealthier countries, the charges strongly reduce utilisation, and thus worsen equity of provision, having a heavier impact upon the poor. There is also some evidence that charges have an adverse effect on health outcomes – and that they carry hidden costs in additional, wasteful managerial and administrative effort (Schieber and Maeda 1997, cited in Robinson 2002: 177).

No moves to control pharmaceutical firms

Rationing the supply of drugs to low-paid workers is a crude and counterproductive way to restrict demand, and appears especially perverse in view of the fact that, even in a period where so much medical advance has been centred on the development of new and powerful drugs, there has been no provision or proposal to nationalise or in any way control the drug manufacturers. With the production of drugs and the research and development process firmly in private hands, the tax-funded NHS was at the mercy of increasingly large and increasingly multinational pharmaceutical corporations, preoccupied with delivering profits to their shareholders. Prescription costs rose by 45 per cent in the first five years of the NHS.

The war had brought a new impetus to medical techniques, and important new drugs were tested and ready to use in 1948. By 1950 half the NHS drugs budget was accounted for by new sulphonamides and antibiotics, and tranquillisers were becoming more widely used, as well as antihistamines. There were new anaesthetics which, unlike earlier varieties, were not inflammable or explosive. There were new drugs available for anaemia, diabetes and high blood pressure, and the late 1950s were to see further development of chemotherapy and radiotherapy for cancer treatment. There were also strong drugs to be used by psychiatrists, notably chlorpromazine (Largactil), and similar strong tranquillisers which, if used in appropriate situations and dosage, can have a calming influence on behaviour and psychotic thoughts, without affecting clarity of consciousness. However, large doses, as well as prolonged usage, can have very undesirable side effects. The potential "market" for drugs to be prescribed for depression was also exploited by the drug companies, as Geoffrey Rivett points out:

> Big business was beginning to realise the large profits to be made out of mental health. All that was necessary was to persuade doctors to prescribe for hundreds of thousands of patients each week.
>
> (Rivett 1998)

Attempts by the Conservative government from 1953 onwards to draw attention to the costs of the drugs involved, and to suggest doctors might cut down on the use of less-effective treatments were resisted by the BMA as an attack on clinical freedom. By 1956, 228 million prescriptions a year were being written, pumping £58 million – almost 10 per cent of the NHS budget – into the coffers of the pharmaceutical giants.

It was not only drug suppliers that stood to gain from the purchasing power of the NHS. Surgical techniques, too, were making big strides, and in the 1960s came kidney dialysis, more sophisticated x-ray and other imaging techniques, new breakthroughs in pathology testing, and tremendous improvements in the care of premature babies. Each of these advances brought with it the need for new and increasingly sophisticated equipment, purchased from the private sector.

In such a dynamic area of science and technique, especially at a time of such rapid technological advance as the post-war period, there was always going to be an upward pressure on NHS spending to keep pace with the latest developments: but the extravagant lust for profits among the private suppliers substantially increased this pressure. Under conditions of tightening budgetary controls, this in turn has a distorting impact on NHS priorities: the expenses of new technology make themselves most forcibly felt in the high-profile acute sector, and headline-grabbing breakthroughs create a public awareness and a pressure to ensure the NHS takes in the latest. But increased spending on these areas can, within a fixed budget, only take place at the expense of the less glamorous services – community health, mental health, care of the elderly.

To this day there remains a massive disparity between the tens or hundreds of millions that can be raised in donations through high-profile campaigns like the Great Ormond Street "Wishing Well" appeal in the 1990s, appeals by the cancer charities and local campaigns for scanners and kidney units on the one hand, and the much smaller-scale resources available to charities concerned with mental health and care of the elderly. In Britain these "lesser" causes have also been hit the hardest by the launch of the National Lottery and its variants.

New hospitals for a modern health service

Bevan had been impatient with the limited size and scope of the old hospital stock, and made clear his preference for larger units, offering more comprehensive services:

> I would rather be kept alive in the efficient, if cold, altruism of a large hospital than expire in a gush of warm sympathy in a small one.
>
> (Foot 1982: 131)

Refurbishment and extension of existing sites was not an easy option. Services had grown up in a variety of small, scattered units, many of them in desperate need of repair. None of the fourteen new towns built since the war had its own hospital, and in other areas hospitals were clearly in the wrong place to deliver accessible care to the new centres of expanding population.

The Guillebaud Report recommended that the NHS capital programme be at least trebled to reach the pre-war equivalent of £30 million a year. As rationing of materials was gradually whittled away in the early 1950s, there was growing interest in the new types of design that would be appropriate for the new hospitals when building became feasible. With no post-war British experience of hospital building, teams were dispatched abroad, notably to the USA, to investigate the latest architectural thinking. They came back with reports describing increasingly sophisticated buildings with centralised facilities, offering big improvements in efficiency and clinical effectiveness (Rivett 1998). Building hospitals on this model to serve the acute service needs of whole districts would enable the closure of smaller, less economic hospitals – with the liberation of capital and a reduction in revenue costs. And with steady reductions already taking place in the average length of stay in hospital, there was the hope that, if community services could be expanded at the same time, fewer beds would be needed.

But it was to be another six years before serious action was taken. Ironically, this was to be led by a Tory minister – Enoch Powell – who until then had been best known for his doubling of prescription charges and his long record of fighting for government spending cuts. Yet the 1962 Hospital Plan for England and Wales which Powell was to take forward changed the shape of the NHS more dramatically than any other single measure.

In 1962 the government was spending just over half the current share of national wealth on the NHS, just 3.4% of GDP – compared with just over 6% in 2000. Within this limited pot of cash, NHS capital budgets in turn consistently accounted for less than 3% each year (though allocations had increased slightly, peaking at £24 million in 1960–1). This was well below the level of around 5% that had been recommended by the Guillebaud Committee. As a result, there was not enough capital to enable any substantial modernisation or even systematic repairs to buildings which were often unsuitable for modern medicine: 70% of hospitals taken over by the NHS in 1948 had fewer than 100 beds, and 20% of the building stock was found to be over 100 years old in 1962 (Ministry of Health 1962).

The situation called for a major change of policy; but perhaps surprisingly, given Enoch Powell's right-wing leanings, the entire 1962 investment programme was to be funded by the government from general taxation – and the completed hospitals would also be assets wholly owned by the NHS. There was no serious discussion of seeking the finance from elsewhere. The only debate within the Tory cabinet was over how much or how little should be invested in the modernisation of the NHS.

By contrast, since 1997 New Labour ministers have repeatedly defended their policy of seeking to build hospitals using the controversial Private Finance Initiative by claiming that PFI has enabled them to embark upon the "biggest ever programme of hospital building in the NHS" (See Chapter nine).

The 1962 Hospital Plan, eventually approved on Powell's urgings, was an extremely ambitious one for its time, spelling out proposals for 90 new hospitals and another 134 major redevelopment programmes. The 280-page Plan also listed a further 356 schemes costing over £100,000 each (equivalent to almost £500,000 today) and also acknowledged the need for many more smaller schemes "which represent a large volume of modernisation and upgrading".

Powell was responding to increasing pressure from health professionals, who pointed to the new possibilities: as the medical capacity to treat and cure increasingly complex diseases and conditions had developed, so too had the requirement for new, specialist facilities which in turn were only economic to provide for a much larger catchment population than had previously been the model. But the Hospital Plan also commenced the shift from institutional to community-based care for mental health, proposing a drastic cut in hospital bed numbers, with a massive 45 per cent reduction in mental health beds (from 3.3 to 1.8 per 1,000) despite a lack of any specific proposals for investment in the necessary alternative services in the community.

Moreover it also took an important step towards setting up a nationwide plan and a coherent policy. It laid down norms for minimum levels of bed provision per head of population for each specialist service, and addressed the issue of staffing levels, both within the NHS as it then was, and within the Local Authority Health and Welfare Services (many of which are now council social services).

Hospitals are extremely complex structures, and the building programme also saw expensive and embarrassing planning fiascos. One was the tower block of the Royal Free Hospital which opened in 1973 at a cost of £20 million before anyone realised that the plans had not included a morgue. Worse, the whole building, shoehorned into a cramped site in Hampstead with extremely difficult access for people with disabilities, was widely seen as out of date before it was opened, and continued cuts in maintenance quickly caused problems. By 1981 a *Times Health Supplement* investigation showed many of the newer hospitals already in need of repair. The Royal Free and Charing Cross hospitals were both to feature in headline-grabbing kitchen hygiene scandals by the mid-1980s.

This type of error is by no means restricted to the public sector and publicly funded schemes. Indeed, the more recent round of PFI-funded hospitals constructed since 1997 have boasted more than their fair share of planning fiascos: poor locations; insufficient beds, with too little space between them; little or no office space or room for storage; "innovative" building designs that leak or cannot cope with extremes of summer and winter temperature; and buildings and fittings of shoddy quality, with high prices levied for repairs and replacements (Lister 2003a).

Modernising mental health care

Enoch Powell's contribution to the NHS was not limited to driving forward the renewal of acute hospital services: he was also the first Minister of Health to nail his colours to the mast of modernising the care of the mentally ill, with his now famous "water tower" speech to the 1961 conference of the National Association for Mental Health (now known as MIND).

The model of mental health care had changed little since the turn of the century, leaving services concentrated in the network of large asylums built on the edges of big cities following the 1845 Lunatic Asylums Act, which obliged all county and borough authorities to establish them. From the outset the investment in these large facilities, some of which had as many as 2,000 beds, represented an ambivalent approach. On the one hand they had been campaigned for by reformers who wanted to improve conditions for mentally distressed people: on the other they were also supported by those who wanted to see "madmen" locked up as far away as possible at the cheapest possible cost.

By the 1920s the Royal Commission on Lunacy and Mental Disorder concluded that mental illness was a public health problem, and pressed for the renaming of asylums as mental hospitals. "Lunatics", the report suggested, should be referred to as "persons of unsound mind". In 1930 new legislation opened up the possibility of voluntary admissions and encouraged the development of outpatient services. While the "continuous warm bath" treatment (immersing the patient for 2–14 days) reported in the *Nursing Times* in 1913, fell into disuse, and the padded rooms were gradually dismantled, the treatment available to inpatients in the 1930s ranged from the bizarre to the barbaric. Alongside the use of the strait-jacket and other forms of restraint, there had been insulin treatment (designed to induce comas in non-diabetic patients), shock treatment (in which an overdose of heart stimulant was used to induce a seizure), and then electro convulsive therapy (ECT). Some patients were even deliberately infected with malaria – with a mosquito breeding centre established at Horton Hospital (Valentine 1996). For some there was also the horror of surgery – pre-frontal leucotomy – which involved removing a part of the brain.

It was not until the advent of the new, powerful post-war tranquillisers, notably Largactil, swiftly followed by the first anti-depressants, that new paths of care could be opened up. Although there were to be considerable problems with these drugs and their side-effects, they opened up a new optimism that mental illness could be treated outside of the hospital environment (Rivett 1998). A Royal Commission established in 1954 reported in 1957, recommending the repeal of all existing legislation, to be replaced by a single new law covering mental illness and mental handicap. There should be less frequent use of compulsory admission. These proposals were swiftly accepted and incorporated into the 1959 Mental Health Act (Rivett 1998).

It was in the context of these recent developments, and amid evidence that numbers of inpatients had already begun to decline, that Enoch Powell in 1961 shocked much of his audience by making a keynote speech that denounced the old Victorian asylums as the "defences we have to storm" in the development of a new model of mental health care:

> There they stand, isolated, majestic, imperious, brooded over by the gigantic water tower and chimney combined, rising unmistakeable and daunting out of the countryside – the asylums which our forefathers built with such immense solidity.
>
> (cited in Timmins 1995: 211)

Influenced by Health Ministry statisticians, themselves carried away by the more optimistic views of psychiatrists on the potential impact of the new drugs which were becoming available, Powell forecast a halving in the numbers of inpatient mental health beds to 75,000 by 1975.

Powell's speech will sound strangely familiar to anyone who has followed the development of mental health policy since that time. The contrast between lofty rhetoric and the grim reality of desperately under-resourced services has been a common feature of official pronouncements for over 35 years, as has the increased reference to the abstract notion of "community care" – in which neither the notion of "community" nor that of "care" is properly defined. Among those who responded with some scepticism was the social scientist Richard Titmuss, who had warned in *Commitment to Welfare* that:

> If English history is any guide, confusion has often been the mother of complacency… What some hope will exist is suddenly thought by many to exist. All kinds of wild and unlovely weeds are changed by statutory magic and comforting appellation into the most attractive and domesticated flowers.
>
> (Titmuss 1968: 104)

The fears of Titmuss and others were well-founded. Powell's speech conspicuously failed to make any corresponding pledge of the funding and training necessary to establish a new, community-based service to replace the lost mental health beds.

Indeed it appears that his enthusiasm to see the closure of the old "bins" may have been motivated as much by his reckoning of the cash savings to be made from pulling out of the crumbling, poorly maintained asylums as by righteous indignation at the pitifully poor standards of care being meted out to long-stay patients in the "back wards".

Instead, with a cavalier spirit which has become the traditional stance of successive Health Ministers dealing with this and other aspects of "community care", Powell called for a "whole new development of local authority services" for people with mental illness. His ten-year plan for Health and Welfare Services, eventually published in 1963, left all of the responsibility in the hands of local government (Timmins 1995). The classic buck-passing suggestion fell on stony ground: more than 30 years later only a third of local authorities were spending more than 10 per cent of their Personal Social Services budget on care for people with mental illness (DoH 1996): by 2004 that share was just 5.5 per cent, with an average allocation in England of just £26 per head of the adult (18–64) population (NHS Health and Social Care Information Centre 2006).

The drive to reduce the reliance on inpatient beds made itself felt on the big psychiatric hospitals. At Horton Hospital a 1963 study found that of the 342 men admitted between January and July, half were diagnosed as schizophrenic, compared with a national average of 36 per cent. But of 1,015 men discharged in the same period, 29 per cent were classed as "undesirable discharges", some of whom left without discussing their case, and some of whom committed suicide (Valentine 1996: 30). By 1969 another study of male patients at Horton found that only 26 per cent were being admitted for the first time: almost three-quarters were among the growing numbers of "revolving door", chronically ill patients whose lives were punctuated by occasional periods in psychiatric beds, and who were finding little, if any, support in the community when discharged (Valentine 1996: 31).

The 1960s after Powell were to see the start of what was not a mass closure, but a steady reduction in mental health beds, averaging 3,000 per year, with a substantial increase in outpatient attendances and short-stay admissions. By the early 1970s there were around 100,000 inpatients in English mental hospitals, 50 per cent of whom had been there for five years or more, and 75 per cent for over a year. By 1989, the inpatient population had fallen to 50,000, only half of whom had been there more than a year, and 30 per cent for over five years (OHE 1989). But in the absence of any capital investment in alternative provision, the reduced numbers of mental health beds were still concentrated in the old asylums. And since they were increasingly catering for the most dependent patients, the average cost per bed went up. By 1986, when the first of the big asylums (the 900-bed Banstead Hospital in Surrey) finally closed, the average revenue cost per inpatient was over five times the cost in 1958 (at constant prices) (OHE 1989).

This concentration of spending in the dwindling hospitals left little if any spare NHS revenue for investment in the necessary network of community services to support the majority of mental illness sufferers in the community. Another trigger towards a 'community' model for health services was the succession of scandals over the quality of care which the big long-stay institutions were providing for elderly, mentally handicapped and mentally ill patients. Secretary of State for Health and Social Security Richard Crossman responded by setting up the Hospital Advisory Service, whose subsequent visits to mental handicap, psychiatric and geriatric hospitals uncovered a wide range of abuses and shortcomings.

But mental health was still not a consistent priority of ministers or the Department of Health and its local managers. Nor was the care of some of the most vulnerable patients who were also housed in large and forbidding institutions. In 1976 it was only strike action by health union COHSE which forced an inquiry into the treatment of patients at the Normansfield mental handicap hospital in South West London, which in turn helped trigger a fundamental rethink on the most appropriate model of care for people with learning difficulties (Rivett 1998).

In the front line for cuts

In the late 1960s the NHS was buffeted by a constant succession of financial pressures as the British economy floundered in international markets. The Labour government which scrapped prescription charges in 1964 was driven to reintroduce them as part of an austerity package in 1968. Having gradually crept up the scale to command almost 4 per cent of GDP, the NHS was therefore predictably at the front of the firing line when a new "radical right" Tory government under Edward Heath was elected in 1970, promising to cut public expenditure in order to maximise tax cuts.

The new Chancellor, Anthony Barber, lost no time in presenting a mini-budget which set the new tone. Centred around a 6d (2.5p) cut in the basic rate of income tax (giving the average industrial worker with two children an extra £7 a year, and top industrialist Lord Stokes an extra £20 per week), it included a doubling of prescription charges and increased charges for spectacles and dental treatment (which would now equal half the actual cost of treatment) (Lister 1988). Three years later another Barber mini-budget was to cut £1.3 billion from social spending, including £111 million from the NHS budget. These were the years in which Margaret Thatcher was to win her first real taste of notoriety – as "Maggie Thatcher, Milk Snatcher", the minister who axed free school milk.

The Commons Public Expenditure Committee declared in 1973 that:

> It is the opinion of our committee that no government has ever provided sufficient money to allow the health service to function and to react to growing needs effectively.

But despite its mission to hack back public spending, and its right-wing rhetoric, the Heath government did not reduce the share of national wealth allocated to the NHS. By 1974 this had risen to 4.8 per cent, a gross budget of £4.2 billion for health (Rivett 1998). The service had become too central, too popular, for the government to be seen to undermine it.

The first reorganisation

The early 1970s also saw the first substantial steps to restructure the NHS and revise the model established by Bevan. Following lengthy debates begun by the Labour government in the late 1960s, two ministries were merged in 1970 to form the Department of Health and Social Security, whose first Secretary of State was the "mad monk" founding father of Thatcherite monetarism, Sir Keith Joseph.

Joseph was keen to establish tighter control over spending, with firmer lines of accountability upwards from local hospitals to the Department (though of course not downwards from the health authorities to their local communities, patients or health workers). He decided that this would best be achieved by a reorganisation of the old Regional Boards and Hospital Management Committees, and in a move carried through with minimal debate or public interest, introduced the NHS Reorganisation Act which laid the basis for a new structure to take effect in April 1974 – which proved to be two months after Labour had again been re-elected.

The new structure set out for the first time to integrate community, domiciliary and preventive health services with acute hospital services, through a network of 90 new Area Health Authorities, which largely followed local authority boundaries. The independent boards of the teaching hospitals were scrapped, and each of the hospitals integrated into a clumsily named "Area Health Authority (Teaching)".

Primary care remained semi-detached, retaining the Family Practitioner Service. There were tokenistic nods towards democracy and the rights of the "consumer" with the establishment of Community Health Councils as (largely toothless) watchdog bodies supposedly scrutinising the activities of the appointed health authorities. Social services remained in the control of local government, and the new system was supposed to promote links between them and the NHS. However, although Joint Consultative Committees were set up between councils and the AHAs, real integration could come only if there were shared financial resources. The non-elected, tax-funded AHAs shared little more than their boundaries with the elected, rate-funded local authorities.

The 90 AHAs ranged in catchment population from 250,000 to 1 million, and their appointed chairs were paid a part-time salary. There was no reason to suppose that this would represent much change from the 1960s, when 11 of the 15 Regional Boards were chaired by company directors or senior business figures. Nor would the AHAs represent any serious break from the panels of worthies that had served on Hospital Management Committees. A survey showed that these included:

> 4 Lord Lieutenants, 20 deputy Lieutenants, 146 JPs, 12 peers or baronets, 5 wives, widows or offspring of peers, 1 ex-Lord Mayor, 8 retired admirals or generals. Of a sample of 92 of the HMCs one-quarter of the chairmen were company directors and not a single one as far as was known was a wage earner.
>
> (Robson 1973)

Joseph's reorganisation was to be roundly criticised by a Royal Commission set up in 1976 (but which did not report until March 1979, shortly before the re-election of the Tories). The scheme had too many tiers of management and too many administrators, said the Commission, which led to a failure to make timely decisions and a waste of NHS resources (DHSS 1979a).

The failed reforms alienated many existing NHS administrators, increased administrative staff by 17,000, and cost at least £9 million to carry out. Behind the facade of the new-fangled health authorities, more power was being given to the full-time Area Teams of Officers and the local District Management Teams, who took all the day-to-day management decisions, and drew up all of the proposals and documents for AHAs, based on the amount of cash made available from the newly renamed Regional Health Authorities.

The new structure was inherited by the returning Labour government in 1974, which proved as unimaginative and tight fisted towards the NHS as its predecessors.

A toothless consensus

By 1976 the NHS had emerged as a service too popular with the electorate for either governing party to challenge its values, but too hungry of resources for either party to summon up the political will to fund it properly, or push through a genuine progressive equalisation of resources. The consensus on the need for a publicly funded, nationally organised service had been cemented in place by the Guillebaud Report, but had not been seriously challenged by other than fringe and extremist elements in the Conservative Party.

However, behind the scenes Health Ministers of both parties – even including Nye Bevan – had sought information on the practicalities of levying charges for hospital "hotel" costs, and prescription charges had been introduced, scrapped, and reintroduced with extensive exemptions – all of which served to underline the political sensitivities of the issue of charges, and the limited possibilities to raise significant amounts through charging what remains a predominantly low-income or no-income section of the population for their drugs or treatment (Klein 2006).

A right-wing Tory health minister (Powell) had driven forward the first systematic effort to allocate hospital investment on the basis of local population and demographics; obtained a cabinet commitment to invest only public funds in a major new building programme; and given a fresh impetus to debate on more civilised and effective methods of delivering mental health care, calling for a switch away from the old Victorian asylums. By contrast a Labour government, consistently struggling against economic adversity, had been relatively tight-fisted on health spending, and in 1976 introduced the first "monetarist" cap on health budgets – cash limits – and followed up with a substantial programme of hospital closures that triggered angry campaigns including protest marches and occupations.

The NHS remained a very different type of organisation from any private sector enterprise or the other industries nationalised by the post-war Labour government. It was the only service explicitly embracing the notion of meeting social needs rather than making a profit or supplying part of the infrastructure for the wider capitalist economy. It had established itself as a national system, and a national employer, creating a career structure for a growing body of NHS consultants, and training many thousands of health professionals: but many of the decisions affecting the quantity and quality of health care for local people were taken at local level by unelected and unaccountable boards and management committees, some of which were also difficult for the Department of Health to monitor or control.

Despite the apparent consensus between the parties, there had been three decades of severe and chronic under-investment under successive governments. Indeed as late as 1997 New Labour ministers noted that more of the NHS estate dated to pre-1948 than post-1948. This under-investment had also left the NHS with many unresolved inequalities and local gaps in care at primary, community and hospital level – and with shockingly obsolete buildings and equipment.

Unequal shares

One of the great strengths of a centrally funded, universal and public sector health care system should have been the opportunity it affords to defy normal "market" principles of focusing resources on the most commercially viable or profitable services, and instead allocate resources according to local levels of need. Yet almost three decades went by in the NHS before any serious attempt was made to identify and address inequalities in health provision or health outcomes.

The problem was not a straightforward matter of party politics – although the Conservative Party, in government and in opposition, proved for several decades resistant to the very notion that social inequalities could generate and exacerbate inequalities in health. The Labour Party did take a different approach, but shied away in the immediate post-war period from any serious attempt to tackle social inequality, and – despite a more radical rhetoric in the 1960s and again in the 1970s – showed itself to be more ready to debate the issue in abstract than to put resources into any radical solutions. The issue is a far-reaching one, since the widening gap in incomes and living standards also generated a consequent widening in health inequalities – a gap which no amount of curative medicine delivered through the NHS could hope to rectify on its own. And there were real doubts over whether NHS funding was correctly allocated to match local health needs.

The new NHS in 1948 had taken over the fragmented and patchy patterns of hospital and primary care provision and the rigid, dictatorial control by doctors which had preserved deep class divisions in health. Funding continued to be allocated on the basis of previous services and spending, leaving health resources concentrated in more prosperous areas, and disproportionately concentrated in the South. There was certainly much more money in the system in the mid-1970s than in 1948: despite the growing and intense pressure on spending, the 1970s had seen a continuing increase in the share of national wealth allocated to the NHS, which exceeded 5 per cent for three years in the decade.[8] However, the increase in the overall budget did not resolve the problem of local inequalities in access to health services.

This unequal reality was for many years concealed by the fact that as a centralised, national service, figures for NHS spending in the first few years were grossed up into national aggregate totals which glossed over regional differences and more local inequalities. This had begun to unravel slightly with the audit of buildings and facilities carried out for the 1962 Hospital Plan, which had exposed some of the gaps, and the Plan attempted for the first time to establish a system for allocating resources (hospitals and bed numbers) on the basis of local population.

But this limited initiative, begun under the Tories, and then taken up by Wilson's economically challenged Labour government, and again under Heath's Tories from 1970, produced at best uneven results. It was not until the mid-1970s that any serious and systematic attempt was made to redress the imbalance in allocation of financial resources when Labour ministers set up a Resources Allocation Working Party (RAWP), tasked with finding a more equitable formula for funding health services across the country by identifying the relative needs of the 14 Regional Health Authorities in England. It produced reports in 1975 and 1976 (DHSS 1976).

The inequalities were real enough. The prosperous South East, which also contained the most powerful concentration of teaching hospitals and consultants, had predictably done rather well, while the regions to the north and west had lost

---

8   The picture was distorted by high levels of cost inflation, which meant that the headline cash
     allocations appeared much higher than the actual purchasing power of the NHS.

out, with much lower health spending per capita of population and less-advanced facilities available. One result was that patients often had to travel long distances – sometimes hundreds of miles to London teaching hospitals – to get certain specialist treatment.

The uneven national pattern of spending was a reflection of Julian Tudor Hart's Inverse Care Law – but the same law also led to stark inequalities within each region and *within* individual Area Health Authorities.

The RAWP proposals were effectively a capitation funding formula – and as such were an early forerunner of the controversial formula to be introduced with the Tory "market" reforms from 1991, and maintained ever since as the basis for "purchasing" or "commissioning" services. RAWP established new "target" levels of resources for each region, which were based on statistical projections of the numbers of people to be served, adjusted for varying proportions of each age and sex; the average death rates (Standardised Mortality Ratios or SMRs) for each age and sex grouping; and the expected levels of need for various hospital, ambulance and other services (Mohan 1995). The strategic goal was to ensure that the regions furthest below the new spending "targets" should receive additional resources, while those furthest above them should receive relatively smaller growth. The assumption was that by preferentially allocating increased funding to the under-target areas, the gap could be closed: Health Secretary Richard Crossman argued that "I can only equalise on an expanding budget" (cited in Klein 2006: 61).

Debates have raged ever since over the ways in which the formula was calculated and the weighting given to each of its component parts. A relatively small change in part of the formula – for example, the weighting given to the older age groups – could have the effect of dramatically altering the target funding level of one type of area, to the detriment of another. But the most immediate problem arising from RAWP was caused by the package of public spending cuts and the new pressures brought to bear on the economy by the International Monetary Fund in the latter months of 1976 (Timmins 1995).

This combined squeeze immediately ruled out any possibility of levelling up the less well-funded health regions: instead RAWP was used as a lever to level *down* the "over-provided" south-eastern regions, which were the only parts of England deemed to be "over-target" – by amounts varying from 5.7 per cent to 10.4 per cent in 1983 (Mohan 1995: 79). The sums to be taken from their funding were sufficient to cause resentment and protests – but not enough to offer much improvement in the "below-target" regions, which were deemed to be between 1.4 per cent and 9.5 per cent under target. To compound the problems, 1976 also saw the imposition by the Labour government – as a move to placate their new creditors in the IMF – of a new system of financing health authorities, which for the first time set maximum spending figures for Hospital and Community Services *in advance* as a "cash limit", and compelling AHAs to remain within this limit, regardless of local health needs.

Only the Family Practitioner Services were exempt from this dramatic new financial discipline, which ended nearly 30 years in which the NHS had been funded flexibly to meet fluctuations in demand. The financial regime was to be progressively tightened in the following two decades. This policy opened up what was to become a growing division between the cash-limited (and increasingly crisis-ridden) secondary care services, and the demand-led primary care services, which increasingly accounted for the lion's share of "growth" in NHS funding through the 1980s. The Tory policy of GP fundholding was the first serious attempt to "cap" this demand-led growth in primary care spending: but it was only in the fiftieth anniversary year of the NHS that the New Labour government's White Paper proposed a fully cash-limited regime for GP services (DoH 1997a).

RAWP became a series of abstract cash targets, which in turn resulted in holding back services in some areas to benefit the others. Even without the overall financial constraints which created even sharper problems, the RAWP approach was conservative in its very conception. There was no suggestion of trying to decentralise the NHS by raising the level of services in under-provided areas – through the building of new teaching hospitals, for example, to serve as what the jargon of the time described as "centres of excellence". As late as the end of the 1980s, the idea of moving either Guy's or St Thomas's Hospital to the south coast was half-heartedly raised – but hastily dropped. Nor were there serious plans for new specialist units to be attached to existing general hospitals that might make services more accessible to local people.

The RAWP formula has also been criticised for basing itself too heavily on premature death (SMRs) as a crude and not especially accurate measure of continuing levels of ill health and need for health services. Some areas have suffered with the financial problems of above-average demand for mental health services in an otherwise relatively youthful population, which does not bring any entitlement to appropriate levels of funding. The regional level comparisons also understate the scale of the differences between health authorities within regions – with the gap between the most over-target and most under-target health authorities in North East Thames standing at 44 per cent in 1983: the pressure to tackle these differences rapidly put huge pressures on some districts in the 1980s (Mohan 1995: 81).

RAWP has also been accused of failing to make adequate allowance for the inflated costs of delivering health care in London, where it has for many years proved impossible to recruit and retain NHS staff on the flat rate of NHS pay, and 'London weighting' has had to be added. To make matters worse, RAWP also implicitly assumed that over-target areas were making excessive use of the NHS in general and hospital beds in particular, despite evidence that "over-target" London had an extremely poor and uneven provision of primary care, and that the higher use of A&E and other hospital services was linked to that underlying weakness (Mohan 1995; King's Fund 1992).

The results were predictably divisive. In what should have been the "losing" regions, the already powerful consultants' lobby, which had been so successful at carving out empires around the big teaching hospitals, took up the fight to protect their services against the new cuts – while ambitious consultants in the outlying areas joined forces with management to press forward projects for their own, more local services. One example was the Dacorum Hospital Campaign which successfully lobbied for the building of a district general hospital in the new town of Hemel Hempstead – one which has had to be defended for the last 20 years against attempts to "downsize" or close it as part of a plan to scale down hospitals across Hertfordshire (Lister 2007c).

There was not enough money on the table to satisfy both lobbies; but the effect of the conflict was for the acute services to grab most of the headlines and even more of the available funding, forcing a new round of cutbacks in community services and smaller hospitals. Driven on by cash pressures, and in some cases by the need to reshape services around new District General Hospitals, the pace of rationalisation plans began to accelerate, again with the heaviest blows initially being struck under a Labour government. Between January 1976 and October 1978, AHAs in England and Wales agreed to the closure or 'change of use' of 217 hospitals. Two-thirds of these (143) went ahead, while local Community Health Councils (CHCs) used their new powers to object to 37 of them. New plans that were drawn up included the loss of 31 per cent of London's hospital beds between 1975 and 1986, with a £110 million cut in spending and the loss of 24,000 NHS jobs (National Union of Public Employees 1978).

There was also an attempt to develop a new theoretical/clinical framework to take the steam out of opposition to cutbacks, by arguing openly for a reduction in the targets for the numbers of hospital beds to be provided. A 1977 document *The Way Forward: Priorities in the Health and Social Services* called for a 17 per cent reduction in the provision of acute beds and a substantial cut in NHS spending on acute and maternity services (DHSS 1977). The *Priorities* report had also suggested small increases in resources for the elderly, the mentally ill, the mentally handicapped, paediatrics and primary care, and actually *increased* target bed quotas for the elderly (never achieved). Far from receiving "priority" care, many elderly patients found themselves rudely and suddenly uprooted from friendly, local community and cottage hospitals – and bundled into large impersonal wards in general hospitals (Politics of Health Group 1979). Once there, they were soon regarded by consultants as a nuisance, "blocking" beds for acute patients. The pressure was mounting for ousting elderly long-stay patients from hospital altogether, and there was a rising tide of Labour government propaganda extolling the supposed advantages of "community care" – despite the absence of structures from either the NHS or social services to support frail elderly people in the community (Radical Statistics Health Group 1976).

With health unions, CHCs and local communities alarmed at the loss of their hospitals, the scene was set for an eruption in campaigns and activity which brought the NHS to the forefront of local political life. Old forms of resistance resurfaced: the workforce at the threatened Elizabeth Garrett Anderson Hospital for Women in central London revived the 1920s technique of occupying a hospital to defend it. They expelled their managers, and mounted what turned out to be a successful three-year "work-in" to prevent its closure (NHS Emergency Action Committee 1985). Across the country, the 30 years to 1979 had seen the closure of 484 (mainly smaller) hospitals, while numbers of patients treated had doubled and the proportion treated in hospital went up by a third, from 90.2 per 1,000 population to 120.4 (Rivett 1998: 475).

Cash-driven rationalisation

The first 30 years of the NHS saw it expand unevenly, with little overall plan, often struggling to compensate for the ill health generated by poverty and social problems. The momentum it had established meant that the return in 1979 of the Tories, now led by Margaret Thatcher, a fervent advocate of privatisation, self-help and cuts in public spending, did not herald the predicted immediate cuts.

Despite inadequate capital investment and appallingly low pay for NHS staff, efficiency had continued to improve, with a steady increase in numbers of patients treated in each bed and reduced average lengths of stay in hospital. Staff numbers had more than doubled since 1948, reaching 822,000 in England, with Wales, Scotland and Northern Ireland bringing the total to over a million. Staff costs were 70 per cent of total NHS spending, and 36 per cent of the NHS workforce were nursing staff (298,000). There had been a three-fold increase in numbers of consultants and hospital doctors, and the hospital sector had increased its share of spending from 55 per cent to 63 per cent.

Community nurses, whose numbers trebled over 30 years, were still outnumbered ten to one by hospital nurses. They faced a daunting increase in workload from the growing elderly population and a continued lack of proper liaison with local authority social services. One factor had remained constant amid all this change and development: preventative services were still the poorest of poor relations in the mid-1970s NHS, with just 0.38 per cent of NHS spending, while health education received a miserable 0.1 per cent. And even 60 years on, there is still no occupational health service.

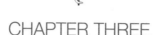

CHAPTER THREE

The end of consensus:
the road back to the market 1979–1988

In areas with more sickness and death, general practitioners have more work, larger lists, less hospital support, and inherit more clinically ineffective traditions of consultation than in the healthiest areas: and hospital doctors shoulder heavier caseloads with less staff and equipment, more obsolete buildings, and suffer recurrent crises in the availability of beds and replacement staff. These trends can be summed up as the Inverse Care Law: that the availability of good medical care tends to vary inversely with the need of the population served. ...

If our health services had evolved as a free market, or even on a fee-for-item-of-service basis prepaid by private insurance, the law would have operated much more completely than it does: our situation might approximate to that in the United States, with the added disadvantages of smaller national wealth.

The force that creates and maintains the Inverse Care Law is the operation of the market... The more health services are removed from the force of the market, the more successful we can be in redistributing care away from its "natural" distribution in a market economy...

(Dr Julian Tudor Hart, *The Lancet*, 27 February 1971)

THE RETURN OF THE TORIES IN 1979 was to open up a new phase in the development of the NHS. Although the Armageddon which many health workers and campaigners feared was not unleashed at once, the stance of the Thatcher government towards the economy as a whole, and the health service in particular, was well illustrated by the reaction of Health and Social Services Secretary Patrick Jenkin to the 1980 Black Report. Sir Douglas Black had been commissioned in 1977 by the Labour government to look into the evidence of a class divide under the broad title of "Inequalities in Health". Labour's Health Secretary David Ennals told the Socialist Medical Association why he had set up the inquiry:

To take the extreme example, in 1971 the death rate for adult men in Social Class V (unskilled workers) was nearly twice that of adult men in Social Class I (professional workers) even when account has been taken of the different age structure of the two classes. When you look at death rates for specific diseases the gap is even wider.

For example, for tuberculosis the death rate in Social Class V is ten times that for Social Class I; for bronchitis it was five times as high and for lung and stomach cancer three times as high...

Maternal mortality – down a long way from the figures of 40 years ago – shows the same pattern; the death rate was twice as high for wives of men in Social Class V as for those in Social Class I.

At age five, Social Class I children are about an inch taller than Social Class V children.

(Ennals 1977)

The Black Report was presented to the government in 1980. Mr Jenkin, no social reformer, expressed his personal distaste for the facts it uncovered in his off-hand "Foreword" to the tatty, duplicated version of the 263-page report which his Department grudgingly published on August bank holiday weekend:

It will come as a disappointment to many that over long periods since the inception of the NHS there is generally little sign of health inequalities in Britain actually diminishing and, in some cases, they may be increasing. It will be seen that the Group has reached the view that the causes of health inequalities are so deep-rooted that only a major and wide-ranging programme of public expenditure is capable of altering the pattern.

I must make it clear that additional expenditure on the scale which could result from the report's recommendations – the amount involved could be upwards of £2 billion a year – is quite unrealistic in present or any foreseeable economic circumstances, quite apart from any judgement that may be formed of the effectiveness of such expenditure in dealing with the problems identified.

(Black D et al. 1980: 1)

The Black Report had indeed trodden on some Tory corns, stressing as it did that 30 years of the NHS had left the health of manual workers and their families lagging even further behind the professional and middle classes. People living in low-income households tended to die younger and suffer worse health at all ages. For every baby boy from the professional classes that died before his first birthday, two died in the skilled working class and four among unskilled manual workers. By 1976, infant mortality had fallen by 45 per cent for the professional class, 49 per cent for the "managerial" middle class, but only 34 per cent for the unskilled manual working class.

The Black Report, which conducted no original research, but merely systematised information already published and available, went beyond these bald figures to look more widely at the problem than simply at the NHS and health services. No matter how good the new systems and methods of treatment, they could not compensate for social conditions which generated a constant stream of accidents and illness.

It found that the children of unskilled workers were ten times more likely to die from fire, fall or drowning, and seven times more likely to be killed by cars than their professional class contemporaries. Unskilled men actually stood a *greater* chance of early death from a number of common causes in 1969 than they had ten years earlier, and the difference in death rates *widened* in the two decades to 1970. In no fewer than 68 out of 92 causes of death, rates were higher for semi- and unskilled workers than for the middle classes.

Manual workers were also less likely to use community health and preventative services than the middle class, who also made the most call on Family Planning and cervical screening services. These problems, too, arose in part from political and economic factors rather than simply the individual decisions and lifestyles of working-class people. The Black Report provided hard figures to support Tudor Hart's Inverse Care Law of 1971 – showing that hospital and community health spending was lowest, and therefore facilities least easy to access, in the regions with the highest proportion of unskilled and semi-skilled manual workers. A working-class person in a deprived working-class area would be less healthy, and less able to find health care than in a socially mixed area.

The Black Report probed the underlying causes of ill health in terms of poverty and housing, and emphasised the increase in poverty over 20 years. Numbers living below or only marginally above supplementary benefit levels had almost doubled from 7.74 million in 1960 (14 per cent) to 14 million (27 per cent) in 1977. A third of these were employed workers or in wage-earning families, while 40 per cent were pensioners. Diet and nutrition were also examined, especially in childhood (pointing to the beneficial impact on children's health of the food policy during the Second World War) and focused on the perils of cigarette smoking, which led to around 50,000 premature deaths a year, and has always been most popular among the manual working class.

Among the recommendations which Patrick Jenkin so contemptuously dismissed were a series of measures to relieve poverty, including an increase in child benefit and the maternity grant; payment of an infant care allowance to mothers of under 5s and a comprehensive disablement allowance. On nutrition, it suggested free school meals for all children. And it suggested free nursery facilities, especially in the most deprived areas, as well as an expansion of sheltered housing for the elderly and disabled.

The whole scheme was costed in 1979 at a total of £1.5 billion a year (little more than half the cost then of the married man's tax allowance). It would have represented a serious investment in health promotion across the age spectrum, and would certainly have produced longer-term cash savings by reducing ill health. Instead the Report and its recommendations were brushed aside by a Thatcher government, which was intent upon policies which were to deepen still further the class divide and increase the numbers in relative and absolute poverty.

The first four years of Thatcher government brought a near 50 per cent increase in numbers living in poverty (from 11.6 million to 16.4 million). Included in this was a 72 per cent increase in numbers of children living on or below poverty levels. While real salaries for the top fifth of wage earners went up 22 per cent in the first eight years of Thatcher's rule, the bottom tenth saw their incomes fall by upwards of 15 per cent. In 1986 alone, the numbers of low-paid workers increase by 400,000. Homelessness rocketed from 57,000 families in 1979 to 94,000 in 1985.

Low-paid workers were the hardest-hit by another Tory policy – massive, above-inflation increases in prescription charges. The Conservatives had pledged in their 1979 manifesto not to increase prescription charges from the 20p per item level set by Labour. But within six months they had raised it a thumping 125 per cent to 45p. In April 1980 the charge went up another 55 per cent to 70p, and by December 1980, when it went up again to £1, patients had suffered a five-fold increase in just 18 months. The break-neck pace of increase continued, reaching £2.60 in April 1988 and £5.75 in 1998 – almost 28 times the cost 20 years previously.[9]

Yet the prescription charge is the epitome of an ideological rather than a practical measure. The token gesture of forcing sick people – irrespective of their ability to pay – to stump up hard cash for their treatment is the driving force behind this relentless rise in charges. With 75 per cent of patients currently exempt, the sums of money recouped from those unlucky enough to pay has only ever been a drop in the ocean of the NHS budget. Each increase, however, has increased the pressure on low-paid workers to avoid going to the doctor, and for those unable to afford several items on a prescription form to choose one or more which they will do without.

A similar approach to charges for dental treatment – most notably the axing of the last vestige of the original free service, the universal entitlement to a free dental examination, which was scrapped a few months after the 1987 general election – has served to deter an increasing number, especially low-income working people, from regular check-ups. This has been coupled with policies which have driven large numbers of dentists out of the NHS altogether, and excluded many modern treatments from the NHS tariff, obliging patients to go privately or do without. Many community dental units have also been scaled down or closed down, leaving many areas of the country with only a faint folk memory of NHS dental services.

Further evidence of the Tory government's determination to head in precisely the opposite direction from the Black Report came with the scrapping of free eye tests, also in November 1987. This came despite Thatcher's specific statement in 1980 that the government had dropped its plan to introduce charges, which "would be wrong in principle and could deter patients from seeking professional advice". In pressing ahead with this policy, the government brushed aside the complaints from the ophthalmic profession that levying a £10 charge would increase problems for the NHS, since it would result in late detection of glaucoma and other potentially serious problems previously spotted during eye tests.

With the progressive social policies of the Black Report rejected, the 18 years from 1979 were to mark a significant, consistent and increasingly rapid shift in government policy away from the traditional concept of collective, inclusive provision of health care. This hard-edged, exclusive, business-style approach

---

9   The rate of increase has slowed under New Labour since 1997, but a single item prescription at time of writing stands at £6.85 in England (November 2007). By contrast, the Welsh Assembly Government has successfully abolished the charge for Welsh residents and the new SNP-led Scottish government has embarked on a similar policy since May 2007.

reduced the patient's status to that of a "customer", and increasingly allowed the methods and logic of the market to predominate over health needs.

The first years of the Thatcher government represented a phoney peace for the NHS. The Tory Chancellor felt obliged by the Party's pre-election promises to uphold the increasing NHS budget allocations pencilled in by the outgoing Labour government – although much of this extra money was in any case to be swallowed up by rampant inflation and an extremely generous increase in pay for nurses and ambulance crews, arising from the 1978–9 pay round (Timmins 1995; Radical Statistics Health Group 1987).[10]

Indeed, though prompt action was taken by Sir Geoffrey Howe's first budget to sever the cherished link between the state pension and average pay – with far-reaching later consequences for millions of elderly people – the main attention of the Thatcher team was not on the welfare state but upon industry, the unions and the privatisation and deregulation of the wider economy (Timmins 1995).

New quangos take shape

This did not prevent significant changes from being prepared. Earlier in the year, a Royal Commission had given a resounding thumbs down to Sir Keith Joseph's botched 1974 reorganisation of the NHS. In response, ministers unveiled a White Paper in December 1979 under the deceptive title of *Patients First* (DHSS 1979b). This proposed scrapping the Area Health Authorities and thus abandoning any pretence of common boundaries for health and local government. Once more, the always fragile links between the NHS and social services were weakened – and at the very moment when health policies were beginning to focus more than ever on the idea of care "in the community".

In place of the 90 AHAs, Regional Health Authorities would now oversee 192 District Health Authorities in England, and seven Special Health Authorities would cover London's postgraduate teaching hospitals. The 1979 White Paper rejected the idea of replacing old-style administrators and the methods of "consensus management" with more business-style chief executives – this was to come four years later. However, it did call for closer working links between hospital management and health authorities.

The White Paper also initially proposed ditching the Community Health Councils. For all the weaknesses many of them displayed, these were the nearest thing to a democratic or accessible voice for local people on health policy and service issues, and possibly the only progressive element of the 1974 reforms. The government was forced to retreat on this, while Health Secretary Patrick Jenkin claimed that his new system would lead to more accountability and local control:

---

10 The nurses' pay award alone was later estimated by the Commons Social Services Committee to account for no less than 37 per cent of the increase in NHS spending between 1979 and 1986.

"I believe it is wrong to treat the NHS as though it were or could be a single giant integrated system," he declared. "Rather we must try to see it as a whole series of local health services serving local communities and managed by local people."

(cited in Klein 2006: 100)

The word "local" proved to be one of the most abused in the evolving health policies from this point onwards, being wheeled in to introduce the 1982 reorganisation, then used as a pretext for dropping national planning norms, and then exploited to the hilt in the (unsuccessful) efforts to win support for the opting out of NHS Trusts from 1989, and the launch of Foundation Trusts in 2003. Of course, the only genuine accountability proposed in 1979, by deliberate policy decision, was still from the District Health Authority *upwards* to the DHSS (with its regime of cash limits). A suggestion from the Royal Commission that RHAs should have greater responsibility and control over their districts was specifically rejected by the government. And of course, there was to be no hint of democracy or accountability downwards to local residents (Mohan 1995).

The new DHAs had fewer members and were no more representative of local people than the disbanded AHAs. As on previous occasions, many establishment worthies merely changed hats and moved across from one quango to another. All members were still appointed by ministers, with a reduced proportion of members coming from local authorities. Political patronage (fiercely denied, of course) was painfully obvious to any outside observer, though a token number of suitably pliable Labour Party members were appointed as DHA chairs, especially in areas where controversial cuts and closures were in the offing. There was still a "trade union seat", but the trade unionist was to be picked not by the local trade union movement, but by the RHA from a panel of nominations. Some RHAs began brazenly to veto trade union nominees who they considered likely to speak up with any independence, while some of the so-called "trade union members" they did appoint proved – as they connived with local cuts – to be obscure figures with little if any support among union members.

As before, the scope for serious decision-making by the DHAs was always slender, since they were entirely dependent for their information on the full-time District Management Teams, which drew up all of the documents for decision: and of course, DHAs had no say or influence over the size of the cash-limited budgets available, which were fixed by ministers and doled out by Regional Health Authorities.

The only obligation of a DHA was to comply with government cash limits. And though, unlike councillors, they ran no personal risk of surcharge if they defied these limits and overspent to protect local services, only a handful even tried to rebel. The whole history of appointed health authorities is remarkable for their almost universal and docile acceptance of virtually every government instruction to cut spending, even where this meant devastating local services, and where the worst that could happen to HA members would be to be removed from office.

One valiant exception to the rule of surrender was the Lambeth, Southwark and Lewisham Health Authority, which in 1979 refused to cut £5 million from its

£138 million budget. Jenkin sent in commissioners to take over from the suspended HA – but was later found to have acted unlawfully (Timmins 1995).

Tighter limits, looser norms

While the structural reorganisation of the White Paper was not to take effect until 1982, the new government took steps to tighten its grip on the existing health authorities with the passing of the Health Services Act in 1980. This made cash limits legally binding – a step that had not been taken when the policy was introduced by Labour in 1976 (Mohan 1995).

Even while they tightened their increasingly rigid financial control over NHS spending, the government was intent upon loosening the planning guidelines which laid down norms for service provision. In 1981, *Care in Action* was published as a policy steer for the DHAs to be established the following year. It advised that health service priorities should be decided 'locally', and abandoned previous efforts to define minimum levels of bed numbers and resources (DHSS 1981a). In a forerunner to the subsequent drive for "income generation", health authorities were also given powers to establish their own local charitable appeals for funds.

Pay battle

1982 was dominated by the long-running campaign of industrial action over pay, which had fallen well behind the national average for all sections of health workers. Between 1975 and 1981, average earnings had risen by 133 per cent, while nurses had received only 118 per cent (representing a real terms reduction in buying power compared with inflation). Ancillary staff had done even worse, with increases equivalent to just 97 per cent over the same period. Three-quarters of all ancillaries and half of all full-time nurses were earning less than the government's official poverty line rate of £82 per week, at which point Family Income Supplement became available (Lister 1988).

The government, possibly in a deliberate trial of strength, or possibly seeking to soften up the best-organised section of health workers for the later imposition of competitive tendering, singled out the NHS for a further real-terms pay cut. With inflation running at 12 per cent, and pay settlements elsewhere averaging 7 per cent, they offered NHS staff an increase of just 4 per cent. Action began in the spring of 1982 and, with a half-baked campaign being reluctantly led by half-hearted union officials, dragged on through the summer and into the autumn with sporadic one-day strikes. Fleeting glimpses of the potential support the health workers could have found had they engaged in more sustained action were visible in the TUC day of action on NHS pay on 22 September, which turned out to be a one-day general strike, with solidarity stoppages widespread: Fleet Street newspapers, 75 per cent of coal mines, many docks, car plants, shipyards, steel plants and many other workplaces and industries in the public and private sector were halted or disrupted by strikes. The Welsh CBI claimed that only 50 per cent of firms had worked normally; 150,000 marched through central London (Timmins 1995).

However, facing an obdurate government and saddled with a hesitant TUC leadership which wanted the dispute ended, the campaign finally wound up in December 1982 with nothing gained by those who had fought the hardest. Ancillary staff faced the added insult of seeing an extra government handout to the nurses who, in the main, had taken no action. Nurses were also promised a pay review body similar to that of the doctors, in the hope that their wage demands would be kept separate from the other sections of health workers. This was the equivalent for health unions of what was to befall the miners in their year-long strike: the defeat set back the development of militant opposition, and gave the government the political confidence to contemplate what would previously have been unthinkable policies (Timmins 1995).

Support services: the cowboys ride in

Two months after the end of the pay battle, the government took a dramatic step towards carving out a slice of the NHS budget for the private sector. Early in 1983 ministers published a circular with the tell-tale title *NHS support services – Contracting Out*. It called on health authorities to commence competitive tendering for hospital domestic, catering and laundry services – but far from offering a genuinely "level playing field", the entire bias of the policy was towards awarding contracts to the private sector (DHSS 1983).

New firms of private contractors sprang up, some of them subsidiaries of major corporations, specifically targeting this new, potentially lucrative market. Although tendering was not legally compulsory, intense government pressure was put onto health authorities to comply, with the threat to remove DHA chairs or appointed members who resisted (Timmins 1995). The consequences for NHS support staff were predictable: in what were already low-wage, labour-intensive jobs, the only way private firms could hope significantly to undercut the cost of the existing NHS service would be to slash back the numbers of staff (thus undermining the quality of service), to cut the wages and conditions of staff (and risk major problems of recruitment and retention), or simply to cut corners on the work that was done (Coyle 1986; Labour Research Department 1987).

Most private tenders incorporated a combination of all three, and the cheapskate firms were aided and abetted by the incompetence and inexperience of hospital management in drawing up detailed specifications of the work to be done and the quality required. Privatisation of services was often swiftly followed by a catastrophic drop in standards of hygiene and patient care. Unfortunately this meant that in order to compete with private bids, in-house tenders, too, began to be based on fewer staff and poorer conditions (Labour Research Department 1987). In the spring of 1984, women cleaners at Barking Hospital walked out on strike against drastic cuts in pay and hours of work imposed by their private employer, Crothalls, as they cut the price of their tender to retain the contract. Left isolated, despite the initial bold words from their union, NUPE, their own heroic efforts to publicise the issue, and the nationwide impact of competitive tendering, the Barking women were to be on strike 18 months before conceding defeat (Lister 1988).

As the government pressed home a policy designed to privatise services hospital by hospital, district by district, there were to be other courageous shows of resistance – notably at Addenbrookes Hospital, Cambridge, Scarsdale Hospital, Chesterfield and Hammersmith Hospital in West London – but few victories. Only in two instances – mental health services in Sunderland and in Oxford – were privatisation attempts successfully beaten back by union resistance. Though the union fight back was weak and localised, it still was not easy for the government to sell privatisation to sceptical health bosses. Health authorities had for years had the option of contracting out, but very few had chosen to do so. Many of them tacitly recognised the points made by London Health Emergency in a detailed examination of the tendering exercise:

> Hospitals are not fast food joints or factories in which "efficiency" can be adequately measured simply by the quantity of patients rushed through in minimum time by a minimum of low-paid staff. Just as it would be ridiculous to suggest that a doubling of class sizes in schools would amount to a doubling of efficiency for each teacher, to whittle down the size of the caring team in our hospitals while boasting of the increase in numbers of patients treated each year is to substitute quantity for quality of care.

> Much of the work undertaken by domestics is labour-intensive, manual work, not readily susceptible to mechanisation. To cut back on the hours of work and numbers of staff employed must necessarily cut back on the level of service, the actual care delivered to the patient. ...such a decline is under way. Indeed the average successful tender under the new system has involved cuts in working hours of as much as 60%, with a 40% cutback commonplace.

> (Newbigging and Lister 1988)

After the initial flurry of privatisations early in 1984, progressively fewer DHAs opted to bring in contractors. By July 1985 a majority of contracts were being awarded in-house. By the end of 1986, private firms had won only 187 out of 1,123 contracts awarded. Only 4 per cent of catering contracts went to private companies. The government claimed total "savings" from the exercise totalling £86 million – less than 0.5 per cent of an NHS budget of £18 billion – but this took no account of the management time consumed by the tendering exercise or the potential knock-on human and financial costs of lowered standards (House of Commons Social Services Committee 1985). By 1988 a number of contractors had pulled out of tendering for NHS domestic service contracts, including Sunlight, Reckitts, OCS and Blue Arrow, whose finance director complained that:

> There is nobody making any money out of the National Health Service.

> (Joint NHS Privatisation Research Unit 1990: 8)

Mediclean, the biggest of the companies that had sprung up to bid for NHS contracts, was sold off to Danish service provider ISS. The contractors may have been gloomy, but so were many of the hospital managers when they tried to get the contract firms to deliver the services specified. Penalty clauses for poor work proved ineffective, and almost every time a health authority managed to break off a failed contract, the government intervened to change the rules to make it harder. The first HA to give a firm its marching orders was Bromley in March 1985, after six months of failure by Hospital Hygiene Services. But one of HHS's directors was prominent Tory backbench MP Marcus Fox, who in a shameless exercise in string-pulling, persuaded Secretary of State for Health Kenneth Clarke to issue new instruction preventing any DHA from ending a contract, no matter how poor the firm's performance. A dissatisfied HA now had to seek Department approval to sack the company (Newbigging and Lister 1988: 10).

Nevertheless, against all the odds, Maidstone HA managed to sack Crothalls early in 1986 – but once again the goalposts were moved to favour the private firms. NHS Chairman Victor Paige fired off a confidential letter to Regional Health Authority chairs setting out new rules, making it even more difficult to get rid of a failed contractor, discouraging "unreasonably punitive" penalty clauses, preventing DHAs from intervening to set maximum workloads for contract personnel, and making it easier to hire duff contractors by preventing DHAs from doing their own vetting of firms. RHAs – which were supposed to do the vetting and compile an approved list of companies – were even told to avoid asking "intrusive" questions on the finance and competence of would-be contractors (Paige 1985).

Such questions were valid, since increasingly desperate companies began resorting to tactics including ludicrously uneconomic "loss leaders" in order to win contracts. ICC won a contract for domestic services at Edgware Hospital in 1987, but having done so immediately asked Barnet Health Authority for higher payments – and managed to be sacked before the contract even started! A trade union survey listed 64 failed contracts between September 1983 to May 1987, and these were only the most glaringly obvious failures (Joint NHS Privatisation Research Unit 1987).

By the spring of 1987, the policy was in such disrepute that even the Royal College of Nursing, which had stood aloof from the problems of support staff, felt obliged to reconsider its policy. At its Glasgow conference, Susie Jewell from City and Hackney reported that the successful in-house tender had resulted in one cleaner being left to look after three wards, serving all the food, ordering supplies and cleaning.

> The result was doctors, nurses and even patients doing most of the cleaning. The wards are squalid to say the least.
>
> (*Nursing Times*, 22 April 1987)

Thousands of ancillary jobs were axed in this process, whether through privatisation or in-house bids. This changed the shape and feel of health services in many hospitals. The number of directly employed ancillary staff fell by a massive 50 per cent between 1981 and 1991. In the process, loyal and dedicated teams were broken up, and experienced health workers, who had played a key role especially on the wards of long-stay hospitals, left the NHS (Mohan 1995: 21).

The new ancillary workforce was effectively casualised, the majority working part time and many only working there while they looked for better-paid work elsewhere. At Oxford's flagship John Radcliffe Hospital, the turnover of staff on the in-house service got so bad in 1988 that less than a third of newly hired domestics stayed longer than one day. The hospital began to offer up to £50 "bounty" payments to domestics who could find a friend willing to work there. Elsewhere, staff turnover levels as high as 550 per cent were reported on private contracts (Newbigging and Lister 1988).

The contract companies, always rootless and unstable, continued a growing trend towards monopoly, with only the largest firms surviving and expanding through takeover bids or mergers, while the smaller, weaker firms went to the wall.

Business methods – and bureaucracy

While ancillary staff numbers went into sharp decline, 1983 also marked the start of a different process of change at the top level of the NHS – and another significant shift towards a market-style approach. Roy Griffiths, managing director of the Sainsbury supermarket chain, was brought in by Secretary of State for Health Kenneth Clarke to conduct an informal inquiry into the structure of NHS management (Timmins 1995).

Griffiths produced a short, superficial, document which centred on a corny old joke: "if Florence Nightingale were carrying her lamp through the corridors of the NHS today, she would almost certainly be searching for the people in charge." She might, of course, equally be looking for help from a vanishing ancillary staff. But Griffiths' report – 24 pages of assertions and recommendations with no supporting evidence – struck a sympathetic chord with a government increasingly keen to install "business methods" in the NHS.

Griffiths proposed that managers should replace administrators: consensus management should go. Consultants should be pulled into line by making them responsible for running budgets, and a separate management board should be established at national level (Griffiths 1983). Here was the first step towards the creation of a new layer of general managers, soon to rename themselves as 'chief executives'; but the impression of greater local management was an illusion. The managers were directly answerable to the national NHS Executive and thus to the government. This meant more central control, but also in turn generated an increase in the bureaucratic apparatus of support staff – managerial, clerical and secretarial. At a time when the government was insisting on a programme of cuts in NHS personnel, numbers of administrative and clerical staff in the NHS rose by a massive 18 per cent in the decade 1981–91, much of this the result of the Griffiths proposals (Mohan 1995).

The system of employing the top managers only on short-term contracts was one most likely to ensure that few if any would be bold enough to speak out against government policies and central directives, no matter how controversial and politically unpopular these might be or what consequences they might have for local services. Ministers were also keen to insist that as many as possible of the 800 new "general managers" (soon to be chief executives) should be drawn not from the NHS but from industry, and faced down the predictable squeals of outrage from the Royal College of Nursing that no nurses were likely to be appointed to these top jobs. However, few of these external recruits were to last very long in the quite different culture of NHS management.

The man appointed as the chair of the new NHS Management Board, Victor Paige, was a good example. Paige previously chaired the Port of London Authority and was Deputy Chair of the National Freight Consortium. This was apparently enough to persuade Kenneth Clarke and Norman Fowler to appoint him to the £70,000 a year post, despite his readiness to admit that he knew nothing about the NHS. On hearing of his appointment, Paige was happy to tell reporters of his long-standing subscription to private health insurance and insisted that he had no intention of cancelling his BUPA policy. "Like most people I am covered by private medical insurance," he blurted out. An embarrassed DHSS was obliged to publish a correction. In fact just 8 per cent – one person in twelve – had any form of private medical cover at that time. Paige, never on the right wavelength for the NHS, eventually resigned after 18 inconclusive months (Lister 1988).

To take his place, Norman Fowler brought in Len Peach, a top figure from the notoriously anti-union IBM Corporation. As might be expected, Mr Peach saw accountability as a vertical structure in which managers were accountable to the NHS Executive, and health authorities were largely irrelevant. In a keynote article in the *Health Service Journal*, Peach praised the new system of Individual Performance Review, through which individual managers could pick up cash bonuses for meeting performance targets – which might include cutting spending to meet cash limits, or even closing hospitals on time (*HSJ* 1988). Nor was Mr Peach any fan of public debate or open meetings to involve ordinary mortals from the general public in decision making:

> Our exchanges are conducted in private. While it may not do much for our street credibility, we all believe it is the way to do business.
>
> (*HSJ*, 14 January 1988)

This type of secrecy, so beloved in business circles, was later to be enshrined in the closed-door meetings of NHS Trusts and the increasingly closed sessions of health authorities after 1990.

But the government's attempt to attract top players like Mr Peach from the private sector also had another effect: it began the upward spiral of senior management salaries in the NHS which was later to lift off even more dramatically after the formation of Trusts in 1991. The traditional arguments wheeled out by top bosses to justify their own pay increases while denying the same treatment to their staff were again brought into play. The public were told that at senior management level (but not among nurses or support staff), "If you pay peanuts, you get monkeys." Cynics might respond that if you pay truffles, you get pigs.

At local level this same emergent managerial layer was to be made even more dominant in the 1990 reforms, when they took seats for the first time as "executive members" of scaled-down health authorities and Trusts. Simultaneously, the lay ("non-executive") members were reduced to a rump of five hand-picked appointees. Another facet of the new "business-style" approach was the introduction in 1984 of Cost Improvement Programmes, through which the health authorities were expected to find year-on-year savings. In many cases these "cost improvements" were little more than thinly disguised cuts in services, in staffing or in maintenance (Mohan 1995).

The NHS was beginning to adopt a shape that has become much more familiar to us since the 1990s, and which has been largely retained throughout ten years of the New Labour government's reforms. This was the point at which the managerial ethos began to change from running a public service to one of restructuring the NHS to run as a business, adopting the language and jargon of management consultants. This was still several years before the fashionable but vacuous theories of the 'New Public Management' were to be imported from the USA as the basis for a further round of reforms designed to bring "entrepreneurialism" into public services (Osborne and Gaebler 1992; Pollitt 2000).

Pressures on Thatcher: thinking the unspeakable

They may have established a long-running process of change, but privatisation of support services and the expansion and restructuring of NHS management were relatively small beer compared with some of the more sweeping changes to the fabric of the service that were being discussed behind closed doors by the radical right of the Tory Party and its hangers-on after the 1983 election. Many of those most committed to the free market model, later to be renamed "neoliberalism" were disappointed at the relatively conservative approach of the Thatcher government, which remained acutely aware of the political consequences of stepping too far outside the popular public consensus in favour of a publicly funded and provided NHS.

In 1984 came the Adam Smith Institute's *Omega Report*, a manifesto for moves towards a privatised, insurance-based health care system. It began by looking at what could be lopped off NHS costs, and which additional services could be contracted out, over and above the core support services already out to tender. But it went on to suggest that health authorities could be run as "independent commercial enterprises". Any NHS buildings and facilities which were unused or under-used should, it suggested, be sold or leased to private health care firms. Impoverished NHS hospitals could in turn hire facilities from the wealthy private sector (Adam Smith Institute 1984).

Expanded private check-up clinics, offering x-rays and other tests, could help speed up the closure of NHS hospital outpatient facilities and give a "boost" to the income of GPs, the report suggested. Ambulance services could be cut back to a minimum, privatised or even replaced by "public transport [!], taxis or cars provided by neighbours or relatives."

It was on the issue of charges that the *Omega Report* went furthest. It suggested charges for GP visits; for (privatised) Family Planning services; and for non-emergency ambulance journeys. There should also be charges for "non-essential" hospital "hotel services" (at around £5 per night at 1981 prices, giving an average fee of £50 per visit – "the equivalent of a TV licence"). Though there might be means-tested exemptions to these charges, they should only be for the very poorest, since "The temptation to exempt too many groups will defeat the whole object of the exercise". The report suggested a "health card" or "Medicard" could be used as the means of covering exemptions. They were especially keen that this notion of "credit", coupled with the introduction of charges, would mean that even the poorest would then be able to play their part in boosting the private sector by using the card as part-payment for private treatment.

The *Omega Report* favoured the provision of different standards of comfort in hospital, depending on how much each patient could afford to pay. Meals would of course cost extra. People without exemption would be encouraged to buy stamps each week to cover the new health service fees – like TV licence stamps. There could be tax rebates as incentives for those rich enough to opt out of health service cover and buy their own comprehensive health insurance. Eventually, mused the *Omega Report*, health insurance would become as obligatory as car insurance (except of course that you can always decide not to buy a car). Redundant NHS hospitals and clinics would be absorbed by an expanding private medical industry. The scheme would have set the clock back 40 years, almost as if the NHS had never existed, and restored a market system despite the preponderance of evidence that nowhere in the world do governments dare to leave health care to an unrestricted private market.

This was also the dream of two Tory MPs who went public at the end of 1984 with their own plans. Edward Leigh suggested a scheme to impose full charges for treatment on "all except OAPs, children and the chronically sick" – apparently unaware that his exemptions would cover a majority of all NHS inpatients. Mid-Sussex MP Timothy Renton went further and proposed a profit-making system (*Conservative Newsline* 1984). In 1986 Sir Keith Joseph's Centre for Policy Studies published a booklet by a former general manager of BUPA, Hugh Elwell. He proposed a combination of the charges and insurance schemes with a delicate extra touch of charity fund-raising thrown in, looking nostalgically back to the golden age of the pre-NHS 1930s:

> Labour MPs especially have decried as "nurses with begging bowls" this form of charitable contribution to the NHS, but views seem to be changing with the demonstrable effectiveness of the hospice movement. Though much money could be raised through fetes or flag days, substantial amounts could come from annual donations allowable against tax by the donor. Charitable contributions might seem like a drop in the ocean against the £18 billion NHS annual budget [!], but many thousands of pounds [!] have been raised for local units like this.
> (Elwell 1986: 7)

Mr Elwell however is forced to admit that even when all the tins have been shaken, hospital charges would be necessary under his plan. But he tries to make it sound pleasant:

> A board and lodging charge would provide the unit with additional funds and would make the patient an active participant [!] in the way the care was provided.

That is like saying that a customer in Sainsbury's is an "active participant in the retail food business". The pamphlet was embarrassing even for the Tory right and was quietly ditched. But the ideological push from the right intensified further after the 1987 election. In November of that year the far-right Carlton Club organised a seminar which began from the premise that "against a background of inadequate Central Government funding, the Health Authorities throughout Britain are technically bankrupt, with aggregate debts approaching £1,000 million."

The great brains of the Carlton Club wrestled with the issues and came up with a rag-bag of ideas that included:

- Privatising more services including Intensive Care Units, pathology, and ambulances
- "Disbanding" the health unions
- Extending the "principles of charging" and "creating a costed service"
- Creating, together with the private sector, a "National Health Insurance Scheme"
- Tax relief on private medical insurance premiums.

(Carlton Club Political Committee 1988: 3)

To give tax relief on private medical premiums would then have cost at least £150 million a year, every penny of which would have gone not to the cash-starved NHS, but into the pockets of the well-to-do.

Cashing in: private medicine

The backwoodsmen were not necessarily as wide of the mark as it may now appear. Behind the scenes in the autumn of 1982 (while health workers staged strikes and demonstrations for a pay increase to at least match inflation) Tory ministers had indeed been debating the possibility of replacing the NHS with private health insurance, and introducing charges for visiting a GP (Timmins 1995: 391).

Other schemes in the same options paper, which was initially supported by Treasury Chief Secretary Leon Brittan, included an end to state funding for higher education and vouchers for primary and secondary schooling. At that stage the ideas went too far for Thatcher's cabinet, and were thrown out before they were leaked to the press. Thatcher herself felt sufficiently concerned about the public impression created by the affair that she went out of her way to insist at the 1982 Tory party conference on her credentials as a defender of the NHS:

> Let me make one thing absolutely clear. The National Health Service is safe with us.

(cited in Timmins 1995: 393)

As Timmins points out, this was only partly true. Many Tories were barely bothering to conceal the fact that they wanted an expansion of private medicine (the 1983 manifesto "welcomed" the growth in private health insurance) as well as the privatisation of parts of the NHS.

The Tory government's 1980 Health Services Act had firmly set signposts for the future by disbanding the Health Services Board which restricted numbers of NHS pay beds[11], scaling down restrictions on private hospital development, and giving the Secretary of State power to decide whether or not a private hospital would interfere with local NHS care. There was now room for a new expansion of NHS pay beds.

By 1985, pay bed numbers had risen by 23% – but the numbers of patients using them had dropped by 22%, leaving a typical occupancy rate of 40–50%. In London, the fall in occupancy rates was especially dramatic: the North West Thames region saw occupancy levels drop by 50%.

These beds were a costly luxury for the NHS. The total of pay bed and outpatient fees paid to the NHS in 1986 was a pitiful £61 million, a drop in the bucket compared with the NHS £18 billion budget.

But under specific policy guidance from the government issued in February 1987, NHS hospitals were forbidden to make a profit on their pay beds. Point 8 of the circular to all health authorities insisted that:

> Authorities should aim to recover the full costs of treating private patients, but not to make a profit.
>
> (DHSS 1987: 1)

---

11 Bevan's early compromise on pay beds with the consultants in 1948 had not seemed especially significant at the time. The new NHS had effectively wiped out the majority of private medicine, and it remained an extremely small and marginalised factor throughout the 1950s and early 1960s. Numbers of NHS pay beds fell from 7,200 in 1948 to 5,100 in 1970 and 4,600 by 1974.

But by 1974 the private sector had taken advantage of the NHS's difficulties to rebuild its base of middle-class subscribers to over 2 million – still only a shadow of its pre-war strength. A series of eye-opening revelations on the extent to which this rump of NHS private beds were siphoning off NHS resources and increasing waiting lists had given the issue a new lease of life in 1971, and the Labour leadership seized upon it, including a pledge to ensure "total separation of private practice from the Health Service" in their 1974 election manifesto (Timmins 1995: 334).

This incurred predictable wrath from the BMA and the right-wing press. A Dr H. Fidler, Chair of the BMA's Private Practice Committee, summed up their view that "If we lose this freedom… the medical profession is finished. Even worse, this country is finished."

Health workers took the opposite view, and from 1973 onwards health unions began a growing boycott of work for private patients in NHS pay beds. Once Labour was elected the campaign spread across London and reached over 100 hospitals in Yorkshire and the north, to the evident embarrassment of Secretary of State Barbara Castle, who declared that "While I can understand the feelings of the staff, I cannot condone the action they are taking" (Lister 1988: 45).

In the event, Castle set up a new quango in 1976, the Health Services Board, with the task of agreeing the pace at which NHS pay beds would be phased out and replaced by beds in private hospitals. 1,600 more pay beds were closed in this way between 1977 and 1979 (Radical Statistics Health Group 1987: 109).

To achieve an exact break-even charge for use of private beds was further complicated by the government stipulation that prices had to be fixed on 1 April of each year, and could not then be increased for 12 months:

> Authorities must before 1 April each year determine charges which apply... throughout the following 12 months. The charges set cannot be added to or amended in any way during the year in which they apply.

This approach stands in stark contrast to the claims that the NHS was adopting "business methods": no big firms were being asked for a 12-month price freeze.

The rules were shaped to give the biggest possible bargain to the private patient:

> Charges should be equitable, that is reasonably closely related to the cost of individual treatment;
>
> Administration costs should be kept to a minimum.

The new regulations came against a background of increasingly public revelations of health authority losses on pay beds. Blackpool DHA had been losing £30,000 a year on private hip operations, while Lewisham and North Southwark DHA lost £376,000 in 1984 on private heart operations.

In May 1987, Bloomsbury DHA's finance director admitted that despite refurbishing its private beds at a cost of £800,000 "We are not recovering our costs at the moment." (In fact the DHA was projecting a loss for the year of £215,000.) The previous year, Bloomsbury had been obliged to write off £500,000 in bad debts from fly-by-night private patients (*Health Emergency* 16, 1987).

The NHS was also losing out heavily on its scale of charges to the private sector. While private hospitals already itemised treatment and services received, charging for every pill, bandage, x-ray, pathology test and charging by the minute for physiotherapy, comparable NHS guideline figures were imprecise and bargain-basement cheap. As *Health Emergency* pointed out:

> At £9 for each attendance, it can be cheaper to get private physiotherapy from an NHS hospital than to take your dog to the vet. Model charges for NHS operating theatres reach a maximum of £81 for anything over 30 minutes...
>
> (*Health Emergency* 16, 1987)

As vital NHS resources were siphoned off in these rock-bottom fees and failed ventures, few health authority members or politicians appeared aware of Section 62 of the NHS (1977) Act, which stated that "pay beds or private outpatient facilities should be withdrawn where their use becomes detrimental to NHS patients for whatever reasons". Among the critics of the government policy on pay beds was Merton and Sutton Health Authority, stuffed though it was with government supporters. Its minutes recorded that:

> Members considered that the regulations worked to the disadvantage of Health Authorities, and that the charges did not reflect the fact that most NHS hospitals provided a much wider range of diagnostic equipment than private hospitals.
>
> (*Health Emergency* 16, 1987)

Private hospitals, too, were finding it hard to get a correct balance between capacity and occupancy. Despite a government committed to the ideology and ethos of privatisation and an NHS facing growing waiting lists, the growth of private medical insurance slowed down in the early 1980s. By 1986 there were still only 5 million people (9 per cent of the population) covered by private policies, most of these through workplace insurance cover purchased for them by employers, and growth had slowed from 30 per cent in 1980 to 5 per cent per year (Mohan 1995).

The NHS "winter crisis" which followed the 1987 general election proved a valuable fillip to the fortunes of the private insurers. PPP announced a 45 per cent increase in public inquiries during January 1988: "It has to be put down to fear, basically" the company told the *Financial Times*. Western Provident Association claimed inquiries had doubled in the same few weeks, while BUPA, according to the *FT*, "says there is a surge of interest very time there is a furore over the NHS." (*Financial Times*, 10 February 1988)

Privatising the elderly

The biggest area of privatisation, which effectively excluded hundreds of thousands of vulnerable patients from NHS care, was in continuing care of the elderly. 1981 saw the publication of a White Paper (*Growing Older*, DHSS 1981b) and a consultative document (*Care in the Community*, DHSS 1981c), both of which centred on the drive to transfer patients and services out from hospital settings into the community.

The consultative document suggested that funds for community-based services would depend upon the sale of surplus land and buildings. These discussions took place under a growing cloud of well-founded suspicion that the NHS was looking to community care as a smokescreen to cover its abdication from responsibility for a growing area of care for the frail elderly and people with chronic mental illness.

The norms for provision of beds for the elderly drawn up by the DHSS in 1976 had been massively and systematically ignored by cash-strapped Regional and District health authorities. By 1984, a survey by Shadow Health Minister Michael Meacher revealed that not one region in England was planning to meet the targets laid down for inpatients or day hospital places. Instead, thousands of beds for the elderly had closed (*Health Emergency* 7, 1985).

Despite a demographic "explosion" which was creating a sharp increase in numbers of elderly people in the vulnerable 75-plus age group, RHA plans across the country were looking to reduce bed numbers to an average of 25 per cent below the 1976 guideline provision – with an even bigger (50 per cent) shortfall in the provision of day hospital places. While the closures of geriatric beds and the shortfall in care for the elderly grabbed headlines, behind the scenes, the biggest shift of policy in care of the elderly – and one which was to have lasting impact on the shape and scope of the NHS – had gone through with little discussion in 1980.

The Social Security Act, endorsing a policy which began to be applied in 1979, gave DHSS offices the discretion to meet the costs of residential or nursing home care for elderly patients from the social security budget. At first, only a trickle of patients from NHS hospitals were to receive care paid for in this way: but they were soon to increase to a flood (Courtney and Walker 1996: 7).

Growing numbers of health authority and hospital chiefs spotted that this was the ideal means of shifting the bill for caring for an expensive group of patients from their cash-limited NHS budgets onto social security: and they followed this by closing down the vacated NHS geriatric beds. And business entrepreneurs with an eye to a profitable investment saw that private nursing and residential homes offered an attractive proposition: numbers of homes and places rocketed during the 1980s,[12] while NHS provision was rapidly reduced – by a third, from 56,000 geriatric beds in 1982 to just 37,000 in 1994 (Courtney and Walker 1996: 7–8).

The procedure under the 1980 Act was made even speedier by a 1982 amendment to the Social Security Act. Until then, Social Security officials had been empowered to make top-up allowances to the board and lodging allowance to cover residential or nursing home fees: the new system made this an entitlement. The process that ensued was one of rapid, unannounced and almost unchallenged privatisation. For the frail elderly, the concept of care free at the point of use and funded from taxation was rapidly disappearing.

More than half of the elderly people in residential homes were paying their own fees. Many of those who moved in to the dwindling number of council-run residential homes (which halved in number from 116,000 to 69,000 places over the same period) were obliged to pay for the privilege: 36 per cent of the costs were being "clawed back" from residents through means-testing – paying charges totalling around £1 billion a year in the mid-1980s, eight times the annual revenue from prescription charges (Lister 1988: 76).

By the end of 1986, the Audit Commission was drawing attention to the scale of this spending, which was running out of control. Secretary of State Norman Fowler called in Sainsbury managing director Roy Griffiths to conduct an inquiry (Timmins 1995: 417).

Mental health

The rundown of bed numbers in psychiatric hospitals accelerated during the 1980s, reducing from 84,000 beds in 1982 to 50,000 in 1992, a reduction of 40 per cent (Department of Health Statistics 1993). There was no evident sign of concern among politicians at national or local level as to what was happening to the patients discharged, or to those chronic patients for whom there was increasingly no appropriate bed available.

---

12 Nursing home places increased from 18,000 in 1982 to 150,000 in 1994; private residential home places expanded from 44,000 in 1982 to 164,000 in 1994.

It is a boring cliché, commonly trotted out by ministers defending real reductions or already inadequate levels of resources, to argue that problems of health care cannot be solved "simply by throwing money at them". Of course, there are many unresolved debates concerning the theory and practice of mental health policy; but it is equally true that *no* policy could have delivered a satisfactory level or standard of mental health care on the level of capital and revenue resources available in the 1980s.

Early in 1985 the Commons Social Services Committee, in a major report, criticised the government's two-faced policy of advocating "community care" without providing the necessary cash, declaring that:

> A decent community-based service for mentally ill... people cannot be provided at the same overall cost as present services. The proposition that community care could be cost neutral is untenable. Even if the present policies of reducing hospital care and building up alternative services were amended, there would in any event be considerable additional costs for mental disability services.
>
> There are growing numbers of mentally disabled people living in the community with older parents; some provision will have to be made for them. The Victorian hospitals in which thousands of mentally ill... people still live, in visibly inadequate conditions, will either have to continue to be shored up, at growing capital and revenue expense, or demolished and replaced by more appropriate housing, at even greater expense.
>
> If the hospitals were to be maintained, it is also inevitable that in most hospitals staffing ratios and the proportion of trained staff would have to be improved.
>
> Proceeding with a policy of community care on a cost-neutral assumption is not simply naive, it is positively inhuman. Community care on the cheap would prove worse in many respects than the pattern of services to date.
>
> There is ample evidence of the decanting of patients from mental illness hospitals in years past without sufficient development of services for them. This has produced a population of chronically mentally ill people with nowhere to go.
>
> (House of Commons Social Services Committee 1985: XIV)

Despite these problems, it seems that many of the scandals that began to hit the headlines arose not from recent premature discharges of 'long-stay' patients into the community, but from earlier phases of the policy, and from the inadequate resourcing of some acute psychiatric units. Others had fallen victim to the way in which mental health services as a whole were shaped around the hospital model, or focused on the discharge and care of the relatively small proportion of mentally ill people who were or had been inpatients, while the large majority of sufferers received little or no specialised help.

There was little evidence to suggest that levels of demand or need for mental health services had decreased. Despite the growing focus on alternative forms of care, there had been a significant *rise* in numbers of short-term admissions to psychiatric hospitals from the mid-1960s, from around 160,000 a year nationally (half of which were 'first time' admissions) to 200,000 a year in the mid-1980s (just 25 per cent of whom were first time admissions, indicating a changing pattern of care but broadly similar numbers) (Office of Health Economics 1989: 15).

Meanwhile, with far fewer available beds, the pressures on services (and staff) increased – driving hospital staff to seek more rapid discharge of patients.

While numbers of psychiatric beds were cut, there was little sign that a new form of 'community care' based on outpatient treatment was emerging: indeed outpatient attendances in England remained almost constant over a ten-year period 1979–89, rising from 1.6 million in 1979 to a peak of 1.8 million in 1985 and 1986, before falling back again to 1.6 million a year since 1987. Even new outpatient attendances, which should have reflected the new policies of treating mental illness outside of hospital admissions, rose only by an average of 0.7 per cent a year from 1979 to 1985.

What *had* been cut substantially is the number in long-stay patients – down from around 50,000 in hospital for five years or more (out of 100,000 inpatients) in the early 1970s to around 17,000 (out of a total of 50,000 inpatients) by the mid-1980s (Office of Health Economics 1989: 17).

By the mid-1980s it was calculated that *half* of all mental illness inpatients were elderly, and that 25 per cent of all referrals to psychiatric departments were aged over 65. In many cases these people are unsuitable for treatment in short-stay acute beds, while the NHS capacity to give long-term care had been drastically reduced, with no sign that local authorities, the voluntary sector, or private enterprise were in any position to take on the responsibility (Mental Health Foundation 1990).

Other figures suggested that at least 3.7 million people each year suffered from *severe* mental illness. Yet only a small proportion of these sufferers were receiving any specialist medical attention. Just 60,000 were receiving treatment as hospital inpatients. Only one in ten severe sufferers (350,000) attended psychiatric outpatient departments. Of the 25 per cent of over 65s suffering from mental illness, only one in fifteen was in any form of institutional care in the mid-1980s (Mental Health Foundation 1990).

Nationally, spending on mental illness treatment and care, at over £2 billion a year, was (and has remained) the biggest single item on the NHS budget – then standing at double the amount spent on cancer treatment, and 30 per cent higher than spending on heart and stroke disorders. Yet almost three-quarters of this allocation (£1.5 billion) was being spent on the hospital care of just 60,000 inpatients, while spending by local authorities came to just £200 million (Mental Health Foundation 1990).

A major problem in the planning of replacement services is that the costs of inpatient treatment tend to *increase* as the number of inpatients goes down. The Commons Social Services Committee discovered in 1990 that while mental illness inpatient numbers fell 27 per cent in the 10 years to 1989, the overall cost of mental illness inpatient services *rose* by 7 per cent, with the cost per case rocketing by almost 50 per cent.

This increase in costs was the result of a number of factors – the inefficient use of large, maintenance-intensive hospital buildings; a greater throughput of patients in each bed, meaning that each required more treatment; the ageing population of those people now resident in long-stay hospitals; and the fact that once those most able to fend for themselves had been discharged, the remainder tended to be the most dependent patients, requiring higher staff members per occupied bed. But what it meant was that there was no automatic release of resources for community care as hospital beds were closed and patients discharged.

To complete the picture of declining services, Department of Health figures also showed a dramatic *fall* in numbers of local authority supported residents in homes and hostels for the mentally ill in England: in the seven years from 1982, the numbers dropped 25 per cent, from 4,880 to just 3,600 in 1989 (Lister 1991: 6). The Social Services Committee argued that to provide a satisfactory level of social care in the community cost £2,752 per person per year. By this reckoning, to provide social care for the 3.7 million sufferers from severe mental illness would have cost £8,256 *million* (£8.256 *billion*) a year – around a third of the whole NHS annual budget, and more than *four times* the current NHS spending on mental health! London's share alone would have been at least £1 billion!

The same committee estimated that it cost about eight times as much (£21,366 a year) to provide a satisfactory level of residential and day care services to people discharged from psychiatric hospitals. This helps explain the lack of government commitment to plug the obvious gaps in the service. To have put right what is wrong in mental health care would have cost far more than the government was prepared to spend (Mental Health Foundation 1990; Lister 1991: 6).

One consistent element of government policy since 1961 has been the verbal, rhetorical commitment to community care. It was reaffirmed in the 1975 Labour government White Paper *Better Services for the Mentally Ill* (DHSS 1975); in 1981 a Tory government consultative paper was issued, entitled *Care in the Community* (DHSS 1981c), and this was followed up by a DHSS circular of the same title in 1983.

But the 1975 White Paper made it quite obvious that there would be no big injection of cash to fund community care. By 1983 the introduction of the new Mental Health Act came alongside a steady rise in the numbers of readmissions to psychiatric hospitals which served to underline the inadequacy of community support for discharged patients.

Not until 1986, 25 years after Enoch Powell's landmark speech, did the first London psychiatric hospital close. Banstead Hospital closed its doors amid complaints that it had been replaced not by community care but by new forms of institutional care – with some smaller institutions set up, and 400 patients simply transferred from Banstead to Horton Hospital (MIND 1986; Lister 1991: 21).

Early in 1985, the Commons Social Services Committee had published its damning critique of the progress so far on community care, insisting that:

The stage has now been reached where the rhetoric of community care has to be matched by action, and where the public are understandably anxious about the consequences.

...The pace of removal of hospital facilities for mental illness has far outrun the provision of services in the community to replace them. It is only now that people are waking up to the legacy of a policy of hospital rundown which began over 20 years ago.

…We do not wish to slow down the exodus from mental illness... hospitals for its own sake. But we do look to see the same degree of Ministerial pressure, and the provision of necessary resources, devoted to the creation of alternative services. Any fool can close a long-stay hospital: it takes more time and trouble to do it properly and compassionately.

(House of Commons Social Services Committee 1990: LIX)

The Committee challenged the lop-sided focus of government and NHS policy – on the apparently 'cost-saving' policy of closing (and asset-stripping) the big long-stay hospitals, while the much bigger task lay elsewhere:

The vast majority of mentally ill people are not and may never be in hospital. The almost obsessive concentration in public policy on the mechanisms for 'getting people out of hospital' has sometimes obscured the fact that most mentally ill people already live in the community, whether with their families, in lodgings, group homes, hostels or private accommodation.

The Committee also pointed out the pitifully small resources available to implement the various plans for community care:

Health authorities at present spend scarcely enough per capita on mentally ill patients to enable a decent community service to be provided at the same price, even if immediate and full transfer of patients or cash or both were possible. Such a transfer is in any event not possible for good practical reasons. Only central funding over a period of several years can help the development of genuine community care over the hump.

Following on the heels of the Social Services Committee came an equally withering and embarrassing report from the Audit Commission, which exposed the shambles of community care services, creating a well of confusion and the potential of a limbo of neglect between the contending responsibilities and cash constraints of the DHSS, health authorities and local council social services.

The Audit Commission drew attention to the fact that while 25,000 psychiatric beds had closed between 1974 and 1984, only 9,000 new day centre and day hospital places had been added: numbers of community psychiatric nurses had risen from just 1,300 in 1980 to a mere 2,200 in 1984. It commented:

It must be a matter for grave concern that although there are 37,000 fewer mentally ill and mentally handicapped patients today than there were 10 years ago, no-one knows what has happened to many of those who have been discharged. Some, of course, have died; others are likely to be in some form of residential care; the rest should be receiving support in the community.... If recent US experience is any guide, it is likely that a significant proportion of those discharged from NHS hospitals will have been before a court and will now be imprisoned; others will have become wanderers, left to their own devices with no support from community-based services.

(Audit Commission 1986: 17)

Into crisis

Despite Thatcher's infamous pledge in 1982, the funding of NHS services had been far from safe in Tory hands. Just three weeks after the 1983 election, Chancellor Lawson announced a one per cent cut in the NHS budget, which triggered a new wave of cuts and hospital closures. The spending squeeze was now on with a vengeance, and the NHS budget stood still in real terms for the five years 1982 to 1987 (Mohan 1995; Radical Statistics Health Group 1987; CIPFA 1988).

Devastating figures were published after the 1987 general election by Colin Reeves, then financial director of North West Thames RHA (later to become financial director of the NHS). A confidential "overview" document kept carefully under wraps until after the votes had been counted showed that real-terms NHS spending had been cut back every year since 1981 – a cumulative reduction of 8.9 per cent (*Health Emergency* 16, 1987). Without extra cash from the government, warned Mr Reeves, the prospect was one of closures "to keep within cash limits." The key was now to cut the numbers of patients treated if big sums of money were to be hacked from spending:

Although rationalisation of wards and hospitals, and indeed closures, have taken place... there has been little change in the overall caseloads being treated.

Nevertheless the hospitals were struggling to cope, especially in London, which had suffered more drastic cuts in spending under the impact of the RAWP formula for the reallocation of resources. By March 1987, hospital waiting lists in the capital were already 22 per cent above the peak level they had reached in the 1982 pay dispute (*Health Emergency* 18, 1988). The burden of the cuts had not fallen evenly across the NHS: Family Practitioner Services were still demand led and exempt from cash limits, meaning that the heaviest pressure was felt by the hospitals and community health services. FPS spending rose by 36 per cent in the ten years to 1988, while Hospital and Community Health Service budgets grew by just 26% (*HSJ*, 20 January 1988). If the budget for hospital services had risen in line with the increased FPS spending, its budget would have been 21 per cent (£2 billion) higher in 1986–7.

The actual situation in the autumn of 1987 was little short of disastrous. Health authorities had begun the financial year deep in debt after succumbing to political pressure to run up bills to suppliers rather than close beds before the election. With £400 million concealed overspend and needing to find another £150 million to make up for government under-funding of the pay award, health authorities were desperate. NHS finance director Ian Mills declared that the service was "technically bankrupt" (Timmins 1995: 454).

Driven by cash limits, plans for sweeping bed closures were formulated and steamrollered through health authority meetings. The closures began in the autumn. Nor was it just the "usual suspects", inner London teaching authorities – although 1987 did bring the closure of 1,400 beds in the capital (*Health Emergency* 18, 1988).

One of the first to hit the skids was the giant West Midlands Region, which was facing a £30 million shortfall, and combined drastic local cuts and closures with a freeze on 49 building projects totalling £256 million (Lister 1988).

At Birmingham's Queen Elizabeth Hospital 146 beds closed to cut admissions by 10 per cent, and doctors were told to treat 1,200 fewer patients. While cancer patients joined the queue, the city's Children's Hospital grabbed the headlines, with the cancellation of heart operations. Cuts also hit Coventry, Worcester, Solihull and Shropshire, where five community hospitals faced the axe. Yorkshire RHA imposed £9 million in cuts, with beds closed and operations cancelled in Wakefield, Doncaster and Leeds. In Newcastle, where the gap was £5 million, the HA decided to close the Fleming Memorial Children's Hospital as well as surgical and ITU beds at the Royal Victoria Infirmary.

Manchester too was hit, with Central Manchester announcing it was £5.6 million in the red and could not pay bills or wages, and seeking 150 redundancies. South and North Manchester and Salford announced heavy closures, while Burnley DHA proposed to close all the acute services at Rossendale Hospital as part of its £3 million cuts package. The South West RHA projected a £10 million shortfall, while Wales was at least £6 million in the red, and reduced in Merthyr to closing a brand new geriatric ward opened less than a year earlier by the Queen Mother (Lister 1988).

By December 1987, 4,000 beds had closed. Consultants were up in arms. A petition launched by Hospital Alert and London Health Emergency gained 1,200 signatures from hospital doctors in 160 hospitals across England, Scotland and Wales in just six weeks. The petition picked up massive press coverage as it was presented to Downing Street on 15 December, with a well-attended press conference in Central Hall, Westminster (*Health Emergency* 18, 1988). Among the consultants who spoke was orthopaedic surgeon Nigel Harris from St Mary's Hospital, who only a few months earlier had shared a platform with Conservative Party health spokesmen, declaring how exaggerated were claims that the NHS was in crisis. He accused Health Minister Tony Newton of being "deceitful" and insisted that if he had known the government's real intentions towards the NHS he would not have lent them his support (Timmins 1995: 457).

Half of the petition's signatories were consultants and 20 were professors, reflecting the deep anxiety running through the medical profession. This was underlined a few days before the petition was to be presented, when an unprecedented statement was issued by three of Britain's top doctors, George Pinker (the Queen's doctor and President of the Royal College of Gynaecologists), Ian Todd (President of the Royal College of Surgeons) and Sir Raymond Hoffenberg (chair of the Royal College of Physicians). Together they warned the government that:

> Acute hospital services have almost reached breaking point. Morale is depressingly low. We call on the government to do something now to save our health service… once the envy of the world.
>
> (Mohan 1995: 16)

The three men went for a meeting with Health Secretary John Moore. But they were not unduly impressed with the government's subsequent announcement of a one-off £100 million injection of cash. Mr George Pinker compared this with "taking a dead man from the ground and telling him he will be going under again on March 31." (*Health Emergency* 18, 1988)

Pinker was far from the only one to be underwhelmed by the Tory response. Health workers, battered by years of increasing workload and dwindling personal purchasing power, were becoming more resentful. As if to rub salt in the wounds, the government was attempting to force through a new series of proposals which would end nurses' entitlement to special duty payments. Early in 1988, anger burst through. On 7 January a group of night shift nurses in Manchester walked out on strike. Though their action forced an almost immediate climb down by the government, it also gave a lead to nurses throughout the country, furious at the cuts, closures and their pitiful pay packets.

Assailed by even pro-Tory newspapers and apparently beleaguered, the Thatcher government turned a hard face to the protests. Questioned hard on BBC's *Panorama* programme on 25 January, Thatcher herself intervened, going over the heads of her health ministers to announce a "review" of the NHS. The same government which had pushed through the Poll Tax was now contemplating reform of the country's most popular public service:

> Just as we considered education, just as we considered the community charge, just as we considered what to do with housing, we are now considering the Health Service. And when we're ready – and it'll be far quicker, I believe, than any Royal Commission – we shall come forward with our proposals for consultation. And should they meet with what people want, then translate them into action.
>
> (*Panorama*, 7 January 1988)

Of course the electorate had been given no inkling of any planned "review" just seven months earlier. In the NHS's fortieth year, Thatcher's strange, secretive review was to herald the most fundamental changes that had been made to the service.

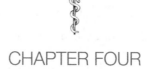

CHAPTER FOUR

The first steps into the marketplace 1988–1997

When the internal market begins to work and signals that there are winners and losers, it's going to be essential that we don't give in to lobbying and bale out the losers.

(William Waldegrave, Health Secretary, *HSJ*, April 1991)

It seems to be part of the government's strategy not to provide all the cash needed for fees [for residential and nursing home care]. Ministers are implying that relatives are part of the income support package. It is a monstrous way of going on.

(Lady Wagner, speaking to a 1991 conference of the British Association of Social Work)

THE FORTIETH ANNIVERSARY YEAR of the NHS opened with a crisis and a strike – by Manchester nurses followed by a continuing rumble of industrial action (including strikes and "work to contract" action) by nurses furious at the arbitrary way their new grading structure was being implemented.

There was also widespread anger among health workers and the wider public at moves to scrap free eye tests and dental check-ups (to save an estimated £170 million), and to lift restrictions on NHS hospitals making profits from private patients and "income generation" schemes – which ministers claimed could net the NHS up to £70 million a year within three years. A new "income generation unit" was set up in February, encouraging hospitals to seek cash from such varied activities as imposing car park charges, running jumble sales and raffles and franchising out space for new shopping malls (Mohan 1995: 182–3).

But events took shape in the shadow of the government's impending review, which had been announced in what appeared to be impromptu fashion by Margaret Thatcher in a January television interview, and which then proceeded behind firmly locked doors amid anxious speculation as to its outcome.

The formal membership of the review team was the Prime Minister plus just four of her ministers – John Moore, returning from his spell of private treatment for pneumonia in the £195-a-night Parkside Hospital in Wimbledon; health minister Tony Newton; Treasury Secretary John Major; and Chancellor Nigel Lawson. It took no formal evidence, invited no participation from the BMA or other professional bodies, ignored the health unions and the representatives of patients, and left MPs as ignorant of its debates as the wider public (Timmins 1995: 456).

Behind the scenes a furtive cabal of advisors included Roy Griffiths, who was still waiting, impatiently, for the government's response to his report on community care, and a group of hand-picked individuals chosen by David Willetts, then employed at the Downing Street policy unit. One of these, Dr Clive Froggatt, was subsequently disgraced after admitting the use of and sale of heroin (Wise 1996).

By February it was already becoming clear that the Thatcher review of the NHS was likely to include the introduction of a form of "internal market". But there was no shortage of outlandish ideas on offer from the backwoods fringes of the Tory Party. Leon Brittan, for example, a former trade and industry secretary, home secretary and chief secretary to the Treasury, let rip in February with a booklet advocating a "National Health Insurance Scheme", transparently designed to promote the growth of the private medical industry (Brittan 1988).

The establishment of a separate "health stamp" might seem like a pointless organisational change, producing no extra cash for the NHS: but its effect would have been to *reduce* income tax contributions – especially for those who might feel rich enough to "opt out" of the state scheme and take out their own private policies – and to *increase* National Insurance contributions by over £9 billion. Critics pointed out that the impact of this would be felt by low-paid workers, who barely pay any income tax, but do pay National Insurance, while those at the top of the salary scale could pocket the difference, and the insurance companies would almost inevitably retain the right to pick and choose those it would take on, leaving the NHS with the bill for the chronic sick, emergency services and mental health.

David Willetts, who played a key orchestrating role in the secretive review proceedings, was also quick off the mark in publishing his views on the way the NHS should be reformed. He praised the model of the American "health maintenance organisations" which manage health care on behalf of their private subscribers. In a booklet for the Centre for Policy Studies in February 1988, Willetts and co-author Dr Michael Goldsmith of the Conservative Medical Society stress that "it is not possible simply to adopt an American model". What they advocated was the separation of the purchasing authority from the providers of health care – with hospitals being detached from health authority control (Willetts and Goldsmith 1988).

Outside the ranks of Tory crackpots, the King's Fund, sometimes described as an independent think tank, published a collection of essays with a preface from chief executive Robert Maxwell suggesting that it might be necessary to recognise that the promise of comprehensive health care was "one on which we simply cannot deliver".

> Some things are going to have to be excluded from the NHS, so that it can do well what it takes on, and so that the public and its staff can have confidence in it.

Among the services to be dropped should be anything the private sector –

possibly with elements of public funding – could do as well as the NHS. However, Maxwell pulled short of advocating a fully market-led approach, warning of "real limitations of the market as an effective and equitable way of providing health care" (Maxwell 1988).

No such reservations were expressed by a broadside in May from the Thatcherite Institute of Economic Affairs, which advocated a voucher system to ensure that "everyone, rich or poor, could become a private patient". The Institute's director Dr David Green proposed a complex procedure in which people could opt out of the health service – renouncing any claim to free services or NHS care even in emergencies – and use their voucher to buy private insurance. But they would not exchange the voucher directly with the private health insurer – instead a "health purchase union" would negotiate on their behalf to find a competitive deal with insurance firms. Health care for the poor would remain a government responsibility (Green 1988).

John Redwood, later more prominent, began to fire off his arsenal of radical right-wing ideas in various directions. In a May pamphlet for the Centre for Policy Studies, written with another rising star in the Conservative Party, Oliver Letwin, he advocated earmarking 50 per cent of income tax as a "national health tax", and allowing individuals and companies rebates if they opted to "contract out" all or part of their risks to a private insurance scheme (Redwood and Letwin 1988). Redwood predicted that such a scheme could lead to 20 million people contracting out, leading to a quadrupling of the share of GDP flowing to private health care – from 0.6 per cent to 2.5 per cent. While this would clearly lighten the load on the Exchequer, it would still leave 30 million people, including the poorest, the oldest and the youngest – the most expensive in health terms – dependent upon the NHS. Nor did Redwood explain how, unless individuals paid more into the system through private insurance, the net result would be an increase in health care provision. In a separate line of argument, Redwood urged the government to combat the rising influence and militancy of the health unions COHSE and NUPE by building up the Royal College of Nursing.

Two months later, Redwood was at it again, this time in a pamphlet jointly produced by the "No Turning Back" group of Conservative MPs, including such luminaries as Neil Hamilton, Edward Leigh, David Heathcoat-Amory, Eric Forth and Michael Fallon. It proposed steps to create competition within the NHS, allowing hospitals to compete against each other, alongside a substantial expansion of the private sector, fuelled by tax relief on private medical insurance. The proposals – which would of course have diverted money from the Exchequer and the NHS into the pockets of well-to-do individuals and private medical corporations – rested on the unsupported assumption that the private sector would be ready and willing to offer a full range of services, and would in this way "siphon at least some of the excess demand away from the NHS." The pamphlet also suggested the establishment of a "Patients Charter" setting out the rights of health consumers (No Turning Back Group, 1988).

Cash pressures

Meanwhile vocal lobby groups outside the Conservative right were demanding a very different way forward. As the NHS ground its way through one winter crisis, there were already fears for the one to come. NHS spending had been squeezed down as a share of GDP from 5.5 per cent in 1981–2 to just 5.1 per cent in the four years 1986–90 (Rivett 1998: 485). Figures grudgingly released in February 1988 by Health Minister Tony Newton revealed that real-terms spending on Hospital and Community Health service revenue had increased by just £66 million since 1982, whereas ministers had previously admitted that spending needed to rise by 2 per cent per year in real terms in order to keep pace with demographic pressures, new technology and the costs of community care programmes (Radical Statistics Health Group 1987: 46).

Government capital allocations for NHS development, too, had actually *reduced* year by year, from £859 million in 1984 to £812 million in 1986–7. The apparent increase in capital was entirely due to cash receipts from asset-stripping sale of "surplus" NHS land – a source of cash which began to dry up with the collapse of property prices in the late 1980s. The dire shortage of capital for new projects, maintenance and refurbishment came at a time when, according to Health Minister Edwina Currie, 81 per cent of hospitals were built before 1918, 5 per cent before 1939 and only 8 per cent had been built since 1964 (*Hansard* 1988).

With spending on primary care services still exempt from cash limits, and growing in real terms year by year, the sharpest problems were being felt in the revenue squeeze on hospitals and community services. Figures published by the Commons Social Services Committee showed the rapid increases in productivity that were being forced onto hospital staff: numbers of inpatient cases per bed had risen by 40 per cent between 1978 and 1986; inpatient and day case numbers were up by almost 26 per cent; and the average length of stay was being steadily reduced (*HSJ*, 26 January 1988).

The BMA in February 1988, warning of a new round of cash problems in the coming financial year, called for a £1.5 billion cash injection into the NHS – the equivalent of 1p on income tax – and for it to remain essentially tax funded (*Independent*, 2 February 1988). The Labour Party mounted a campaign involving Shadow Chancellor John Smith and shadow social services spokesman Robin Cook calling for an extra £2 billion (*HSJ*, 25 February 1988). This effort was reinforced by a Gallup poll in the *Daily Telegraph* in which over two-thirds of those asked said they would be prepared to pay at least an extra £1 per week in taxes for the NHS. At local level, too, doctors and others were campaigning. In Redbridge, NE London, 140 GPs and 30 hospital consultants placed newspaper adverts warning that they were no longer able to treat patients to the best of their ability or within a reasonable time. One GP said:

> Forty percent of our surgical beds are closed, half the operating theatres are closed, and even if we could recruit nurses we could not afford to pay them. My advice is that people should not come and live in this district.
>
> (*HSJ*, 25 February 1988)

In Birmingham a pressure group of 150 consultants "for the rescue of the NHS" was formed after 250 doctors signed a protest letter to West Midlands Regional Health Authority. The consultants called for an extra £13 million to halt rising waiting lists in England's second city, and complained that only one of the four new operating theatres had opened at Sutton Coldfield's Good Hope Hospital. Their stand inspired the formation of a similar organisation in Manchester (*Independent*, 22 April 1988; *HSJ*, 18 February 1988).

The anxiety over funding grew as the year went on. In August the National Association of Health Authorities warned that many HAs were heading towards a fresh winter crisis with many beds still closed from 1987, and a new projected overspend totalling over £500 million. More bed closures were also being triggered by growing shortages of nursing staff. The squeeze on beds and services was having a predictable impact on waiting lists, which rose throughout 1988. By early 1989 the combined total for inpatients and day cases was rising by 6,000 a month, and had reached the dizzy heights of 928,000, with growing numbers waiting over a year for treatment (*Health Emergency* 23, 1989).

In early July 1988 the massive Department of Health and Social Security was split into two separate departments, with Kenneth Clarke taking over as Health Secretary. Within weeks even more alarming figures were to be revealed, as an internal memo was leaked, showing that the government was not fully funding the apparently generous 15.3 per cent pay award to nurses, linked to the introduction of the new clinical grading structure. Ministers were forced to agree to pay the full £803 million cost of this, but refused to underwrite the cost of pay awards to other staff including admin and clerical, ancillaries and laboratory technicians, none of whom had settled for less than 5.5 per cent: the government had only allocated an extra 4.5 per cent to cover NHS inflation (*Independent*, 22 April 1988). To make matters worse, NHS managers dragged their feet in implementing the regrading exercise, while others attempted to cut costs by allocating nursing staff to lower grades. It became increasingly obvious that Kenneth Clarke's pledge to have the money in nurses' pay packets by Christmas was a hollow one. Frustrated at this new setback, nursing staff at the Maudsley psychiatric hospital walked out in September on a 12-day strike (*Health Emergency* 20, 1988).

Militancy was again growing into a "hot autumn" across the country, as angry down-graded nursing staff protested by the effective tactic of "working-to-contract", exposing the holes in the management case. All 19 health districts in the North West were affected: in Burnley health chiefs agreed to reconsider 800 gradings after the health authority meeting was besieged by 1,000 angry nurses. In Yorkshire there was action in Leeds, Bradford, Hull and Rotherham, while Wakefield saw a 95 per cent vote for work to grade action by COHSE members. In the West Midlands, 50 hospitals were affected by the industrial action, including Walsall, where 300 out of 340 nurses lodged appeals against their grading. In London, NUPE nurses at St George's hospital staged a three-day strike, and both NUPE and COHSE found strong support for days of action (*Health Emergency* 21, 1988).

White Papers

Clarke faced growing impatience from Tory backbenchers, who were irritated by leaks suggesting that the outcome of the review was going to be far less radical than some had hoped. They were going to have to wait almost six more months for its findings, which skipped a traditional stage in the formulation of new policy, by publishing not a Green Paper for general discussion but a White Paper, *Working for Patients* (DoH 1989a).

Having done their deliberating, Thatcher and her government machine were now pressing forward the process of change. No concessions were likely to be made to those who opposed its central thrust (Timmins 1995). Six months later, in July 1989, came *Caring for People*, the long-delayed government response to the Griffiths Report on community care (DoH 1989b). Both lines of policy were to be grafted together in the NHS and Community Care Bill.

The most far-reaching changes were those spelled out in the January White Paper, which was launched with a lavish £1.25 million nationwide press and TV extravaganza, including a promotional video featuring Margaret Thatcher. It was swiftly renamed "Working for Peanuts" by staff and "Working for Profits" by campaigners. The new plan embodied elements of many of the nostrums put forward by backwoodsmen and think tanks, but relied heavily on the concept of an "internal market" which had been advocated in a 1985 paper by an influential figure in American health care, Alain Enthoven, suggesting "some reforms that might be politically feasible" (Enthoven 1985).

Central to Enthoven's approach was the allocation to health authorities of budgets calculated on a per capita basis: the HAs would then be free to buy services for local residents – either from each other, or from the private sector. His model was the US Health Maintenance Organisation, a device to regulate the ruinously expensive private health care sector which appeared to succeed in that objective for a few years in the mid-1990s (Ranade 1998).

Indeed, Enthoven was one of the many economists, politicians and academics seeking ways of "managing" the chaotic and ruinously expensive private market in health care in the USA. His proposals aimed to restrict the costs of private medical insurance – and therefore reduce premium payments for individuals and for corporations – through the introduction of "managed care", offering a restricted choice in the form of a defined range of funded treatments from a preselected range of "preferred providers" with whom specific deals would be done. Enthoven later went further, and argued that excessive market freedom in the hands of health service users could undermine the market tools in the hands of the insurance companies, who would use their power to purchase in bulk as a means to hold down prices:

Free choice of provider: "destroys the bargaining power of insurers".

(Enthoven 1997: 196)

For a while it looked as if Enthoven and regulation might have succeeded in holding down price increases and forcing up operational efficiency in the US, where a more competitive regime had lamentably failed. US hospitals had apparently become *less* efficient at treating and discharging patients in the ten years 1982–92, when 'throughput' per bed dropped from 35.9 patients per bed per year to 33.7. However, they managed a near 10 per cent increase in throughput in the five years from 1992–7, the period in which "managed care" was seeking to regulate the market (Enthoven 1997). The Thatcher review plumped for an even more radical version of this, though stopping well short of the root and branch "privatisation" or attack on the essence of the NHS that some had feared.

The market

There would be an "internal market", in which purchasers and providers would be separated, though both remaining within the framework of the NHS. For secondary care, the main purchasers would be health authorities, with funding allocated on a complex formula to take account of the age profile and social circumstances of their population. Health authorities themselves would be drastically reshaped: numbers of HA members would be cut from an average 18 to just 11 – but this reduced number would include five "executive members" (NHS managers, who had not previously had formal positions on health authorities). Among those excluded would be the four nominees from the local authority, the "trade union" seat and the Community Health Council – leaving the new DHAs even less connected than before to the local community.

Each HA would have a chair appointed by the Secretary of State, and paid £20,000 a year for part-time involvement, and five "non-executive" members, paid £5,000 a year, also selected by ministers. These payments strengthened the government's control over the network of quangos through the power of patronage: the reform succeeded in halting any further shows of dissent or independence by health authorities, which have since 1990 without exception obediently complied with cash limits and policy guidelines.

A second line of purchasers would be GPs: bigger practices would be urged to take responsibility for cash-limited budgets, from which they would buy non-emergency hospital treatment for their patients – from local NHS hospitals or if they chose, from the private sector. GP budget-holders were swiftly renamed as "fundholders" to avoid concerns that their budgets would run out.

The "providers" – the hospitals and community services – would initially be separately managed in an arm's length relationship with the health authorities, but they would increasingly be encouraged to "opt out" of health authority control as "self-governing" hospitals (later renamed "NHS Trusts" in an attempt to overcome complaints that they were effectively "opting out of the NHS").

Hospitals would be obliged to compete against each other for contracts from health authorities and GP fundholders. The claim was that in this way money would "follow the patient", rewarding the hospitals which best succeeded in meeting local requirements, with an all-round extension of "choice" and a downward pressure on costs.

Competition

The notion of competition was not popular in the NHS. Many hospitals were still showing the scars from the "competitive tendering" of ancillary services, in which the lowest-priced tender had almost always been taken. There were legitimate fears that, as with the tendering exercise, the "competition" would make only ritual nods in the direction of *quality of* care, and overwhelmingly centre on the issue of price: it would also lead to a further round of cost-cutting, which in turn, with labour costs still representing 70 per cent of NHS spending, implied a fresh attack on staffing levels, pay and conditions.

Any comparison between the "competition" that prevails in the retail market and that between NHS hospitals was obviously inappropriate. While the big supermarket chains make a profit on each transaction, and thus have a vested interest in increasing their sales and their customer base, and can borrow money or recycle their profits in order to expand, quite the opposite was true of the NHS. Its services were restricted by arbitrary cash limits, and each item of care was not a potential profit but a charge against the limited resources available. Far from the seemingly endless expansion of supermarket chains, as NHS managers sought to reduce their spending, they were seeking an ever smaller, more centralised, rationalised network of hospitals, with development plans hobbled by a lack of NHS capital. A better comparison would be with the crazy fixed quotas of goods traditionally supplied to retail outlets by old-style Stalinist states. In a Polish supermarket, regardless of the level of consumer demand, supplies would run out before the end of trading, and rationing took place through queuing.

Competition is also the enemy of planning: in the wider marketplace it commonly leads to problems of over-supply and over-production. For NHS hospitals to be able genuinely to compete with each other for market share, it would be necessary to increase frontline resources, since for any real "choice" to be offered a patient would have to be able to find treatment not only in one, but in *more* than one hospital. This was ever less likely to be the case in an NHS where bed numbers, driven by cash crises, were rapidly falling.

But competition also brings losers as well as winners. Less-favoured hospitals which lost out to rivals for major contracts would also lose contract revenue. Those determined to steal away contract income from rival hospitals might decide to concentrate on a few, potentially lucrative services, at the expense of closing others. With health authorities already beginning to run down their provision of elderly care and mental health beds, it did not take a genius to work out the likely areas that were going to be scaled down.

Bureaucracy

Behind the rhetoric of business methods, competition and efficiency lay a concealed raft of additional bureaucratic costs. Separating the management of hospitals from health authorities would mean expanding the ranks of senior managers.

But establishing competition between hospitals also meant that every form of treatment would have to be "priced", contracts costed and monitored, and bills prepared for individual cases sent for treatment (or admitted as emergencies) in hospitals where their local health authority had no regular contract.

None of this bureaucracy had been necessary in the NHS, and the simplicity of the system was one reason why administrative costs in Britain had been so dramatically lower than those in other insurance-based health care systems in Europe or the "free market" system in the USA. The scene was set for the runaway expansion of NHS administrative bureaucracy. Critics of the proposals asked whether it was purely by coincidence that the new system was to establish a comprehensive apparatus for pricing and billing for individual episodes of treatment – or so that this same apparatus could be subsequently used by a future government to impose means-tested charges for care, in a possible move towards an insurance-based, privatised service (Hands Off Our Hospitals 1989).

Fundholding

The proposal of GP fundholding was initially restricted to the largest group practices, with over 11,000 patients on their register. But behind the initial facade of generous cash handouts and "clinical freedom" lurked the imposition for the first time of cash limits on primary care services.

While opponents of the scheme asked what would happen when a fundholding practice ran out of money, a handful of GPs were lured by the lavish cash incentives. Enticements included the chance to break away from the narrow confines of services dictated by their local health authority, the opportunity to negotiate preferential deals for their patients to secure more rapid treatment at selected hospitals (opening up a two-tier service within the NHS), and in some cases the possibility of buying services from the private sector. Another attraction for the most grasping of fundholding fans was that they would be able to retain within the practice any surplus left over from each year's budget (Paterson and Walker 1997).

Hospital Trusts

The most drastic step towards the fragmentation of the NHS was in the "opting out" of self-governing hospitals, an idea which originated with the nostalgia for the old Hospital Boards of Ian McColl, a confidant of the Tory inner circle, who was then Professor of Surgery at Guy's Hospital (Timmins 1995). At that point there were 320 larger hospitals (with over 250 beds), which might be expected to opt out: any one District Health Authority might find itself trying to negotiate contracts with two or more local Trusts, and possibly with more in neighbouring districts or further afield.

The opting-out procedure deliberately side-stepped any form of democratic consultation. There would be no ballots or votes (Timmins 1995). Local residents, hospital patients, local charities (many of which had raised large sums for their hospital), local authorities which needed to liaise with hospital staff on the discharge of elderly patients, and of course health workers whose jobs and working conditions were potentially at risk – all these were excluded from having a voice on the decision to "opt out", which could be proposed by senior management and rubber-stamped by the Secretary of State. Self-governing hospitals were each to be run by an appointed board of directors structured in the same way as the new health authorities – five executive members, with a chair and five lay members appointed by the Secretary of State. Despite the flowery rhetoric, which waxed lyrical about how "local" the new bodies would be, the entire structure was answerable only to central government. Trusts, as rival "businesses" competing for NHS contracts would guard their business secrets by meeting behind closed doors, with only one public meeting a year.

The vast assets of land, buildings and equipment would be "owned" by the Trust boards, which would have the power to sell off surplus assets. A big selling point to frustrated managers whose redevelopment plans had been stuck for years in the queue for the dwindling pool of NHS capital was the suggestion that self-governing hospitals would have the freedom to borrow money from the government or from the private sector. This proved to be one of the most misleading promises, as Trusts found themselves constrained from day one by rigid cash limits (Mohan 1995). To make matters worse, Trusts were required to pay interest ("capital charges") on half of the book value of their assets. This was promoted as creating more business-style awareness of the value of assets, and as more of a "level playing field" with the private sector, but served primarily as an incentive to push Trusts into selling off spare property assets in order to escape capital charges.

Other promised "freedoms" for Trusts included the right to expand private wings and numbers of pay beds, and the right to decide "local" pay and conditions for Trust employees – tearing up the long-established Whitley Council system of national-level agreements underpinning all grades of staff. In return, Trusts were to be obliged only to balance their books and show a return on assets of six per cent each year: any retained surpluses could be ploughed back into services. But of course any losses would also be the sole responsibility of the Trust, and the reforms carried the underlying threat that a failing Trust could go bankrupt. Ministers insisted from early on that they would not bail out Trusts which failed financially.

Opposition

The package represented a massive change to the workings of the NHS. None of the new proposals had even been hinted at in the Conservatives' 1987 election manifesto, and the plans proved immediately and almost universally unpopular. But the government was committed to push the plans through at break-neck speed, to get Trusts up and running before the next election.

The resistance to the proposals was quickly off the ground. The scheme was opposed by the Labour Party, by the health unions, and by the BMA, which saw it as a measure which would not only fragment but also lay the "groundwork for the future dismantlement of the NHS." Its leaders embarked on a massive advertising campaign, including bill-board posters with the memorable slogan "What do you call a man who ignores medical advice? Mr Clarke" (Rivett 1998).

Another source of BMA grievance were the simultaneous government moves to force through a new GP contract which most GPs saw (correctly) as increasing their workload and reducing the amount of time they would be able to spend with each patient. Health Secretary Kenneth Clarke offered only the most minimal concessions to the BMA before deciding to impose the deal on GPs, who had voted three to one to reject it in a ballot with a staggering 82 per cent response. He made little secret of his eagerness to squash the residual power of the BMA, just as the government had beaten back the miners in 1984 and the health unions in 1982 (Timmins 1995).

The BMA campaign was not matched by any comparable effort from the health unions. Although health workers were the most likely victims of the new market-led regime, there was no coordinated campaign. A pamphlet (*Hands Off Our Hospitals*) by London Health Emergency, together with LHE car stickers, leaflets, and badges sold in their thousands to local campaigns and union branches throughout the country for want of any official material from the health union headquarters or the Labour Party. The Thatcher government was not one to hold back for fear of public opinion, and the polls showing almost 75 per cent of voters and more than half of all Tory voters to be opposed to the reforms did not prevent the proposals being pushed through Parliament as the NHS and Community Care Bill.

Community care

The community care proposals in the Bill followed closely on from the 1988 recommendations in the Griffiths Report that continuing care of the frail elderly should be switched from the control of the NHS to social services. Thatcher, no fan of local authorities, had taken some persuading to agree to this switch, despite the fact that it would bring a substantial reduction in government spending.

An ever-increasing share of continuing care had already been privatised during the 1980s, with elderly patients claiming DHSS payments to help cover the fees. Nursing homes had become a massive area of business growth. In 1979 it had cost the DHSS £10 million to finance 11,000 clients in nursing homes. By 1993, 281,000 people were receiving state-funded care in private homes, at a cost of £2.575 billion (Courtney and Walker 1996).

The 1988 "Griffiths Report" (*Community Care: Agenda for Action*) proposed what amounted to the consolidation of privatisation and means-testing, with an end to the direct use of social security funding, and the transfer of responsibility for continuing care of the elderly from the NHS (where it was still provided free of charge at time of use) to local government (where it would be subject to means-tested charges). A London Health Emergency pamphlet in 1988 warned that "We can hear the till bells ringing and the knife sharpening" as it responded to the Report, emphasising that means-testing (and thus cutting NHS expenditure at the price of increased charges on individuals, their savings and property assets) was the main driving force behind the Griffiths proposals (Lister and Martin 1988).

Health Minister Edwina Currie had not long before suggested that people should forego foreign holidays to finance private health care, and that elderly patients might take out loans or mortgages on their houses to pay for private treatment. The key words from Griffiths, whose report was quite explicit in its call for means-tested charges, argued that:

> Many of the elderly have higher incomes and levels of savings than in the past... This growth of individually held resources could provide a contribution to meeting community care needs.
>
> (Griffiths 1988: 6.61)

As if to underline the financial agenda which informed his whole approach to the community care issue, Griffiths had little of substance to say about mental health services, which were to be left under the lead control of the NHS. It is a painful fact not lost on Griffiths that while many pensioners have savings and property assets which could be used to pay their own way, few psychiatric patients have sufficient wealth to make a similar approach worthwhile.

The Griffiths proposals implied even more wholesale privatisation, as they aimed to subject every aspect of community care services – whether residential or domiciliary – to "competitive tenders or other means of testing the market". They would also confine social services departments to the role of "purchaser" of continuing care. Eighty per cent of the government money flowing to social services had to be spent in the "independent" (private or voluntary) sector. There were measures to deter councils from providing their own residential care services for the elderly.

Strangely enough, however, these policies, commissioned and published by a government with a track record of attacking local authorities, had been enthusiastically greeted by many Labour-led councils and chairs of social services. They seemed oblivious to the perils of what would later be described (in a rare political insight by shadow health spokesperson David Blunkett) as a "poisoned chalice", which would involve Labour councils in means-testing pensioners and forcing many of them to sell their houses to pay for care in profit-seeking private homes. Indeed, a bizarre local government pressure group called "Griffiths Now" (dubbed "Turkeys for Christmas" by London Health Emergency) joined forces to lobby for the reforms to be introduced *sooner*! Shadow Health Secretary Robin Cook raised questions in the Commons pressing for swift implementation of the Griffiths proposals.

Few within the health or local government unions had followed the issue closely enough to recognise the danger. The policy was widely presented in the press (notably the *Guardian*) as a progressive package of reforms. LHE, which openly criticised the councils' campaign, and which spoke at meetings of health workers and pensioners warning of the implications of the Griffiths reforms, came under pressure for its hard line of outright opposition to every part of the package. Once the community care reforms were incorporated into the Bill, Labour's already tepid opposition to the market was further defused by its acceptance of half of the new legislation.

Kenneth Clarke described his community care proposals, which had only with difficulty won the endorsement of Margaret Thatcher, as "80% Griffiths". The missing 20 per cent was significant. Dropped were Griffiths' proposals for a separate minister for community care, and for the money transferred from social security to local government budgets to help pay for placements to be "ring-fenced" to ensure transparency and prevent it being used for other purposes. Gone was Griffiths' call for additional cash for community care (*Health Emergency* 23, 1989).

Also dropped, however, were some of the worst Griffiths proposals, notably the idea of using youth on job-creation schemes as a source of cheap labour for domiciliary services. In the event, the government recognised the potential disruption that could be caused if the reforms were introduced in 1991, alongside the new internal market. Although the legislation was pushed through Parliament, the date for implementation was pushed back to 1993, meaning that the first new means-tested charges would be imposed comfortably after the election.

NHS and Community Care Act

The Bill was steamrollered through Parliament, nearing the end of its committee stage in March 1990, and receiving the Royal assent in the summer. The way was opened to the appointment of the new, slimmed-down health authorities, and the applications of the first wave of NHS Trusts and fundholding GPs.

The new model health authorities held fewer meetings, taking even more decisions behind closed doors. A 1990 survey by the West Midlands NHS Monitoring Unit of 129 non-executive members appointed to health authorities in the region, summed them up as "male, middle class and white". Just one was a trade unionist, only two were black, a mere 22 per cent were women, while 53 came from business and 17 from "professional backgrounds". South Warwickshire was saddled with two property speculators, a merchant banker and the managing director of a plastic roofing firm.

Squeeze on Trusts

With the green light to implement the reforms in the NHS and Community Care Act, the first priority for ministers was to line up the first wave of opted-out NHS Trusts and fundholding GP practices. Nobody had any firm idea of how many hospitals would put in applications. Campaigners warned that many of those which put their names on Health Secretary Kenneth Clarke's "short list" were deep in financial crisis: 14 of the front-running contenders – including King's College Hospital in Camberwell and Northwick Park Hospital in Harrow – subsequently withdrew their bids before the decision date (*Guardian*, 9 May 1990).

In an analysis of 50 of the 65 applications for Trust status throughout England, London Health Emergency pointed out that combined assets totalling £4–5 billion were likely to be handed over to appointed quango boards which would not be in any way accountable to local people. The limited financial details in the published bids gave serious grounds for concern over their viability (Lister 1990).

Some "expect to succeed, but only if they manage to attract substantial inflows of patients (and therefore revenue) from surrounding districts, with potentially serious impact on other hospitals."

> Many Trusts base their financial projections on a substantial increase in income from private patients, with many planning to build or extend existing private wings.

Other bids "are based on ludicrously optimistic financial assumptions... including unrealistic inflation figures, high caseload figures, crazy income generation schemes, and... the notion that the Trusts will only be required to pay interest on 33% of the assets they take over". In fact interest had to be paid on 50 per cent of assets (Lister 1990).

Even though the opting-out process for Trusts – unlike that which the government had introduced for the establishment of grant maintained schools – had carefully avoided any mechanism such as a ballot or referendum through which local people could express their views, the scale of public opposition to the measures and the new culture of the internal market was making some impact on senior NHS managers. The deputy chief executive of the NHS, Peter Griffiths, later to become the chief executive of the Guy's Hospital Trust, warned health managers:

> Don't talk about business plans. Don't talk about marketing. Don't talk about market share and segmentation. Don't talk in the kind of commercial language that switches off every member of staff.
>
> (*Guardian*, 8 June 1990)

He was already far too late. Few NHS managers had used any other type of language for the previous 18 months. Their jargon, littered with the buzz-words of the reforms, including liberal use of the word "local", was almost daily becoming less intelligible to any wider public. One health authority general manager, Dr Elaine Murphy, resigned, complaining to the *Guardian* that:

> At a time when waiting lists are growing... and services are pretty stretched and not of a high quality in inner London we are spending all our time as general managers engaged in implementing the White Paper, in the organisation of contracts and in shifting stuff around.
>
> (*Guardian*, 18 May 1990)

"Steady state"

But ministers were already getting cold feet on the possible impact of the new market system in destabilising services in the run-up to the coming general election. Although the Trusts lifted off on schedule, in April 1991, the market itself was to be heavily controlled, with instructions to health authorities to maintain a "steady state".

William Waldegrave, heralding the brave new world, began with bravado, declaring in April that:

> It is essential that we let the internal market indicate what is needed in London, and we will then have to respond to those signals, which will force us politicians to take some decisions which have been postponed for much too long.
>
> (*HSJ*, 26 March 1991)

However, this line soon changed as he, like Clarke before him, was warned of the impact on London's health authorities in particular of the hefty reductions in funding arising from the new capitation formula which underpinned the internal market. Civil servants had predicted that the reforms would lead to the closure of another 2,000 acute beds and the loss of at least one teaching hospital as a result both of the London squeeze, and of health authorities in the home counties seeking to save money by switching contracts for routine treatment to cheaper provider hospitals outside of the capital (*Guardian*, 8 and 9 August 1990). Closures on this scale would have been an electoral disaster in London, so 'transitional funding' was surreptitiously pumped in to avert any embarrassing rapid collapse: but a political fig-leaf was required to cover both the delay and the eventual painful closures of busy and well-loved hospitals.

At the 1991 Conservative Party conference Waldegrave decided to tackle both problems by announcing a "review" of London's hospital services. This was to be conducted by a safe pair of hands, Professor Sir Bernard Tomlinson, a long-standing appointed chair of the Northern Regional Health Authority, who had been knighted in 1988.

The inquiry published its terms of reference, and was seen by some as setting a framework within which the "over-provision" of hospitals, beds and resources in London could be redressed (Klein 2006: 165): but it was clear to government opponents that its main functions were to postpone awkward decisions for at least 12 months – and to draw up a "hit list" of hospitals for closure (COHSE 1992a).

Extra cash

Additional cash suddenly became available – to serve the twin purposes of boosting the ranks of NHS management and administration to the level needed to implement the reforms, and to avert any fresh cuts crisis in the run-up to the election. NHS spending rose sharply by £1.8 billion – up as a share of GDP from 5.2 per cent in 1990–1 to 5.7 per cent in 1991–2; and again by another £1.8 billion in 1992–3, to reach 6 per cent of GDP. This was the highest level achieved until the Blair–Brown government began its programme of increased spending after 2000 (Rivett 1998: 485).

However, the extra costs of the market system meant that the cash uplift was not enough to avert another bout of bed closures and a winter crisis in 1990. As early as November, 20 major hospitals in London announced that they would only take emergency admissions if instructed to do so by the Emergency Bed Service. London Health Emergency revealed that over 2,000 beds in the capital had closed or failed to reopen after "temporary" closure in the previous year (*Health Emergency* 26, 1990).

As the new, carefully controlled, market creaked into action some early anomalies were pointed out by London Health Emergency in October 1991. Among them:

- Guy's Hospital Trust, the "flagship" of opting out, had hit immediate cash problems, announcing job losses to retrieve a massive £6.8 million deficit. Senior managers had fallen out, resulting in a £200,000-plus-BMW pay-off to departing finance director Peter Burroughs.

- Twelve other first-wave Trusts, including 8 of the 13 in London, had already admitted to being in financial difficulties just six months into their first year, with shortfalls ranging from £200,000 at Oxford's Nuffield Orthopaedic Centre to £7 million in Bradford.

- Orthopaedic patients imported from Exeter were jumping growing queues of local people needing treatment in Riverside's hospitals (West London).

- Consultants at St Mary's Hospital, Paddington, had been told to wait four days for authorisation from clerical staff before promising non-emergency patients they could have the treatment they needed – to check that their health authority was willing and able to pay the bill.

- Managers at Bloomsbury and Islington Health Authority had complained of "an increasing number of [health authority] purchasers who are refusing to pay invoices".

- The specialist child heart-surgery unit at Guy's Hospital had already used up its contract income for local patients, meaning that children from South East London would have to wait until the following April, while those from other areas could be treated sooner.

Behind the scenes, an extra £200 million was being pumped in to the NHS to prop up hospitals facing deficits as a result of the new market system. The National Association of Health Authorities and Trusts (NAHAT) found that 82 per cent of hospitals were facing problems, many because they were treating more patients than expected – but not being paid extra because they had agreed to fixed price contracts (*Health Emergency* 29, 1992).

Elderly care under fire

The new community care policies may have been postponed for two years, but the legislation had made it very clear which way the wind was blowing. Long-term care of the elderly, a relatively costly service with few financial rewards for the acute service Trusts, was already under the axe (a survey by the Association of Community Health Councils in 1991 found that 75 per cent of health authorities had cut back numbers of long-stay beds for the elderly in the previous three years). Department of Health figures showed that over 13,000 geriatric beds (24 per cent) had closed in ten years, 9,000 of them in the previous four years (DoH Statistics 1993). This type of treatment was increasingly to be squeezed out of the NHS.

From 1991 onwards more health authorities began to jump aboard the "community care" bandwagon by closing down their remaining beds for the elderly. First out of the blocks was West Berkshire HA, with a plan unveiled in late summer 1991 to shut down all 200 of its continuing care beds and hive off care – including services for the elderly mentally ill – to the private sector. The scheme hinged on the HA being able to "top up" social security payments of £245 per person per week – a policy whose legality was called into question by the Department of Health (*Health Emergency* 28, 1991). A revised scheme scaled down the closures to 153 NHS beds; but the West Berkshire plan was not care in the community, it was to sponsor the building of large (60-bed) nursing homes. It ran into a hail of sustained opposition from the local Community Health Council, along with relatives groups, health unions, councillors and others (COHSE 1992b; *Health Emergency* 29, 1992).

The second wave

There had been plenty of stormy meetings in opposition to the second wave of Trust opt-outs, too, some of them more militant than the first round. Many prospective Labour parliamentary candidates – some of them displaying little knowledge of the NHS or health policies – were keen to get in on the act as the election drew closer.

This did not stop another clutch of Trusts getting the rubber stamp, several of which ran into trouble from day one. Barnet's Wellhouse Trust was subsequently admitted to have "got its sums wrong" after it turned out that it was starting life with a deficit of £1.7 million – more than eight times larger than the projected £200,000. Other Trusts lifted off with business plans reflecting management hopes of scraping by with wafer-thin surpluses, only to plunge rapidly into the red (*Health Emergency* 31, 1992).

The Labour Party's national campaign in the 1992 general election made little or no reference to the popular line of scrapping Trusts, however, and its handling of the NHS issue was blown off course from the outset by the disastrously ill-conceived "Jennifer's Ear" political broadcast. This focused not on the unpopular market reforms but on the (still relatively marginal) increase in private medicine – and made the additional blunder of hanging the whole case on an identifiable individual family, which proved to be politically unreliable and divided in its loyalties. The Labour leadership was almost immediately forced onto the defensive on this issue, which rumbled on and served to discredit them on health policy (Black N 1992).

This was far from the only weakness in Labour's 1992 campaign – but it did effectively neutralise the NHS as an electoral weapon against John Major's attempts to win a record-breaking fourth electoral victory for the Tories (Kettle 2005). The returned Tory government was obliged to carry through the unfinished business of Thatcher's reforms. In the autumn came the publication of the Tomlinson Report, predictably calling for the closure of 10 hospitals – including four teaching hospitals (Bart's, Charing Cross, the Middlesex and either Guy's or St Thomas's) – and 4,000 beds in London (Tomlinson 1992).

London crisis

The capital had always had a paradoxical position in the NHS. Externally the impression was of the power and privilege of the big, historic teaching hospitals which trained over 40 per cent of medical staff. But in practice, London's NHS had always been deliberately divided up, and for the previous 20 years, despite its unique and pressing problems of poverty and ill health, London had been on the losing end of every new formula that had been devised for the allocation of NHS resources. It was always easy to whip up an "anti-London" sentiment among ill-informed MPs from outside, especially those representing rural constituencies or poorly provided industrial towns and cities: the same superficial response is also echoed in Klein's account, which argues that London was "over-funded", with an "over-supply of acute beds", and refers without supporting evidence to "redundant beds and institutions" (Klein 2006: 164).

Historically, London's concentration of a dozen mighty teaching hospitals was seen by Bevan and his successors as so potentially powerful within the new NHS that they (and London's health care planning) were to be kept separated. This was the main reason why the Greater London area was initially carved up into four separate Thames Regions, each of which reached far beyond the capital – deep into the Home Counties to the north, or down to the south coast. Throughout the process of redevelopment and rationalisation since the 1960s, London has at times had as many as 30 different health authorities, each of them tied to its own cash limits and constraints, and with no overall body to plan or coordinate NHS services across the capital.

London has also fallen victim to some of the most half-baked policy-making, superficial reports and inappropriate proposals as governments have attempted to deal with the obvious contradictions of care in the capital. The attempts to reallocate NHS resources throughout the country on a more equitable basis since the RAWP formula in 1976 have led, in the context of a continuing squeeze on health spending, to a process of levelling down London's NHS budget rather than levelling up the under-resourced regions. This in turn led to a succession of plans and proposals for the reduction of health care in London. In 1979 a "London Health Planning Consortium" (LHPC) surveyed services and called for London to lose over 6,000 acute beds over the next ten years (out of a 1977 total of 50,000 beds in the Thames Regions). While health authorities outside London were to *increase* their bed provision by 1,100, non-teaching districts in the capital were to lose 3,900 beds (24 per cent) and the teaching districts 2,300 beds (23 per cent).

In March 1988 London Health Emergency leaked a top-level, confidential draft report that had been compiled by DHSS officials with assistance from the Thames regions and London health authorities. Entitled *London Study*, it was replete with out-of-date statistics (some bed numbers were over three years out of date, and some other statistics five years old), most of which failed to square with the facts on the ground. It also ignored the majority of outer London districts. One valid point the *London Study* did make was on the pace of closure of acute beds, which was admitted to be going at *double* the planned rate. "These plans envisaged an annual reduction of over 300 local acute beds per year (equivalent to closing a medium sized District General Hospital) in inner London. Over the first three years of the strategic period the pace of change has been twice that rate…" (DHSS 1988: 61–2).

The DHSS researchers concluded that: "were it to continue at that pace over the ten year period, two-thirds of the local acute beds in London would have disappeared over the ten years." (DHSS 1988: 62) Early in 1992 came a report by the King's Fund Commission which was also studded with out of date and inaccurate information, partial figures, maps that missed out key hospitals (including a teaching hospital!), and a series of conclusions – including a reduction of another 5,000 acute hospital beds by 2010 – based on the wildest, most optimistic projections of the extent to which primary care services could replace hospitals (King's Fund 1992).

Enter Sir Bernard

The Tomlinson Report was to prove even more of a travesty: it had consulted no representative organisations in London, held no open sessions, and proceeded furtively in secret. Sir Bernard Tomlinson himself, on a rare visit to London, had admitted in a GLR radio interview that he began from the assumption that despite the rapid closures of frontline beds, the capital was still "over-bedded" (COHSE 1992). This assumption was strongly challenged by Professor Brian Jarman and others who also produced Department of Health figures to show that London had dramatically fewer nursing homes and suitable beds for the elderly than the national average. They argued that this resulted in extra pressure on the remaining acute beds (Jarman 1993, 1994).

Far from looking at health services throughout the capital, Tomlinson had looked only at *inner* London, completely ignoring the outer districts where two-thirds of the city's population live. Several key outer London hospitals and one whole health district (Barking and Havering, with 400,000 residents) were left off the maps included in the Report. Local residents in the forgotten areas tempered their anger with relief that their health services had not been directly singled out for closures. Tomlinson assumed that all the 200,000 patients from outer London and the shire counties who were still being treated in inner London hospitals were "elective" (waiting list) cases. In fact more than half of them were emergencies (Lister 1992a, b).

Even inner London was examined by Tomlinson in such a way as to ignore all of the unique features of the capital city and its deprived central areas. The "throughput" rates of inner London hospital beds were unfavourably compared with national averages, without taking any account of the extra pressures on health care in Europe's largest city. There was no attempt to compare like with like – for example, by examining the similarities between the performance of inner London hospitals and hospitals in other inner-city areas.

The unique pressures in the capital include:

- London's massive commuter population
- the sheer scale of the population caught in inner-city poverty
- London's unique ethnic mix
- the concentration of homelessness and poor housing
- the concentration of severe mental illness and drug and alcohol abusers
- the concentration of AIDS sufferers (70 per cent of the English total were being treated in London)
- social service cuts hitting London boroughs
- and sharply increased mortality rates in inner London.

(Lister 1992b)

"Primary care led NHS"

Tomlinson also brushed aside the special pressures on the capital's teaching hospitals (together with the cost implications arising out of them), which train over 40 per cent of the country's doctors. Borrowing arguments put forward earlier in 1992 by the King's Fund – in a similarly flawed report (King's Fund 1992) – Tomlinson suggested without a shred of evidence that if long-awaited improvements could be made in primary care services, this would reduce the demand for acute hospital beds:

> The developments in primary and community health services which we have recommended could reduce the pressure on acute hospital facilities in three ways: first, by promoting a healthier population not needing such frequent hospital admission; secondly by providing health care in more appropriate settings in the community; and thirdly by enabling "blocked" beds to be released more rapidly.
>
> (Tomlinson 1992: 21)

We may note in passing that the creation of a "healthier population" calls for public health policies and economic policies far more radical and wide-reaching than the changes proposed for London's NHS. The ill health and inequalities in health that generate larger than average use of London's A&E and hospital services are generated from underlying social inequalities – although these factors were repeatedly denied by Tory ministers into the early 1990s.

With reality pushed to one side, on the basis of applying the most optimistic projections, based on London's hospitals somehow exceeding even the most rapid levels of throughput of patients in other areas, Tomlinson calculated how many beds could close in the capital. The uncritical response to his report from the government, and from much of the media, led to health authorities in other allegedly "over-bedded" cities – including Glasgow, Edinburgh, Cardiff and Liverpool – seeking to invoke the authority of what was a deeply flawed investigation, and launch their own "Tomlinson-style" plans for wholesale rationalisation.

The enthusiasm was not shared by health workers or users of London's health services. The Tomlinson Report itself – leaked to the press the night before publication by London Health Emergency – caused public outrage, with thousands queuing to sign protest petitions and brisk business on a "Hands Off Our Hospitals" hotline set up by LHE. Riding roughshod over the views and needs of Londoners, new Health Secretary Virginia Bottomley responded to Tomlinson in February 1993 with a document *Making London Better* (DoH 1993b), which actually *extended* the list of possible closures, raising questions over the future of hospitals in South West London (Queen Mary's, Roehampton) and North West London (Edgware) which Tomlinson had not even mentioned: both were to run down and close. Only Charing Cross Hospital from the original hit list managed to escape the axe: there was an active all-party campaign in its defence, but there was also the powerful and well-connected pressure behind the scenes from the medical school.

Bottomley again echoed the old, outdated assumption that London had too many beds:

> We can't afford to have people lingering around for a recuperative holiday. We are not catering for people who do not have a home or who have nowhere else to go. Now people have telephones, central heating, GP services and remarkable drugs. The whole structure of health care has changed, and beds are not what we want. We want the minimum beds necessary. We still probably have got more than we need.
>
> (Virginia Bottomley, interviewed by *Hampstead and Highgate Express*, quoted in *Health Emergency* 30, 1993)

The evidence suggested otherwise. The London Bridge train crash in November 1992 had been dealt with by ambulances shuttling patients to three central London hospitals – Bart's, Guy's and St Thomas's – two of which were now due to close. And on 29 December 1992, not a single hospital emergency bed was available in the capital.

Nevertheless, Bottomley's plan forced forward the "merger" of the Guy's and St Thomas's hospital Trusts, leaving it to the resultant internal power struggle to decide which hospital should close. She also set up a series of "Specialty Reviews" to examine how key specialist services might also be rationalised across the capital, although few of the recommendations of these subsequent reports have yet been implemented. The closure package was to be overseen by a new London-wide quango, the London Implementation Group (LIG), to be headed by a trusted former Tory MP and RHA chair, Tim Chessells (Rivett 1998).

Money down the drain

Bottomley also announced an ambitious £170 million investment programme – later boosted to £200 million – in primary care, to be targeted at the inner area of London, the so-called "London Initiative Zone" (Rivett 1998). Despite the apparent generosity of this move it was soon obvious that there was no serious strategy for improving the dire infrastructure of primary care, which was still dogged by an excess of single-handed GPs, too many elderly GPs, sub-standard practice premises, and a lack of practice nurses, practice managers and outreach staff.

Few of the short-term schemes promoted by LIG addressed these issues. LIG was a closed group of seconded NHS administrators, meeting in secret, and predictably including no members from any representative organisation of Londoners, let alone any health professionals from either primary or secondary care. It proved to be an expensive flop, unable either to instruct or persuade health authorities or the RHAs, and incapable of delivering any significant improvement in policy or in services. LIG was wound up after just 18 months of ignominious failure, leaving large amounts of cash sloshing around but no overall body in charge (*Health Emergency* 35, 1994).

A year later London Health Emergency found that early LIG schemes were proposing to spend £6 million over three years to close 156 hospital beds – most of them in mental health, alcohol abuse or long-term care of the elderly. The average cost of closing each bed was £12,500 a year – until the money ran out (*Health Emergency* 37, 1994).

Elsewhere, money was simply wasted through financial mismanagement and incompetence. Late in 1994, City and East London Family Health Services Authority admitted to a list of blunders totalling over £1 million in bad loans, failed projects and bungled computer schemes. By 1995, over £125 million "LIZ money" had been allocated throughout London to over 900 different schemes, with next to no evidence that any of them had been of benefit to patients (King's Fund 1995: 20).

There had been no significant increase in the numbers of GPs in inner London, and according to information obtained by Tessa Jowell MP, one inner London GP in every six still had a list of over 2,500. By 1998, official figures showed 1 per cent fewer GPs in the capital in 1996 than in 1990 – compared with an increase of 6 per cent in England (DoH 1998a: 33), while London still had more than double the English average of single-handed GPs. Perhaps the biggest failure was in the attempt to modernise GP premises: by 1997, fewer than half London's GP premises were deemed to exceed minimum standards, despite the expenditure of over £100 million. The worst-hit area was Barking and Havering, where a shocking 92% of premises fell below acceptable standards, with Redbridge and Waltham Forest not far behind with 86% (King's Fund 1995: 36–7). A third of GP practice premises were below minimum standards in inner London, compared with none in Manchester, 5% in Birmingham and 15% in Liverpool.

The money was flowing out, but nobody was in charge. Even the King's Fund, a noted protagonist of the idea of a primary-care-led NHS criticised the absence of any mechanism to gather and evaluate the evidence on whether these schemes had succeeded or failed. Meanwhile in a little-noticed statement in evidence to the Commons Health Committee, Virginia Bottomley was forced to admit that she knew of "no definitive work" to support her view that improved GP services would lead to a reduction in demand for hospital care (*Health Emergency* 38, 1995). But whether or not there was evidence to support it, she was intent on reducing hospital bed numbers.

Accidents and emergencies

Pressure to rationalise the provision of accident and emergency services onto fewer, larger sites, has not just come from the tightening NHS cash limits: it has also been driven by the medical profession. In 1988 the Royal College of Surgeons published the findings of a working party that there had been "significant deficiencies in the management of seriously injured patients": it claimed that a third of the deaths of 514 major trauma patients admitted to A&E departments could have been avoided (Royal College of Surgeons of England 1988).

Drawing lessons from the USA, the RCS paper recommended the establishment of Regional Trauma Centres, which would marshal together specialists in all of the key aspects of trauma care, including A&E medicine, anaesthetics, neurosurgery and orthopaedics. By drawing on large catchment regions, these centres would treat a high volume of seriously injured patients (between 10 and 20 per week). Under pressure from the Royal College, the Department of Health agreed to set up a pilot trauma unit for evaluation over a four year period 1990–3: the North Staffordshire Royal Infirmary was chosen for this, because of the large potential regional catchment area and the already high volume of activity in its A&E department.

The choice of an American model of service was particularly inappropriate for trauma care, since much of the workload of US trauma centres consists of people suffering from gunshot wounds and knife injuries, problems thankfully rare in Britain. But even while the study was under way, half-digested fragments of this policy were used by District and Regional Health Authorities as arguments for the rationalisation of their A&E units.

The findings from the Stoke study, published late in 1995, was that "there was no evidence of any reduction in avoidable death rates", and that it was "not a cost-effective service for major trauma" (Nicholl, Turner and Dixon 1995). An insuperable problem facing the £500,000-a-year project was the chronic shortage of sufficiently sick patients: the volume of major trauma treated in the centre was "less than 20 per cent of the volume recommended for level 1 trauma centres in the USA".

The 1990s have seen other arguments brought forward for fewer, larger A&E units. Changes in the career structure, training and working hours of junior doctors, and the problems these have created for staffing smaller A&E

departments, have been invoked alongside economic arguments by health authorities and Trusts seeking cash savings.

A 1995 study for the London Implementation Group – never published – found that the ideal size for a cost-effective, high-quality A&E department was between 50,000 and 100,000 attendances a year (DoH 1998b: 59). In 1996 the Audit Commission published a major investigation, *By Accident or Design*, which argued for fewer, bigger units. It pointed out that most of the 227 A&E departments in England and Wales treat an average of between 70 and 200 new patients each day, while only a few "giants" see over 300. Insisting that its suggestions were based on quality of care rather than cost, the Commission admitted however that "there is no conclusive proof that amalgamating medium-sized departments would really release resources." (Audit Commission 1996)

But it went on nevertheless to recommend "reviews" of "all small A&E departments (with, say, fewer than 50,000 new attendances per year) where there is good access to alternative facilities (say, within ten miles). ...If these reviews were to result in the amalgamation of 50 per cent of such small departments, this would mean closing 31 A&E units in England and Wales" (Audit Commission 1996: 67).

In fairness to the Audit Commission, its report did underline the need to take account of the numbers that would require admission to hospital from the A&E, warning that: "There would either be greater fluctuations in bed occupancy, which might mean more beds were required, or an increase in the numbers of patients who had to be transferred to other hospitals after admission." (Audit Commission 1996: 67)

However, many health authorities seized upon this latest report as another argument for rationalisation. Alongside the call for fewer A&E units came efforts to detach the more minor cases from A&E departments, to reduce the apparent caseload. Following the lead of the earlier King's Fund Commission report, Tomlinson had focused attention on the varying proportion of patients who attend A&E units for relatively minor problems – some of which might appropriately be dealt with by a GP – if indeed they were registered with one, and able to access services promptly.

A study carried out in the A&E unit at King's College Hospital, serving a deprived inner-city area with poor primary care services, large numbers of homeless people and many not registered with a GP, found up to 40 per cent of A&E attendees had health needs that could have been met by a GP. This very specific report, focused on one London locality, was soon to be widely misquoted and inappropriately used as the basis for changes in many very different Trusts and districts. Health authority bosses in Brent and Harrow Health Authority went even further, claiming that "up to 75% of the caseload in accident and emergency departments can be dealt with by nurse practitioners" (Brent and Harrow Health Authority and Barnet Health Authority 1994: 32).

In London, a rapid run-down of accident and emergency units from 1990 came against a pattern of steadily rising numbers of patients attending A&E and requiring emergency admission. In 1990, government figures showed 60 A&E units serving Greater London. By February 1994, the equivalent government figures showed that a fifth of these units had closed, leaving just 48 (*Health Emergency* 35, 1994). Two years later, the NHS Executive's *Fact Sheet* showed just 35 fully fledged A&E departments surviving, two of which were outside London and mainly serving a Home Counties catchment. Four more A&E units have since closed – at Mount Vernon, Edgware, Queen Mary's, Roehampton and Guy's Hospital, leaving more than 2.3 million people who attend an A&E with just 31 units to choose from. As this study is completed (2007), a fresh round of rationalisation is posing questions over the future of A&E services at Central Middlesex, Chase Farm (Enfield), King George's Hospital in Ilford, Queen Mary's in Sidcup and Epsom General Hospital (Lister 2007d).

Other big cities have also faced a drastic reduction in numbers of A&E units, leaving the centre of Birmingham without any frontline emergency hospital service: county areas too have seen the pressure to rationalise and centralise, with repeated moves to slim down hospital services in Hertfordshire, Kent, Sussex and many more.

While full-scale A&E departments have been axed, it was fashionable for a while for many health authorities and Trusts to trumpet the opening of new Minor Injury Units (MIUs, also known as Minor Accident Treatment Services (MATS) or Urgent Treatment Centres (UTC)). These are aimed at the most minor end of the "emergency" spectrum: the one common factor is that they do not receive 999 ambulances.

This model of service has been widely copied by health managers across the country in what appears to be a determined and consistent effort to focus the greatest energy and management resources on that category of patient which has least need of health care.

A common menu of services from a Minor Injuries Unit would include:

- Minor burns and scalds less than 2 per cent
- Bruises and abrasions
- Minor sprains and strains (knees to be excluded unless very minor)
- Lacerations which need only steristrips, dressing or suturing
- Dog bites not on hands or face
- Fresh insect bites and stings
- Very minor head injuries
- Foreign bodies in ears, noses or eyes.

(Hertfordshire Councils 1995: 18)

While these services may be welcome to the worried well in need of little more than Elastoplast or ointment, it is clear that MIUs offer no relief to the growing demand on A&E units and hospital beds from patients requiring emergency admission. In many cases they represent an expensive form of care, since their caseload tends to be very low: poorly publicised MIUs can even be a stepping stone to full-scale closure – as happened in Birmingham.

There are other concerns, too, about MIUs. As one A&E director complained:

> I do not think people should be conned into thinking that minor injuries units are anything other than the scaling down of A&E. I think it is a dangerous policy because they cannot provide a safe and cost-effective service for patients. If a minor injuries unit is to cope with the unexpected they need resuscitation units and the skills to use them, x-ray equipment and somebody with diagnostic skills. So they might as well have kept an A&E department in the first place.
>
> (*HSJ*, 1 December 1994)

In 1995 Hertfordshire Health Agency published detailed figures on the St Albans minor injuries unit, and concluded that:

> It appears to be a relatively expensive service to operate, as
> * the re-attendance rate is over 25%;
> * there are no nursing cost savings;
> * overheads have tended to be high as the unit replaced an A&E department and continues to use the large floor area and most of the facilities;
> * the number of attendances was not up to the capacity in the first year.
>
> (Hertfordshire Health Agency 1995: 14)

Fewer, bigger hospitals?

While the debate has raged in many parts of the country over the closure of A&E units, the pressure for a more comprehensive rationalisation of acute hospitals has been steadily building, again driven both by cash problems and by the medical profession, notably the Royal Colleges.

As early as 1969 the Bonham Carter Report had questioned the desirable size of the catchment population for district general hospitals, suggesting that they should be twice as big, covering a catchment of up to 300,000 people, with 1,000–2,000 beds (Central Health Services Council 1969). This had been dismissed by Labour's Richard Crossman as leading to hospitals which would be expensive, impersonal megaliths, and which would in all probability fail to deliver the promised economies of scale (Rivett 1998: 245).

But when the same arguments resurfaced in the 1990s, the bed numbers being proposed to cover the same target population were much more modest.

The 1993 Calman Report which restructured the training of doctors, leading to a shorter and more structured path to qualification as a consultant, has proved to be a major factor in destabilising many district general hospitals. By shortening the training period (alongside a welcome, if belated, reduction in junior doctors' hours) the new system restricted the availability of junior staff to treat patients. But it also increased the need for a high caseload in hospitals where junior doctors are trained, to ensure that they get a sufficiently broad experience in the shorter time they spend in each specialty.

The Royal Colleges, which have the power to grant or withdraw accreditation for the training of junior doctors, have begun to argue that bigger catchment populations are necessary to ensure sufficient caseload for most specialties, with even larger catchments for more highly specialised work such as vascular surgery.

The Royal College of Surgeons went on to call for emergency surgical services to be organised and financed for a population of 450–500,000, which "might be expected to generate approximately 90,000 to 100,000 new patient attendances per year." (Royal College of Surgeons of England 1997: 6)

Its report did concede that a smaller unit (serving a 200–250,000 population) is:

> considered optimal for the provision of a general medical service, and is regarded as more easily managed and patient friendly than a larger unit.
>
> (Royal College of Surgeons of England 1997: 6)

But for the RCS, the views and interests of patients, NHS managers and even their physician colleagues clearly come a poor second to the views of the surgeons themselves. The RCS is conspicuously silent on the numbers of beds that would be required to handle this expanded caseload in fewer, bigger hospitals.

A BMA report in 1997 went further, looking at the implications of rationalising hospital services, including the logical end-point – the building of a single regional hospital to cover a population of two million. The BMA took a sample area and added up the total hospital resources and activity which would need to be provided and came to the conclusion that a single regional hospital could expect to handle over 400,000 inpatients and day cases a year, requiring 758 consultants and 6,900 beds! Apart from the logistical nightmare of patients getting to and from this grotesque factory-sized hospital, there was another stumbling block: "The estimated cost of a new build single site hospital with 6,900 beds would be approximately £860 million"[13] (BMA Health Policy and Economic Research Unit 1997).

The BMA report also examined alternative schemes, in which the same population of two million would be served by five general hospitals each with a catchment of 400–450,000. But it pointed out that to accommodate the necessary bed numbers such a scheme would require extensive redevelopment costing over £400 million.

These discussions on models of service, in each case one-sided and impractical, have since been misquoted and exploited by health authorities and Trusts seeking primarily to save money by cutting rather than rationalising services (for example, Worcestershire Health Authority 1998 and West Hertfordshire Health Authority 1998). It is common for health chiefs to latch on

---

13 In today's crazy, inflated world of Private Finance Initiative hospital schemes, in which the average cost of a new hospital a fraction the size now exceeds £300 million, the BMA estimate is hopelessly optimistic on the likely actual cost of such a mega-hospital.

to the idea of fewer hospitals covering a larger catchment population without taking on board the need for sufficient beds to enable them to function effectively – and the cost implications of this both for capital and revenue, or the impact on patients whose local hospital services close down.

Community care

The community care reforms took effect from April 1993. The Institute of Health Services Management warned that the system would be little more than "crisis management on an individual basis", while the *Health Service Journal* in a scathing editorial denounced the policy as "such a grotesque caricature of the promise and potential that today's launch of the community care reforms appears almost like a cynical April Fool's day joke perpetrated on the most needy members of society." (*HSJ*, 1 April 1993)

A BMA poll found that 92 per cent of GPs were unaware of any formal policies on hospital discharge of elderly patients, and 80 per cent were unaware of any mechanism for collaboration between the NHS and social services. By the autumn, the Association of London Authorities was warning that councils would need an extra £1 billion to run their share of the new community care system in 1994–5.

It was becoming very obvious that, with social service departments across the country facing spending cuts, the result was going to be a proliferation of "bed blocking" by frail elderly patients who could not be discharged from acute hospitals.

The NHS was rapidly pulling out of any involvement. A *Guardian* survey of two health regions found that NHS elderly care beds had been cut by 46 per cent over ten years, with a 40 per cent reduction in the previous five, at a time when the population of over 75s was rapidly increasing. A subsequent survey in December found that half of the hospitals in the 48 districts covered had cut the number of beds for elderly people with long-term illness (*Guardian*, 7 December 1993). The Alzheimer's Disease Society found that 72 per cent of the districts they surveyed provided fewer than the recommended allocation of continuing care beds for people with dementia (Alzheimer's Disease Society 1993).

By the autumn of 1994, the Isle of Wight and Gloucestershire became the first councils to run out of money for community care, as the full impact of the reforms began to make itself felt. In the summer of 1995 a BMA survey found that less than a quarter of GPs believed community care services had improved in the first 18 months of the reforms. Two-thirds said that home help services had actually deteriorated, and 40 per cent said it had become more difficult to get elderly patients admitted to nursing homes.

Ever since, 40,000 or more elderly people a year have been forced to sell their houses to pay means-tested charges for nursing home care, with anyone with savings in excess of a fixed threshold having to pay the full cost of care from their own pockets (Doughty 2007; Phillips 2007). In some areas there was a growing problem of patients refusing to move from NHS beds to nursing homes: in many more there were conflicts between cash-limited health authorities and council-tax-capped councils over who should be responsible for the care of particular patients or groups of patients. Some health authorities had gone much further than others in the closure of their long-stay beds for the elderly. In one highly publicised case health chiefs in Leeds were criticised for attempting to discharge a severely disabled stroke victim, saddling his family with a massive bill for care.

Elsewhere, the failure of the private sector to offer sufficient nursing home places, within the "benchmark" limit set by councils as the top limit to fees, led to shortages of places for the discharge of elderly patients. Many of these had been admitted to hospitals as emergencies and were occupying acute beds (Lister 1996a).

From increasingly desperate Trusts complaining of a rising number of frontline beds "blocked" by these frail elderly patients, and from health authorities impatient to transfer the costs of caring for these expensive patients, came a demand for the government to spell out a coherent policy (*Cambridge Evening News*, 29 November 1995; *HSJ*, 30 November 1995 and 8 May 1997).

Trusts and HAs wanted guidance which would establish the principle that no patient would have the "right" to occupy an NHS bed indefinitely, and which would set out criteria by which patients could be deemed ineligible for continuing care funded by the NHS. This would create a framework through which hospitals could legally get shot of patients who they considered no longer required health care. This was to be the formal end to the NHS philosophy of "cradle to grave" care for all, funded from taxation – the biggest exercise in privatisation in the 50 years of the health service.

In the autumn of 1995 the Department of Health responded to these demands by issuing a draft circular, misleadingly entitled 'NHS Responsibilities for Meeting Continuing Health Care Needs' (DoH 1995a). In fact it was a document designed to define where the NHS would recognise no such responsibility. Significantly, the Department pulled back from issuing firm and detailed national guidelines. Instead it called on each health authority to review locally the arrangements for the delivery and funding of continuing care, and on the basis of this to draw up local "eligibility criteria" explaining the basis on which patients would be offered – or refused – NHS treatment (Lister 1996b, c).

The Department's document was carefully drafted to avoid taking responsibility for any subsequent withdrawal of local services. It spelled out a raft of new responsibilities for health authorities without offering any extra funding to enable them to carry these out. It presumed a harmony of interest between the NHS and social services which has never existed – and which cannot exist as long as both organisations are wrestling with inadequate and cash-limited budgets. And it handed over responsibility for policy-making to local health authorities, opening up the prospect of major variations from one area to another, without establishing any mechanism to monitor the outcome.

The local eligibility criteria were to be published by each health authority and opened up to a process of "consultation" before being adopted and implemented by April 1996. In many areas the consultation on what appeared to many to be a complex and obscure issue was even lower in media profile and less subject to public debate than the average health authority consultation exercise. With a handful of notable exceptions, few people recognised that the implications of the new policy proposals were easily as great as the closure of a local hospital. Those least likely to be able to respond to the documents drafted by their local health authority were of course those most at risk of losing NHS services – the frail elderly users of continuing care services (Lister 1997a).

Perhaps even more surprising was the near-total silence of local councillors, including those sitting on social services committees which were being expected to pick up the bill and the responsibility for caring for a large number of patients abandoned by the NHS. With few councils remaining in the hands of the Tories, it might have been expected that some more perspicacious Labour councillors would spot the way in which they were being left to carry the can, while any attempts to raise resources through increases in council tax were denounced, ridiculed or simply blocked by Tory ministers.

How many of these silent Labour councillors were still carried away by the delusions of the "Griffiths Now!" lobby five years earlier, and how many were simply too slow-witted to understand what was happening is not clear (although many will doubtless have fallen into the second category). Labour had been heavily compromised by its backing for the Griffiths reforms, effectively dropping any opposition to the Tory privatisation of care of the elderly. The party's policy had been reduced by the mid-1990s to the minimalist call for a Royal Commission to look into the issue.

More vocal were Tory backbenchers embarrassed by the complaints of prosperous families forced to sell up the family home to pay sky-high fees for nursing home care: some noticed that this sat badly with the expressed Tory objective of a "property-owning democracy", in which wealth should in theory cascade down the generations.

Many health authorities drew up extremely strict new guidelines designed to minimise the numbers of patients who would be deemed eligible for NHS-provided or NHS-funded continuing care. Some – notably in Cambridge and Huntingdon Health Authority (CHHA) – were downright draconian, with the explicit objective of closing the remaining local continuing care beds. Among the criteria set out in the CHHA draft policy was that a patient would only be considered for long-term NHS care if – in addition to other major health problems – it also required "more than two skilled persons" (i.e. a minimum of three) to move them (Cambridge and Huntingdon Health Commission 1995). Eligibility required extreme levels of disability:

> Patients who need more than two [i.e. three or more, JL] skilled persons to move or transfer and in addition are severely affected by at least one of the following conditions:
>
> - double incontinence complicated by severe pressure sores
> - complex management of pressure sores or large leg ulcers which are down to muscle, tendon or bone

- inoperable fractured neck of femur needing continued traction.

(Cambridge and Huntingdon Health Commission 1995: 38)

Another Cambridge criterion for admission of those diagnosed as terminally ill specified that they should be "likely to die within two weeks!" (Ibid.) The outcome of these criteria, which were rubber-stamped with only minimal alterations by the health authority, was that NHS continuing care in Cambridge was effectively reduced to a palliative care service for the dying – while the lack of suitable nursing home places in the Cambridge area led to a recurrent problem of bed blocking at Addenbrookes Hospital (Lister 1997a).

Other health authorities were less rigid and brutal in their approach than Cambridge, but one common factor ran throughout the eligibility criteria implemented from April 1996: the health authorities' abdication from responsibility for these patients rested on the assumption that social services were ready, willing and resourced to step into the breach and offer the required additional care to patients unable to fend for themselves.

This soon ran into problems. By November 1996, a survey by the Association of Metropolitan Authorities found that three-quarters of the councils which responded recognised a local problem of "bed blocking", with at least 1,000 people inappropriately occupying hospital beds. A quarter of the councils admitted to being at loggerheads with the local health authority over this issue (*Guardian*, 28 December 1998).

Another problem which the health authorities had hoped would not raise its head was the extent to which this new model of "community care" was dumping extra work onto GPs, who were expected to give ongoing medical support to patients discharged to nursing homes. In November 1996 the BMA advised GPs to refuse to treat any new patients in nursing homes from the following April, unless they received more money for doing so (*Daily Telegraph, Guardian, Independent, Financial Times*, 7 November 1996).

Ever since 1993 local councils have been subjected to constantly tightening cash limits, as well as the restrictive provisions of the Community Care Act, which included the requirement that councils must spend at least 85 per cent of the government funds they receive for community care in the "independent" [i.e. in most cases private] sector. The cash squeeze has compelled many councils to resort to imposing their own "eligibility criteria" for social services, resulting in a targeting of resources which increasingly excludes all but the most severely disabled. This process continued into 1997, with councils across the country being compelled to cut social service budgets to keep spending below the "cap" imposed by the government. An estimated £200 million was to be cut from social services in 1997–8, with the closure of over 1,000 places in residential and day centres and hundreds of social service jobs axed (*Community Care*, 13 March 1997).

The pressures on councils increased further in the autumn of 1996 when Chancellor Kenneth Clarke responded to the growing pressure from his own backbenchers, worried at the number of relatively prosperous constituents who were being forced to sell their homes to pay nursing home fees. Clarke raised the threshold of savings and assets above which patients have to pay the full cost of their care to £16,000: those with less than £10,000 should not be liable to pay any charges. Since fees not paid by the client would have to be paid by social services, the Chancellor's generosity effectively dumped a hefty extra bill onto councils already struggling to cope.

Early in 1997 a High Court judgement summed up the impasse created by the community care reforms. Gloucestershire County Council, supported by the government, won a ruling that allowed any council to use its own financial difficulties as a reason to withdraw or refuse social services to local residents who are disabled or chronically sick (*Guardian* editorial, 21 March 1997). A week later Sefton council won a ruling that it had no duty to provide residential care to anyone who has savings or assets of more than £1,500 – the estimated price of a funeral (*Community Care*, 3 April 1997). This effectively overturned the legal right to care which had prevailed for many of these clients under the 1970 Chronic Sick and Disabled Persons Act, which compelled councils to take account of the needs of the individual, and imposed a 'duty of care' on social service departments.

Mental health

Although attracting even less public debate, mental health services – the sector largely bypassed by the Griffiths reforms – underwent rapid changes in the 1990s. Following the closure of Banstead Hospital, which in 1986 had been the first old-fashioned "water tower" asylum to close its doors following Enoch Powell's 1961 speech denouncing large and impersonal institutions, more hospitals and beds were closing. But health authority budgets were unable to afford sufficient community-based services to support many people suffering severe and chronic mental illness, for whom there were ever fewer long-term beds (Lister 1997b, 1999).

In many areas mental health services were now provided by specialist NHS Trusts: in others they were combined with community services, or occasionally with acute services in "district-wide" Trusts. Whichever permutation had prevailed, the new market system did not appear to offer any greater share of spending for this most under-resourced of "Cinderella" services. Mental health was still awash with well-intentioned rhetoric and impractical policies. Sir Roy Griffiths had suggested that local authorities should work together with health authorities in assessing the health needs of individual mental health patients, with a specific "case manager" put in charge of their care (Griffiths 1988).

However, this was not linked to the provision of any extra funding to make this possible. Instead, councils and health authorities were urged to make "realistic" assessments of the level of services they could afford to provide within existing cash limits. The "assessment" process was viewed by most as a means of limiting the obligations of authorities to provide care: no individual had any right to be assessed, or any right to appeal against an assessment which offered them unsatisfactory or inadequate care. The subsequent (1991) introduction of the "Care Programme Approach" resulted in many cases in an extra load of paper work but little additional support for patients discharged into the community (*Community Care*, 25 July 1996).

A new "mental health specific grant" to encourage local councils to take responsibility for the social care of mental health sufferers was unveiled by the government to muted applause: it amounted to just £21 million nationally in 1991. The puny amounts available to each council had to be matched by additional local funds from the council's kitty. By February 1996 the nationwide total of the mental health specific grant had risen to just £54 million.

Meanwhile, the pressures on frontline mental health services were intensified by the findings of the Reed Report on the treatment of mentally disordered offenders (Department of Health and Home Office 1991). This called, among other things, for an increase in the number of NHS secure beds, to ensure that those with psychiatric problems were treated in hospital rather than imprisoned.

Progress along these lines was extremely slow, hampered by cash shortages. In February 1996 the NHS Executive predicted that 1,200 purpose-built medium secure beds would be in place by March 1997. The lack of appropriate NHS beds for these demanding patients led to an escalating spiral of spending on placements in costly private units, creating huge and growing financial problems, especially for health authorities and mental health Trusts in deprived inner-city areas (*Evening Standard*, 26 April 1996; Lister 1999).

Pressure was also increased by a succession of highly publicised scandals exposing the gaps in the infrastructure that was supposed to provide "community care". In August 1993, in the aftermath of the stabbing of Jonathan Zito by discharged psychiatric patient Christopher Clunis, and the episode in which Ben Silcock climbed into the lions' enclosure in London Zoo, Virginia Bottomley unveiled a new ten-point plan, including controversial proposals for the "supervised discharge" of psychiatric patients who needed ongoing support outside hospital.

Six months later the report of the official inquiry into the care and treatment of Christopher Clunis lifted the lid on a fragmented and chaotic patchwork of services, in which the predominant ethos had become that of buck-passing between over-stretched and under-funded agencies, departments and authorities (Ritchie et al. 1994). Despite this evidence that the system could not cope with its existing workload, it was announced that supervision registers would be introduced for "at risk" mentally ill people from April 1994 (NHS Executive 1994a).

No extra money was made available to fund this increased workload. By the autumn of 1995, a Thames Regional Health Authority report revealed that less than ten per cent of the patients put on supervision registers had been seen by community psychiatric nurses even once a month between April and June. There was also a glaring disparity in the numbers of patients put on the registers: nine health authorities had put none on the register – suggesting perhaps that they were conscious of the lack of resources to follow them up (North Thames RHA 1995).

In May 1994 the government again toughened the guidelines on the discharge of mental patients, placing "particular emphasis on the need for risk assessment prior to discharge". It stressed that patients should be discharged "only when and if they are ready to leave hospital… so that any risk to the public or to the patients themselves is minimal and is managed effectively" (DoH 1994).

Again the words were hollow. The pressure on the remaining beds was becoming so intense that consultants were obliged to discharge patients as soon as possible in order to free the bed for another desperate case. Some patients discharged home temporarily on leave returned to find their beds taken. Some patients who had been compulsorily detained on "section" under the Mental Health Act were sent home on leave to make room for those judged even more sick.

Late in 1995 the Mental Health Act Commission published a report on the grim national toll of 240 suicides by psychiatric patients and 39 homicides. It concluded that bed occupancy levels then averaging 90 per cent across the country – but frequently reaching as high as 130 per cent in inner-city districts – could "quite easily" lead to staff inappropriately giving leave to some patients.

Another report by the Royal College of Psychiatrists, which had been commissioned by the government, warned:

> Overcrowded wards, excessive disturbance and unsuitable community facilities militated against participation in treatment. It seems unlikely that effective care can be given in acute wards with over 30 beds and with only three or four staff on duty.
>
> (Royal College of Psychiatrists 1996)

Following these and other reports (NHS Trust Federation 1996a), Health Secretary Stephen Dorrell in February 1996 announced another revamp of government policy, this time deliberately avoiding the use of the phrase "community care". He coined the new term "Spectrum of Care" to describe a policy which appeared to back-track from the programme of rapid bed-closures, and to call instead for the provision of a new system of "24-hour nursed care" (NHS Executive 1996). Critics were quick to point out that the spectrum ranged from nothing at all to not enough.

The starting point of this new guidance to health authorities was the astonishing, though understated, confession that there was a large and growing area of unmet need. This gap in care had been created (or at the very least exacerbated) by the bed closures forced through by government policy and by cash pressures in the preceding 15 years, together with the evident failure of health authorities or councils to ensure that adequate new community-based services were developed.

The NHS Executive guideline document pointed out the way in which thousands of seriously ill people had been left in limbo by bed closures:

Mental health planning has by and large been reasonably successful in providing accommodation for the old, long-stay clients emerging from the old, large institutions. However few health authorities have made adequate provision for new long-stay clients with severe and enduring mental illness, who may never have been in a large institution, but who will require daily supervision of medication and daily monitoring of their mental state for many years. ...

Recent inquiry reports have demonstrated the lack of such highly supported accommodation and care for new long-stay patients. Such patients tend either to be inadequately supported in the community or are inappropriately occupying an acute hospital bed.

The consequence of this "bed blocking" by chronic sufferers was the soaring levels of occupancy of acute psychiatric wards:

Audit shows that up to 40% of people in acute mental illness hospital beds do not need to be there, with the result that they themselves receive sub-optimal care, the bed is not available for another patient who needs it, and their inpatient care has to be provided through an extra-contractual referral.

(NHS Executive 1996 Annex, para 3)

A closer examination of the breakdown of beds closed in psychiatric hospitals confirms that while many were beds for the elderly mentally ill, thousands had been continuing care beds for adult patients (Lister 1997b, 1999).

The NHS guidance concluded that the needs of these patients – numbers of whom were estimated (conservatively) at 5,000 nationally – would best be met through the provision of 24-hour nursed accommodation: it urged health authorities to set up such services in small units of no more than 12 beds, and helpfully provided detailed costings and suggested staffing levels.

But, predictably, perhaps, the government did not back these very reasonable suggestions with the capital to build the new units, or the revenue to run them. The national bill for 5,000 places along the lines proposed totted up to some £400 million in capital, and up to £250 million a year in revenue costs. In the absence of anything approaching these amounts, the policy has remained little more than another display of empty rhetoric, a dead letter.

Problems with primary care

Elsewhere, despite the rhetoric of a 'primary care-led NHS', all was not well among the GPs. In the summer of 1994 it became clear that fewer doctors were entering general practice, and health academics warned that "Ministers must recognise there is a problem of morale" (*Guardian*, 24 June 1994).

The new NHS chief executive Alan Langlands admitted that GPs faced a "paper overload" in the new, market-style NHS. Dr Ian Bogle, chair of the BMA's GP committee warned that doctors were being turned into a "demoralised and demotivated workforce".

A consolation for GPs was that there were promising pickings if they decided to become fundholders. The figures were starting to become available. It emerged that the government had been handing out £16,500 a time in lump sums as a down payment to any GP who expressed an interest in fundholding – money that was theirs to keep. Several practices had reportedly picked up this largesse more than once, and no less than £2.3 million had been handed over in this way in 1991–2. It would be followed by another cheque for £30,000 as a start-up gift for any that joined the scheme (*Sunday Express*, 23 January 1994).

There was an added incentive in that practices could retain any unspent surplus from their annual budget. Figures obtained by Alan Milburn MP showed that 585 fundholding practices had retained a total of £28 million in 1993–4. Health authorities had no power to retrieve unspent allocations, which averaged £48,000 per fundholder in the second year of the scheme. In the North East Thames region, fundholding GPs held onto more than £1 for every £6 allocated, equivalent to £77,000 per doctor (*Guardian*, 23 December 1993 and 28 February 1994).

There was growing anger, too, at revelations of the predicted "two tier" service emerging within the NHS. A BMA survey of 173 hospitals in 1994 found 73 of them were offering preferential services to fundholders' patients, 41 of them promising "fast-track", more rapid admission (*Guardian*, 10 December 1993).

The administration of the contracts between a growing number of fundholding practices and the NHS Trusts from whom they purchased services also became increasingly complex and expensive. By 1997, a report researched by the NHS Support Federation estimated that each Trust was spending up to £1 million a year on the bureaucracy of deals with fundholders – suggesting a national bill as high as £500 million – a "hidden" cost of fundholding (Paterson and Walker 1997: 17; NHS Trust Federation 1996b).

The mounting bill for the bureaucracy of the NHS market was also causing some embarrassment to ministers. In 1995 Stephen Dorrell as Health Secretary had demanded a reduction in management costs, and required Trusts to publish in each year's Annual Report what percentage of their revenue budget was being spent on management. Results were patchy, and the biggest reduction in senior management posts took place in 1996, when 4,000 nursing managers with professional qualifications were reclassified as "nurses" – apparently reducing management and boosting nurse numbers at a stroke, while changing nothing! (*HSJ*, 9 May 1996)

The costs were further boosted by an explosion in salaries for top Trust directors, who were quick to exploit the new "freedoms" of Trusts to fix pay scales, while – as many had cynically predicted – the wages of most of their lowest-paid staff continued to rise at less than inflation. The first £100,000-plus chief executive was Peter Griffiths at the Guy's Hospital Trust, where his package reportedly also involved two cars – one for him and one for his wife! In Wales the chief executive of the tiny Pembrokeshire NHS Trust picked up a salary of £73,000 plus a Porsche 994S coupé (*Health Emergency* 35, 1994).

The inflation of management pay was not restricted to Trusts: in Waltham Forest in North East London, the Community Health Council complained bitterly at a top-heavy management structure in which the local health authority had a chief executive and eight directors (each paid between £45,000 and £80,000 a year) as well as no fewer than 24 "Associate Directors", each of them paid over £30,000 a year.

Out of control

With the end of the "steady state" from 1993, the NHS market system itself was beginning to take a toll of losers. The fight for contract income was uncovered when leaked documents showed the bitter conflict between acute Trusts in East Anglia (James Paget Hospital NHS Trust 1994).

In London, Charing Cross Hospital bosses were exposed plotting to destabilise a competitor in the specialist cancer market by "poaching" a top consultant from the Royal Marsden Hospital three miles away. A leaked letter declared that the plan would not only boost Charing Cross but "would have the additional benefit of weakening one of our strongest competitors" (*Evening Standard*, 5 July 1994; *HSJ*, 14 July 1994).

Closures of acute hospital beds continued, with the effects masked by a succession of mild winters and the use of "waiting list initiative" funding to reduce the numbers of patients waiting over a year for treatment. But the sharp winter of 1995–6 triggered a "trolleys crisis" in London and other big cities. In South West London, medical directors from six acute service NHS Trusts broke the official silence and published a letter they had sent to Health Secretary Dorrell protesting at the impact of the bed shortage. They pointed out that in one hospital the lack of beds had left 52 patients to spend a whole night on trolleys.

Because there were insufficient beds to deal with medical emergency admissions:

> These patients first fill the medical beds and then have to overflow into unsuitable beds in surgical wards... When all beds are full, the emergencies (often very sick) log-jam back into A&E, "overnighting" on trolleys which are insufficiently supervised, uncomfortable and stressful for both patients and staff. ...Neighbouring Trusts are unable to help as they face the same problems.
>
> (O'Sullivan et al. 1995: 1)

The consultants went on to complain that purchasing health authorities were refusing to pay for the extra emergency work – and even threatening to penalise Trusts which were forced to cancel waiting list admissions for lack of beds.

When they received no reply from Dorrell, a similar letter to him was signed in February by the medical directors of all the acute Trusts in the South Thames region. This contained an even more scathing root and branch criticism of the internal market system and the policies of community care and "primary care-led NHS" (South West Thames Medical Directors 1996).

The pressure on beds – intensified by the renewed government spending squeeze – continued through 1996, with many Trusts warning that emergency admissions across the normally quieter summer period had continued at near-winter levels. As many had warned, the 1996–7 winter saw even worse problems, with several hospitals running out of trolleys as well as beds, and one hospital reduced to treating emergency patients in the backs of ambulances parked outside a packed A&E department. Hillingdon Hospital in West London, struggling to cope with many of its beds "blocked" by elderly patients after the closure of A&E services at the nearby Mount Vernon Hospital, hit the headlines when it announced it could admit no more patients aged over 75 until social services found nursing home places for some of those who should be discharged (*Evening Standard*, 17 December 1996 and 9 January 1997).

This was not the first time Trusts in London and in Brighton had been caught restricting services for patients deemed to be "too old". There were accusations of ageism and rationing care to the elderly – but there was a difference: the Hillingdon policy had flowed naturally from the dislocation of local services and the lack of any genuine infrastructure of community care.

The debate over "rationing" some forms of health care had begun to grab the headlines. It gained the widest currency in 1996 with the unsuccessful legal challenge by the father of "Child B" (Jaymee Bowen) to Cambridge and Huntingdon Health Authority's decision not to fund further treatment of her rare form of leukaemia. The health authority had reportedly discussed for a whole hour and a half before voting to withhold treatment and allow the child to die. Explaining their decision, there were references to the cost in comparison to other forms of treatment for which patients were waiting. Health chiefs also said that they thought the chances of success from the treatment were too slim (*HSJ*, 16 March 1995).

The media latched on to this, and publicised a controversial report sponsored by drug companies and promoted by former NHS chief executive Sir Duncan Nichol which concluded that the rationing of NHS services was "inevitable" (*Guardian*, 19 and 20 September 1995).

As the May 1997 election drew closer, the evident chaos in the provision of acute hospital services, community care and mental health services made even Labour's vague and conservative proposals for the replacement of the internal market with some form of "local commisioning" appear an attractive alternative for many health workers and for concerned voters. But the NHS yet again played a remarkably small part in Labour's national campaign – being largely reserved to Tony Blair's memorable and often quoted warning that voters had "24 hours to save the NHS".

Nevertheless, the pattern of polling showed much stronger support for Labour in areas where hospital services were seen as being under threat – notably in London, where the overall swing to Labour was well above the national average, and especially in the areas surrounding three hospitals – Oldchurch (Romford), Edgware and Queen Mary's, Roehampton – where sitting Tory MPs fell to candidates who had been given only outside odds of winning.

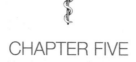

CHAPTER FIVE

New Labour – new market?
Picking up the pieces 1997–2000

Many GPs seem to see the white paper as a triumph of primary care over the rest of the NHS and the creation of a new nirvana for them. Sorry comrades – this is the beginning of the management of primary care within a cash-limited budget.

(Professor Alan Maynard, *HSJ*, 29 January 1998)

We are talking about taking half a billion pounds of spending power out of the system. I think that is a very real problem, because if you have to try to explain to the public that you are making cuts in services to improve the balance sheet it is a very difficult message to get across.

(Jaki Meekings, Chair of the Healthcare
Financial Management Association, December 1997)

Only Spain, Portugal, Greece and Turkey devote a lower proportion of their national wealth to health care. In 1995 Britain spent $1,300 (£824) per person on health care compared to an OECD average of $2,071. Such parsimony has turned the NHS into a third rate service.

(*Economist*, 13 March 1997)

THE NEW LABOUR GOVERNMENT elected with a landslide majority in May 1997 carried with it the hopes and expectations of millions of health workers, patients, carers and campaigners for the NHS. In opposition, Labour's shadow team had promised a moratorium on hospital closures in London and a reprieve for particular hospitals – Edgware General and Bart's. Labour had pledged to sweep away the Tory market system, and thus make massive savings on the cost of "bureaucracy", the first results of which would be to reduce waiting lists, which had topped the million mark in England (DoH Press Release, 22 May 1997).

In government, however, the new ministerial team, headed by Frank Dobson as Health Secretary, were much more cautious. A team was set up with the ominous task of reviewing the financing of the NHS, and another began a detailed reappraisal of the formula for allocating funds on a per capita basis.

Far from being saved, Edgware Hospital, which had been cynically run down in the few weeks immediately prior to the election by the local Barnet Health Authority and Wellhouse Trust, was swiftly dispatched. Its A&E unit was closed along with the remaining acute beds, with the closure rubber-stamped by Health

Secretary Alan Milburn, to the anger of the vocal, broad-based campaign which had battled for over three years to defend their hospital. Milburn, however, also urged the health authority to come back with proposals for the development of a "community hospital" on the Edgware site (DoH Press Release, 23 May 1997): this was eventually built, with NHS funding.

Soon after Edgware lost its acute services, Dobson announced a moratorium on the closure of hospitals in London, with words carefully chosen to allow scope for substantial closures of beds and specialist services. And in July, Milburn announced the establishment of an independent review of health services in the capital, to be headed by Sir Leslie Turnberg, and including a noted critic of the Tomlinson Report, Professor Brian Jarman. The review was given just three months to accumulate the necessary information and make its recommendations. This may have seemed like an exercise in locking the stable door after the horse has died, but unlike the Tomlinson team, the Turnberg inquiry was genuinely independent and relatively open: it immediately invited submissions from a wide cross section of organisations and concerned individuals (Turnberg 1997).

Funding

Also in July, the new Chancellor Gordon Brown drew cheers of delight from the Labour benches when he announced in his budget that there would be an extra £1.2 billion for the NHS in 1998–9. This sounded far more generous than it turned out: Labour had taken over, pledged to reduce waiting lists, but also committed to stick to Tory spending limits and levels of direct taxation. The financial plight of the NHS was already dire. Shocked health ministers were soon leaking their initial findings – that NHS Trusts and health authorities had carried over a massive £300 million in deficits from the 1996–7 financial year, and were piling up debts at £1 million per day.

Brown's "extra" money proved to be a very limited uplift from the amount already allocated by outgoing Tory Chancellor Kenneth Clarke, who had fixed impossibly tight cash limits for the health service in his final budget the previous November: spending was due to increase by just 0.3 per cent in real terms over the three years to 1999. Even the impeccably right-wing *Economist* magazine pointed out that this was "far less than the 3 per cent annual rise in NHS spending over the past 20 years" (*Economist*, 15 March 1997).

Before the election, the Institute of Fiscal Studies had sounded the alarm, warning that by endorsing Clarke's spending plans for the next three years, Brown was committing a Labour government to the toughest spending limits for at least 30 years, with health spending rising more slowly than at any time since the NHS was set up in 1948. The increase for 1997–8 was to be just £1.8 billion – well below the likely level of inflation in costs and wages – and then frozen for two years. If Brown – unlike his Tory predecessors, who had repeatedly given way under pressure – attempted to tough it out and resisted calls for more spending to relieve pressures on the NHS, it could open up a new £2 billion "gap" between actual spending and the 2 per cent per year real terms increase needed to keep pace with growing numbers of elderly patients and the cost of medical technology.

Spending on health care in Britain, at a total of just 6.9% of gross domestic product (5.9% of it in the NHS, 1% in the private sector) compared with an average of 10.4% in most developed countries. The *Economist* pointed out that:

> Only Spain, Portugal, Greece and Turkey devote a lower proportion of their national wealth to health care. In 1995 Britain spent $1,300 (£824) per person on health care compared to an OECD average of $2,071. Such parsimony has turned the NHS into a third rate service.
>
> (*Economist*, 13 March 1997)

Brown's announcement appeared to offer limited relief for the following year, but did nothing to resolve the mounting immediate financial problems that were facing Trusts and health authorities. Price inflation was running at 0.75% above projected levels, and with emergency admissions remaining high through the summer of 1997, and the grim experience of two successive, worsening winter crises, there were fears that acute services would be simply unable to cope with another combination of freezing weather and a flu epidemic (BMA Press Release, 14 October 1997).

This was the context in which Frank Dobson successfully negotiated an additional one-off cash injection of £300 million to stave off some of the pressures on hospitals through New Labour's first winter. This ran alongside clear directives that emergency admissions were to be given priority over waiting list cases, with a warning to acute Trusts to ensure they avoided embarrassing "trolley" waits (DoH Press Release, 12 June 1997). Many Trusts had already moved towards an emergencies-only service, either because they had run short of funding for elective treatment, or because they were keen to avoid the chaos of last-minute cancellations across the coming winter period (*HSJ*, 12 June 1997).

The extra £300 million – to be spent in the three to four months ending March 1998 – was to be allocated not on the basis of the general capitation funding formula, but in response to specific bids by health authorities and Trusts. It was said from the outset that some of the money was to be passed on to cash-strapped social service departments to facilitate the swifter discharge of elderly patients from "blocked" hospital beds to continuing care in nursing homes. There was a real irony to this aspect of the policy, since one of the first decisions made by John Prescott as Secretary for the Environment and Transport had been to uphold the Tory "cap" on council tax in Oxfordshire, a policy which was leading to hefty cuts in social service budgets. Other councils throughout the country had also been forced to cut back on social service spending, with cuts averaging £2.5 million per authority (*The Times*, 12 July 1997; *HSJ*, 19 June 1997).

However, the new money channelled into these services through the NHS proved a mixed blessing to some local authorities, which as a result were obliged to find places for frail elderly patients – places for which the councils would have to pick up the bill after the NHS funding ran out the following April. Some social service directors warned that they could wind up worse off as a result of accepting this limited amount of money. In Gloucestershire, extra "bed blocking" funds for social services ran out by the end of January (*Community Care*, 5 February 1998).

In Colchester, 21 out of 24 beds freed up by the discharge of older patients using the winter crisis money were blocked again within a week. At the end of December, 10 per cent of the acute beds in Essex Rivers Trust were filled with people waiting for social care (Lister 1998a: 6). In Oxfordshire, where at least 45 elderly people remained marooned in acute hospital beds, despite an extra £1.4 million being allocated to social services across the winter period, assistant social services director Lorna Brown told the *Oxford Times*:

> If there is a set amount of money, like £1.4 million, what happens when it runs out? If you place someone in a nursing home they could still be there in two years' time. Short-term money doesn't solve long-term issues.
>
> (*Oxford Times*, 30 January 1998)

Surveys at the end of 1997 underlined the contradictions and problems of the NHS. One commissioned by Age Concern, looking at 83 social services departments, concluded that inconsistent eligibility criteria for continuing care were turning it into a "national lottery" (*HSJ*, 20 November 1997). Another, for Help the Aged, warned that the lack of services for older people had reached "crisis point", with many vulnerable people stuck in "a downward spiral of increasing dependency" (*HSJ*, 27 November 1997).

The apparent success of the new government in averting a winter crisis was made more straightforward by the absence of the usual winter cold snap. A combination of one of the warmest winters for years, with the absence of any major flu epidemic, and the planned reduction of many acute hospitals to an emergencies-only service created a false semblance of calm.

Beneath the surface, however, acute hospital beds in many areas were reduced to a level which could not cope with the pressures of a 'normal' cold British winter.

Rationalisation: the drive towards mergers

The period after the 1990 NHS reforms had brought a dramatic reduction in the numbers of health authorities, with the purchasing bodies merging into ever-larger and less locally accessible organisations. The 192 English health authorities established in 1982 had been reduced to 146 by early 1994. The numbers of providers also sharply reduced in the same period: 245 hospitals closed in England and Wales between 1990 and 1994 (Talbot-Smith and Pollock 2006: 6).

Numbers of beds had also declined very sharply. Acute beds, key to delivering reduced waiting times and improved emergency care, fell in number by over 7,000 in just four years from 1990, a 6 per cent reduction; but from 1994 onwards, under Tories and New Labour alike, acute bed numbers were to remain almost constant for a decade as hospitals identified a basic minimum requirement to cope with peaks of demand for medical, surgical and specialist care. However, the Reid/Hewitt crises of 2005 to 2007 forced a fresh, dramatic downsizing of acute hospitals.

In some cases the reduction in inpatient beds was compensated by a rapid expansion of day-only beds for the expanding system of day surgery, which also contributed to substantial reductions in length of stay for surgical treatment. Day case beds expanded in number by over 60 per cent (from a small base) in the four years from 1990, and by a massive 132 per cent, to reach a total of over 7,000, by 1998. However, day beds and day case treatment are not suitable or useful for the growing numbers of (mainly elderly) patients requiring emergency admission for medical rather than surgical treatment: and many older people, especially if they live alone or suffer from other complicating conditions, are among those excluded from day surgery. For them, while it may lessen the overall waiting times and delays, the switch from inpatient to day case surgery is of little or no direct benefit.

Other categories of hospital beds were even more drastically reduced after 1990. By 1998, the NHS had lost 15,662 geriatric beds – equivalent to 34 per cent of the 1990 stock in just eight years. This in turn placed far greater pressure on the remaining frontline acute beds. And the same period saw the closure of 18,638 mental health beds, again 34 per cent of the 1990 provision (all figures from DoH Hospital Activity Statistics website, 2007), but with nowhere near a 34 per cent expansion in alternative community-based services to take their place. In September 1998, Frank Dobson set up an inquiry into NHS bed numbers – headed by Clive Smee, the Department of Health's chief economist. The report was eventually published in February 2000 (see Chapter six).

Restructuring the purchasers

In April 1996, the Conservative government had pushed through another restructuring of the NHS, in which the 70 English Family Health Services Authorities were merged with the District Health Authorities, to form just 100 unified health authorities to oversee hospital, community and family health services. The halving of the number of health authorities ran alongside the reduction in numbers of lay members sitting on each authority, and the loss of any residual notion of local accountability (Rivett 1998: 431).

This followed the reduction of the previous 14 Regional Health Authorities in England to just eight mega-regions in 1994, each one served no longer by an authority with meetings and members, but by a regional office of the NHS management executive (ibid.). Far from reversing this process, the Labour government's 1997 White Paper *The New NHS: Modern, Dependable* suggested that more health authorities – and even more Trusts – should merge in the next few years, offering one way in which the government hoped to achieve its ambitious targets in the reduction of bureaucracy (DoH 1997a).

The NHS has never been subject to any local democracy, and none of its repeated organisational restructuring in its first 50 years had given local residents and users of the service any more influence or control than a customer in a supermarket. The limitations were encapsulated in John Major's "Patient's Charter" (1991), which appeared to set out a series of limited consumer "rights" (Klein 2006: 168–9); but if these were not delivered, the consumer, like any dissatisfied customer, had no more than the right to complain.

There were 450 NHS Trusts at the end of 1997, ranging from small Trusts providing community services, mental health or single specialty services, to major Trusts with £250 million budgets, based on big teaching hospitals or covering the whole spectrum of services in a particular district. Each was equipped with its own board of executive and non-executive directors, its own team of accountants and management hierarchy: splitting the NHS up in this way was a huge and costly exercise.

However, the early impetus towards separation gave way, in the harsh competitive regime of the internal market, to an increasing drive towards *mergers* – even in some areas towards the development of monopolies as larger Trusts devoured their smaller and weaker competitors. The first casualty of this process was the Anglian Harbours Trust, which delivered community and mental health services to residents of Norfolk and Suffolk until both health authorities combined forces simultaneously to withdraw vital contracts. The resulting loss of income triggered the first Trust collapse since the market reforms. Its work was shared out between other Trusts in the two counties –some of its services to the elderly were even handed over to the Allington Trust, based many miles away in Ipswich. The cost of winding up the doomed Trust's affairs, which landed up with the Secretary of State, was estimated to be as high as £4 million (Dawe 1996; Martin 1997).

Another floundering Trust gobbled up by predators was the Horton General Hospital Trust in Banbury. The Horton, a poor relation in a county dominated by the powerful Oxford teaching hospitals, had been dogged by persistent cash deficits, and was eventually taken over by the Oxford Radcliffe Trust. Local people have campaigned ever since to defend the Horton's accident and emergency unit against cutbacks which may be decided by a Trust management based 30 miles away (*Oxford Times*, 6 February 1998). Other major Trust mergers followed, notably in Leeds, and in Derby, where the plan was linked with the proposal to shift acute services out from the city centre Royal Infirmary to a new hospital on the Derby City General site.[14]

By the spring of 1998, *Health Emergency* was able to identify "dozens of hospitals and thousands of beds at risk from a new round of mergers and rationalisation", quoting a report in the *Independent* which warned that up to 80 hospitals were on a government "hit list" for closure, with 32 Trusts set to merge from 1 April (*Health Emergency* 46, 1998).

---

14 To be funded under the Private Finance Initiative, in a scheme eventually signed off at £333 million: see Chapter nine.

Ambulance Trusts also began a continuing series of mergers which have lasted half way into the current decade, although always pulling up short of the trade union aspiration of a single national ambulance service with a common system of training and standards of staffing (Lister 2006b).

A survey of 500 senior NHS managers for the Institute of Health Care Managers showed that almost three-quarters of them thought there were too many Trusts, and 85 per cent thought services must again be reconfigured. But almost 75 per cent thought that most mergers in themselves would save less than £1 million a time in annual revenue costs (*HSJ*, 15 January 1998). There was also a new wave of cash-crisis-driven "collaboration" between Trusts. The "collaboration" between Kingston Hospital Trust and its neighbouring Richmond, Twickenham and Roehampton Trust was the predictable prelude to a rapid rundown and closure of acute services at Queen Mary's Hospital, Roehampton (*Health Emergency* 45, 1997).

White Paper 1997

While various limited changes were made in day-to-day policy, there was great interest in the government's strategic plans for what system should replace the Tories' internal market. During what seemed like a very long delay, many of the previous commitments made by Labour in opposition had been discarded, and for those who had looked for a root and branch dismantling of the market system, the abolition of fundholding, the scrapping of Trusts and an injection of funding to rebuild the NHS, *The new NHS: Modern, Dependable*, was a serious disappointment. As the *Economist* pointed out, ministers had shrunk from the challenge and opted to live with the market rather than abolish it:

> Rather than being scrapped, the market is being modified, in some ways for the better, in others for the worse.
>
> (*Economist*, 15 December 1997)

Klein disagrees, focusing instead on the contradictory government rhetoric of the time, which argued that the internal market "was to go, though the separation of purchasers and providers would remain" (Klein 2006: 193) – but he shows no evidence to back up this view.

There were a few morsels for diehard government supporters to trumpet as good proposals – notably the consolidation of existing government policy demanding that Trust boards should meet and discuss in public, and publish their papers, with no more routine management information to be classified as "commercial in confidence". This did open up some health authorities and Trusts, but soon others found new pretexts for keeping key financial and other data secret.

The White Paper also argued the need for community hospitals and local services, and rehearsed some solid arguments against local decisions to impose rationing on certain treatments and areas of health services. It pointed out correctly that the costs of what were once pioneering medical techniques were steadily falling as they became more common, while the efficiency of the tax-funded NHS compared with other health care systems around the world was itself a factor keeping costs (and taxes) down (DoH 1997a: 9).

But even as it made these valid points, the White Paper failed to address the contemporary reality of the NHS, in which health authorities up and down the country – facing combined deficits projected at upwards of £500 million by the following April – were busily *closing down* many of the surviving community hospitals, *cutting back* local services, and debating which services ought to be rationed to meet Gordon Brown's stringent cash limits (*Health Emergency* 44 (July) and 45 (November), 1997).

The White Paper's biggest ideological and political retreat was on the central issue of the market system. Although ministers had proudly proclaimed the end of the Tories' "internal market", and a new era in which "competition" was to be replaced by cooperation, New Labour left many key elements of the Tory reforms intact.

The root of much of the bureaucratic waste ushered in by the Thatcher–Clarke reforms in 1990–1 had been the "purchaser–provider split", in which cash was allocated to quango "purchasing authorities", which were then charged with buying health care services from opted-out NHS Trusts – the so-called "provider units". Each side of this new divide needed to develop its own separate management structure, administration, accounts and finance departments, and each Trust was obliged to negotiate not only with health authorities but also with a growing proliferation of fundholding GP practices (Klein 2006: 175).

The NHS under New Labour's proposed new system would still be run by a network of unelected, unaccountable quangos – health authorities. These would act as planners and purchasers, while key local decisions would be taken by even less accountable new commissioning groups – Primary Care Groups (PCGs) – consisting of GPs, community nurses and possibly social workers, but with no public access or involvement.

Health authorities – many of which would be merged with neighbouring authorities to form fewer, larger, even less accountable bodies – would be charged with drawing up strategic three-to-five-year Health Improvement Programmes. These would have to take account of the needs of their local population – but also, of course, the amount of money available. Ten areas of deprivation (later increasing to 27) would be singled out for the establishment of Health Action Zones (HAZs), which would aim to link up all of the various public sector and other organisations with a role of play in improving public health (social services, transport, housing etc., in addition to the NHS) (DoH 1997a: 77). Despite ambitious targets for these new hybrid embodiments of the current buzz-phrase of "joined up government", HAZs never really got going in England.[15] Many proved unable even to spend their allocated budgets, and by

---

15 However, they appear to have been more successful in Northern Ireland, where the
    programme has been funded through to 2008 (Investing for Health).

2004 they were being evaluated in the past tense by the Health Development Agency, which admitted:

> Changes in national policy, including the NHS reforms and the emergence of local strategic partnerships, changes in HAZ priorities, and uncertainty about their future reduced the HAZs' ability to influence local policies.
>
> (HDA 2004)

Another organisational innovation introduced in the White Paper was the establishment of a new National Institute for Clinical Excellence (NICE) which would "give a strong lead on clinical and cost-effectiveness", tasked with deciding whether or not new techniques should be rolled out across the NHS (DoH 1997a). Taken alongside plans for a new series of National Service Frameworks, setting out the basic building blocks of services for mental health, elderly and other specific services, and a new Commission for Health Improvement – an embryonic inspectorate of hospitals – it seemed that ministers were biting the bullet and moving back towards national planning and combating the "postcode lottery" that had begun to emerge under the Tory market reforms (Klein 2006: 197).

However, there were weaknesses from the beginning: NICE was given the responsibility to decide whether a drug or treatment should be made available, but had no budget or means to ensure that local cash-limited health authorities were in a position to afford new treatments, or that NHS Trusts had the necessary pump-priming cash to invest in setting up a new service. NICE was also a body widely perceived as a means to limit rather than generalise access to high-cost drugs – but at the same time it was also seen as having been swiftly "captured" by drug companies, whose industry was represented on NICE's government body (Pollock 2004: 81).

Cash limits were also a major obstacle to transforming the National Service Frameworks into anything more than an abstract wish-list and a blueprint for good practice: many of the mental health NSF targets, especially for improved access to acute psychiatric beds and to crisis intervention services have still not been fully met, if at all, in many areas across the country as this book is completed. Instead, mental health services have too often been seen as a "soft target" for spending cuts while more media-friendly acute hospital services remain largely intact. And the uneven quality of inspectors and the varying circumstances of Trusts have severely limited the effectiveness of the CHI monitoring and inspection process, which has now been repeatedly reorganised and merged into today's Healthcare Commission.

Overall, it is clear that there is a contradiction. On the one hand, national standards, national targets and national inspection are established, measuring the local effectiveness of one Trust against another; and on the other, a market system is developed in which NHS Trusts, "third sector" organisations and the private sector are encouraged to operate with minimal regulation. The government, operating the New Public Management principle of "steering, not rowing", retains few powers to intervene directly.

Bureaucracy

While they left a fragmented and unequal NHS, in which life-saving drugs authorised by NICE are still available for patients in one area but not for similar patients in another, the New Labour proposals did at least aim to reduce the number of negotiations and transactions, and promised to cut the numbers of invoices and the volume of administrative work, partly by cutting the number of purchasers ("commissioning bodies") from 3,600 to around 500 through the end of GP fundholding. But they did not eliminate any of the existing tiers of NHS management, and the promise of savings totalling £1 billion from reduced bureaucracy appeared massively over-optimistic.

The White Paper argued that the number of transactions would also be reduced by replacing the annual round of contract negotiations, which had bogged down Trusts and HAs since the 1991 Tory reforms, with longer-term agreements lasting a minimum of three, but possibly five or even ten years. This was a worthy objective, but unfortunately it depended on persuading the Chancellor (then Gordon Brown) and his Treasury team to fix NHS cash allocations for similar periods. If this did not happen, cash-strapped Health Authorities would still be obliged to reassess each year how much, if any, of their long-term plan they could afford to carry out – and therefore what economy measures had to be imposed on the Trusts providing frontline care (*Health Emergency* 46, 1998).

After years in which Labour's shadow health secretaries had denounced – and promised to scrap – the "two-tier" inequality and corresponding bureaucracy involved in the Tory system of GP fundholding, the White Paper was suddenly at pains to explain that its proposals aimed to adapt, rather than overturn the scheme. The government wanted:

> to keep what has worked about fundholding, but discard what has not... The argument between fundholding and non-fundholding is yesterday's debate. The time has come to move on...
>
> (DoH 1997a: 33)

The difference was that *all* GPs, along with community nursing staff, would be able to participate in the new Primary Care Groups, and to have a voice on how local budgets were spent for each "natural community" of around 100,000 people. In this way, Labour adopted without question the Tory vision of a "primary care-led NHS", in which GPs had increasingly (though in most cases unwittingly) been enlisted as allies in the rationalisation and run-down of hospital services.

The only proposal in the White Paper to override the purchaser–provider split and establish a genuinely integrated local body was the suggestion that new "Primary Care Trusts" might be established, with a responsibility both to purchase and provide primary and community care services. It was to be another eight years before ministers began to press for these services to be hived off to the private sector or "arms-length" bodies, leaving the PCTs as purely commissioning bodies (see later chapters).

Cash limits

The catch was that as a result of the same reforms, primary care budgets were to be fully cash limited for the first time since the NHS was founded, almost 50 years previously. For all the fine words about partnership and quality services, the underlying agenda driving forward the White Paper reforms was the imposition of cash limits to the area of the NHS which had escaped them up to now – primary care as a whole, and not just the GP fundholders.

York University's Professor Alan Maynard underlined the significance of this change:

> Many GPs seem to see the white paper as a triumph of primary care over the rest of the NHS and the creation of a new nirvana for them. Sorry comrades – this is the beginning of the management of primary care within a cash-limited budget.
>
> (Maynard 1998; *Doctor*, 12 March 1998)

In reality many GPs did not want to add yet another set of meetings and more managerial responsibilities to their already pressurised working days. They abstained from involvement in PCGs, while others decided to employ managers or delegated others to participate on their behalf. Alan Maynard predicted the inevitable line of march:

> The primary care groups will eventually be trusts with a chief executive, a finance officer and a full board. A clear majority of these managers will not be GPs. …They will seek to manage drug expenditure, hospital referrals (and GPs' breathing) to stay within budget. They will exploit skill-mix opportunities, replacing doctors with nurses.
>
> (Maynard 1998)

Cooperation

There was a great deal of ministerial rhetoric about establishing a statutory duty of the new "leaner" HAs to cooperate with local authorities: but the key issue of resources was avoided. This meant the net result would be little more than a pooling of deficits, as HAs and social service departments found themselves simultaneously starved of cash. Nor did the new cooperation involve any extension of democracy: local authority chief executives, rather than elected councillors, were to be the ones given the right to participate in health authority meetings.

In this context of increasing quangoisation, the regional framework established by Virginia Bottomley was also to be retained. She had first merged, then scaled down and then abolished the old Regional Health Authorities – with their meetings held in public session, their published list of lay appointees, published papers and published minutes. Instead, she appointed trusted lay "Regional Chairs" to front up a system of "Regional Offices" of the NHS Executive, where they preside over rump teams of anonymous civil servants, holding no meetings, and publishing as little information as they can get away with (Rivett 1998).

The fundamental split of the market system remained, as did Trusts (which Labour had for years promised to scrap and return frontline services to health authority control), although Trusts faced a new wave of mergers. And, despite the claim that the new system would be even more "local" in its approach, the White Paper made clear that any assessment of the special needs and local pressures on hospitals would take a back seat to a new, national system of "reference costs", under which hospitals would have to reduce their running costs to match the lowest figures achieved anywhere. Since around 70 per cent of most Trust spending was on pay, this also implied a new round of job losses and attacks on pay and conditions.

The White Paper was also decorated with a few superficial distractions: one was the promise of a new 24-hour telephone 'hotline' service, NHS Direct, which was to be staffed by nurses, offering advice to patients who could not get to see their GP. This scheme has never proved cheap or effective, and has subsequently faced cash crises and cutbacks.

PFI – Profits From Illness?

So the essentials of the Tory market system seemed set to remain intact into the millennium. But at the same time another Tory policy, the Private Finance Initiative (PFI), which had fallen flat on its face in the final four years of John Major's government and brought hospital building schemes to a grinding halt from the time of its introduction in 1993, was dusted off and repackaged by the New Labour government. Under PFI, large-scale building projects, which would previously have been publicly funded by the Treasury, were to be put out to tender, inviting consortia of private banks, building firms, developers and service providers to put up the investment, build the new hospital or facility, and lease the finished building back to the NHS – generally with additional non-clinical support services (maintenance, porters, cleaning, catering, laundry, etc.).

Lease agreements for PFI hospitals are long-term and binding commitments, normally at least 25 years. The NHS Trust involved, which would normally pay capital charges on its NHS assets, instead pays a "unitary charge" to the PFI consortium, which would cover construction costs, rent, support services, interest payments on the loans involved, and a further margin to cover the "risks" transferred to the private sector.

The big difference from capital charges is that not only are the costs much higher, but PFI "unitary payments", rather than circulating back within the NHS, flow into the coffers of the private companies, from where they are issued as dividends to shareholders.

The appeal of PFI both to the Tories and to the Labour government has always been that it enabled new hospitals and facilities to be built "off balance sheet", without the investment appearing as a lump sum addition to the Public Sector Borrowing Requirement. The government could therefore appear to be funding the "biggest ever programme of hospital building in the NHS", while in practice injecting less public capital than ever. In fact, only six major NHS-funded schemes, totalling less than £300 million, were given the go-ahead between 1997 and 2001 (Lister 2001).

The new line on PFI represented a major change in established Labour policy. As recently as 1995 Margaret Beckett, Shadow Health Secretary, told the *Health Service Journal*:

> As far as I am concerned PFI is totally unacceptable. It is the thin end of the wedge of privatisation.
>
> (*HSJ*, 1 June 1995)

But in the summer of 1996, Shadow Treasury Minister Mike O'Brien announced the key change of policy:

> This idea must not be allowed to fail. Labour has a clear programme to rescue PFI.
>
> (*HSJ*, 22 August 1996)

This flew in the face of growing concern even among NHS managers over the implications of PFI: a 1996 Gallup poll among Trust bosses showed that 70 per cent of chief executives thought PFI was not cost effective in the long run, and 90 per cent believed that the private sector would take no risks and only get involved if profits were guaranteed (UNISON 1996).

By the spring of 1998, PFI was:

> A key part of the Government's 10 year modernisation programme for the health service.
>
> (DoH Press Release, 7 April 1998)

The scheme was indeed one of the very few priorities receiving instant attention after the May 1997 election. With 43 PFI projects waiting Department of Health approval, Health Secretary Alan Milburn took on the task of pushing some of these to completion, and the *only* specific NHS commitment in the Queen's Speech in 1997 was for a short bill which would again shift the goalposts in favour of private firms in PFI deals.

The new law compels a future Secretary of State to pick up any outstanding bills for Trusts which default on PFI contract payments. It stood in stark contrast to Gordon Brown's insistence on limiting government spending.

Despite its new popularity with Tony Blair and his ministers, and especially with the Treasury team, PFI still incurred the vociferous opposition of the BMA, the Royal College of Nursing, almost all trade unions, local campaigners in affected towns and cities, and a growing body of academics. *Guardian* financial columnist Larry Elliott summed up a widespread view, denouncing PFI as "a scam":

> Of all the scams pulled by the Conservatives in 18 years of power – and there were plenty – the Private Finance Initiative was perhaps the most blatant. ...If ever a piece of ideological baggage cried out to be dumped on day one of a Labour government it was PFI.
>
> (*Guardian*, 26 October 1998)

Nonetheless PFI was now proclaimed by Labour's team as the basis of "the biggest hospital building programme in the history of the NHS". It has become such a central feature of the NHS in the twenty-first century that it is explored in more detail in Chapter nine.

Elderly hived off

Another area where the Labour government was more than happy to roll out the red carpet for the private sector was in continuing care of the elderly. The muted Labour criticism of the Tory "community care" reforms was followed after May 1997 by a substantial delay in establishing the promised Royal Commission.

Frank Dobson hit the headlines by announcing that he was determined to "bang heads together" and force health authorities and social services to speed the discharge of growing numbers of elderly patients in acute beds, who had been variously termed "bed-blockers", "social care waiters" or Patients Awaiting Appropriate Facilities Elsewhere (PAAFEs!) (*Health Emergency* 45, 1997).

But there was mounting evidence that the problem needed far more than head-banging to solve it. The system was severely deficient, failing to deliver adequate numbers of beds providing suitable or affordable care in many areas of the country. A Department of Health survey suggested that as many as 7,000 elderly patients were unnecessarily in hospital for lack of suitable arrangements to support them at home or in residential or nursing homes. Four-fifths of social services departments had made cuts in the 1997–8 financial year.

One spin-off from these cuts was that local authorities had been unable to raise the "benchmark" figure which limits the amount they will pay for nursing or residential home placements – and this in turn piled pressure on to the private-sector home owners. Figures published in 1997 showed that a typical 50-bed nursing home could offer a financial return as low as 50p per bed per day – well below £10,000 a year – for its proprietor. The problem was compounded by growing numbers of empty beds as cash-limited councils struggled to meet the rising costs: occupancy levels had fallen from well over 90 per cent to 84 per cent in 1997 (Laing and Buisson 1997).

Private-sector analysts warned that if the margins were squeezed further, proprietors would begin to vote with their feet and close down unprofitable homes. Either more money had to be forthcoming from central government to raise local authority fee levels, or there would have to be a reduction in the capacity of the sector. There was certainly no scope for further savings in the running costs of nursing homes, many of which were already heavily dependent on unskilled, low-paid staff. Care home owners, some of the most notorious low-payers, had repeatedly warned Labour ministers against setting a minimum wage without increasing funds for community care, arguing that it would lead to job losses and the closure of nursing homes.

The drop in standards of care had even led to a warning from the nurses' professional standards watchdog, the United Kingdom Central Council, which published a major report *The Continuing Care of Older People* in December

1997. It pointed out that while 21,000 private and voluntary sector homes employed a total of more than 120,000 qualified nursing staff, "very little is known about this workforce". Worse, despite the growing level of dependency of clients in these nursing homes:

> There are currently no requirements for staff in nursing homes to have any specific qualifications in caring for older people.

The chances of obtaining such a qualification were obviously declining, since the NHS, which is (still in 2007) the only body training nurses, was steadily reducing its numbers of specialist geriatric beds and its continuing care services for the elderly. But newly qualified nurses could easily find themselves the *only* qualified member of staff if they took a post in a nursing home – where poor rates of pay and conditions helped to maintain staff turnover levels averaging as high as 20 per cent. The UKCC report warned:

> The large proportion of unqualified support workers in continuing care settings raises considerable issues in terms of training, supervision and accountability. …The full impact of the market in continuing care has yet to be seen. Conflicts of interest may increase …There have already been cases where a desire to cut down on overheads has led to the inadequate provision of food or heating for residents.
>
> (United Kingdom Central Council 1997: 41)

But there were also wider problems facing professionals. Guidance from Health Secretary Stephen Dorrell and the Department of Health had tried to dissuade health authorities from inspecting the standards of care at nursing homes more than twice a year (one announced visit, one "unannounced") – making it difficult to raise or enforce standards of care. In any case health authorities and social service departments, eager to place patients in nursing homes, were reluctant to take steps which might force the closure of potential places.

The UKCC also warned of the downward pressure on professional standards among staff in community health teams:

> Practitioners who have budgetary responsibilities under care management may also be under pressure to assess clients in relation to the resources available rather than the client's health and social needs in order to meet their financial targets.
>
> (United Kingdom Central Council 1997: 41)

The downward pressure on fees and quality of care was most acutely felt in those homes which catered for state-funded clients. For those targeting more wealthy "self-funders", and aiming to deliver more of a prestige service, there were fewer restrictions on charges. Bills of £1,500 a month were not unusual, and health insurer PPP complained that many homes were charging far more than this, and raising their fees faster than inflation. In the run-up to the 1997 election, Dorrell had floated various schemes to persuade elderly people and those of working age to take out insurance policies to cover private nursing home fees. But the costs were heavy – well beyond the means of the average pensioner.

For a 60-year-old woman to buy a policy from BUPA paying out just £1,000 a month, she would need to fork out £66 a month in premiums. But even then she would have been at least £500 a month short of the likely fees if she had needed nursing home care. A 35-year-old woman would have had to pay £30 per month for the same benefit – equivalent to at least £9,000 in premiums before retirement age. But only one in five elderly people require continuing care, making any type of insurance scheme a poor gamble (Courtney and Walker 1996).

While the smaller home owners suffered the squeeze, the larger chains were witnessing an expansion. The successful £273 million BUPA bid for the nursing home market leader Care First established the private medical giant as the predominant force in this area of continuing care, with 16,000 beds – although this was still only three per cent of the total market (*Guardian*, 3 December 1997). As the Royal Commission began its work, long-term care of the elderly – entering its fifth year outside the NHS – was exhibiting many of the least attractive features of a privatised service run for profit. Its inadequate and poorly distributed provision offered two tiers of care according to personal ability to pay: a cheap and cheerless bog-standard service with minimal staffing levels for those funded by the state, and a soaraway sky-high deluxe service for those rich enough to ignore the means-test and the queues for social care.

Mental health: no end to the nightmare

Another area of developing crisis for New Labour in 1997 was mental health services, where none of the problems identified by Stephen Dorrell early in 1996 has been resolved. Indeed, the striking aspect of Health Secretary Frank Dobson's pronouncements on community care early in 1998 was how similar they were to previous statements by his Tory predecessor and by other commentators back into the 1980s.

Like them, Dobson was of course keen to dissociate himself from the scandals arising from under-funded, poorly planned and under-staffed community-based services masquerading as "community care". Like them, he raised once again the question of slowing or pausing the process of closing beds in the psychiatric hospitals. Like Dorrell, Dobson touched upon the need for more places offering 24-hour nursed accommodation to people suffering severe and enduring mental illness. But unlike Dorrell, Dobson put no costings on this provision, choosing simply to evade the nitty gritty question of the funding required to develop a service that could really work.

More scandals – some publicised, many going unnoticed – took place after Labour inherited the Tory run-down of mental health care. Bed occupancy levels in acute wards climbed even higher: one psychiatric ward in Guy's Hospital recorded a staggering 230% occupancy rate in the autumn of 1997, with Trust bosses admitting that this was excessive (Guy's and Lewisham MH Trust 1997). But occupancy levels of 150% and above were far from rare in acute wards in inner-city mental health trusts.

Department of Health statistics in 1997 showed 56 Trusts recording acute mental health beds as 100% or thereabouts (upwards of 97%) occupied during 1996–7 (DoH statistics 1997). Services and staff were struggling to cope. Chronic sufferers were being cared for in the wrong wards – or in many cases not at all.

It was not enough for the government to make general pronouncements and to have set up yet another "review" – the one established on mental health services involved so many people from organisations with conflicting policies and views it was hard to see how any coherent line could emerge (Lister 1997b, 1999).

Without an injection of fresh money, the decline of mental health services was certain to accelerate. And in the process, a side-effect was that ever larger sums were being spent each year by hard-pressed health authorities and Trusts purchasing poor-quality and poorly monitored care from the private sector – often miles away from the patient's home and the support services that would be needed to arrange a proper discharge (Lister 1999).

All change for London's NHS?

The report of the independent inquiry set up by Health Secretary Frank Dobson was published in February 1998 (DoH 1998b).

The Turnberg report – the main lines of which were accepted by Labour ministers – represented an apparent shift of emphasis. It refuted the view that London has too many hospitals and too many beds and drew attention to the massive run-down of hospital services in the capital in the 1990s – with the loss of over 9,000 beds, including 2,700 acute beds (handling waiting list and emergency cases), almost 4,000 mental health beds, and 1,300 beds for elderly people (DoH 1998b: 17).

It also argued that up to 2,800 of London's remaining 17,400 acute hospital beds were being used by people who did not live in the capital. As a result of this it concludes that:

> London probably has fewer beds available to its population than the average and that further bed closures should not be planned.
>
> (DoH 1998b: 19)

To make matters worse there was a growing shortage of nursing staff, with many Trusts facing vacancy rates of 20 per cent (DoH 1998b: 15).

Turnberg made an explicit call for specialist health services to continue at Bart's Hospital, which Virginia Bottomley had set out to kill off five years earlier. There was also a suggestion that some additional services should be based at the threatened Guy's Hospital, where a run-down had already left ten floors of the tower block and an area equivalent to two general hospitals vacant. However, the closure of Guy's busy accident and emergency unit was to press ahead.

The inquiry also suggested new investment in the Whittington Hospital (Islington), Newham General Hospital, and in London's far east it overturned the long-standing plans of the health authority and urged the building of a single site hospital in the more deprived Romford, rather than endorse controversial plans for it to be located in the prosperous Harold Wood, close to the M25.

But even while the report was being drafted, desperate NHS Trusts in London and elsewhere had been attempting to cut spending by closing down even more beds: it was clear that without an injection of more new money, the change of rhetoric in the government's response to the Turnberg Report was unlikely to herald any lasting reprieve for hospitals or services. There was little extra cash on offer. In the face of the report's evidence of continued severe neglect of primary care services in the capital, a modest £140 million was allocated over four years for the improvement of primary care and mental health services.

Almost all the rest of the "£1 billion investment programme" announced by Frank Dobson in his response to the report consisted of a series of privately financed hospital building schemes which would leave the NHS in hock to banks and consortia for decades to come.

Even the Tory-commissioned Tomlinson Report of 1992 had urged an increase in the provision of mental health beds, and the Turnberg Report also singled out mental health as the area "widely regarded as being the most under strain". It specifically called for extra beds, suggesting that once the necessary extra services were opened up in the community, notably 24-hour nursed accommodation for chronic sufferers, "the ultimate requirement for acute beds may be reduced in the longer term."

The inquiry also lifted the lid on the underlying financial instability of London's Trusts in the internal market, and the completely ineffective mechanisms put in place by the Tories to direct health planning. It reported that a staggering £600 million of "transitional support funds" had been pumped in to prop up London's health services over the previous three years – but did not point out that this had failed to prevent health authorities and Trusts facing massive and growing cash deficits.

And it totted up a massive £403 million sunk into a proliferation of primary care improvement projects since 1993 – showing that these had done little to bring London's services up to the national average. There were fewer GPs in London in 1998 than in 1990, and less than half of the 1,900 GP premises in London were judged to be above minimum standards in 1977. One factor in this was the lack of any strategic planning body for health services in the capital. The half-baked "London Implementation Group", a secretive quango set up by Virginia Bottomley in 1993, had proved an ignominious failure, and was wound up after only 18 months.

The new report urged the need for effective planning across London and the creation of a "single London Regional Office". Although this body, effectively a team of civil servants with an appointed lay "Chairman", would fall far short of the accountable London Regional Health Authority which health unions and campaigners have demanded, it would represent a qualitative step forward from the historic division of London into two or four regions. The new government did indeed bring a new approach to London's health care: but with the tide of closures, cuts and rationing of services gathering pace as health chiefs wrestled with Tory cash limits, the change looked more dramatic on paper than on the wards.

Charging in?

The change of government did not silence the undercurrent of debate on the future funding of the NHS. The autumn of 1997 saw rampant speculation that ministers were really "thinking the unthinkable" and contemplating the introduction of charges for visiting or calling out a GP. In the run-up to the BMA conference in October, dubious surveys were produced, one claiming that 27 per cent of the sample would be prepared to pay a fee of £9 to visit a GP, while 48 per cent would allegedly fork out £13 for a home visit from their doctor at night. The right-wing media proudly referred to the popularity of a walk-in private GP surgery at London's Victoria Station charging a staggering £32 for a consultation, and claimed that more were about to open (*Guardian*, 3 October 1997).

BMA leaders took a chance, arguing devil's advocate style, that the NHS funding gap was so wide that if charges were to be imposed for GP services or for inpatient stays in hospital, they would have to be hefty (*HSJ*, 9 October 1997). All of the old arguments were again rehearsed: it was plain that it would be impossible to impose charges for primary care without also imposing them for attendance at A&E units or for hospital treatment. One foot on this path could rapidly slide down the slippery path to a service in which heavy charges for care would compel increasing numbers to take out private medical insurance.

In the event BMA delegates showed good sense and overwhelmingly threw out the resolution which suggested a policy of charging. But in a climate in which the unthinkable was becoming the new orthodoxy, variants of the same idea remained in circulation: one idea was that women should be charged for the contraceptive pill –instead of it being provided free for those who wanted it. The potential saving was a miserable £50 million on a drugs bill of £4 billion – to be set against an inevitable increase in NHS spending on the increased numbers of unwanted pregnancies. A 1995 study showed that the NHS saved £1,100 for every £100 it spent on contraceptive services (*Guardian*, 1 January 1998).

A rash of rationing

As they weighed their options for balancing the books, a growing number of health authorities were openly discussing the exclusion of a growing number of elective treatments from the NHS. These debates took place despite the government's firm rejection of local rationing in the 1997 White Paper.

One of the most far-reaching lists of services which health chiefs felt should be obtainable by local people only in the most exceptional circumstances was adopted in January by Merton, Sutton and Wandsworth Health Authority as it wrestled with a £23 million deficit. It imposed a near-blanket ban on:

- Vasectomies
- Sinus surgery

- Varicose vein surgery
- Some hernias
- Some cataracts
- Cruciate ligament reconstruction
- Some hip and knee replacements
- Plastic surgery for post burn or scalding
- Hysterectomy for fibroids
- Sterilisation.

In their Service Framework for 1998–9, the health authority described all of the above as "low priority" and stated bluntly that they would only be funded in "exceptional circumstances" (Merton Sutton and Wandsworth HA 1998).

The imposition of this blanket ban on key services meant that the concept of comprehensive health care, free at the point of need, had been wiped out in South West London. The clear implication was that services no longer provided by the NHS would have to be bought from the private sector by those patients who could afford them: others would have to do without – and suffer the consequences.

Other health authorities, too, notably in North and South Essex and West Hertfordshire, were also resorting to widespread rationing of care, singling out comparatively rare and expensive treatments, such as cochlear implants, and those notoriously unpopular with the public (such as tattoo removal), while also targeting varicose veins (West Hertfordshire HA 1997; North Essex HA 1997; South Essex HA 1997).

Acute crisis

The driving force compelling top NHS managers, consultants and others to contemplate policies that would do such damage the NHS as a comprehensive service available on the basis of clinical need rather than ability to pay was the continued financial crisis.

The situation was summed up in early December 1997 by the NHS finance director Colin Reeves. He told the conference of the Healthcare Financial Management Association that the NHS faced a £460 million deficit in its income and expenditure; £190 million of this had to be cleared by April 1998, with the remaining £250 million cut back by April 1999. The chair of the HFMA, Jaki Meekings responded by pointing out that a deficit on this scale meant that "excess" activity was being purchased. "We are talking about taking half a billion pounds of spending power out of the system", she said. "I think that is a very real problem, because if you have to try to explain to the public that you are making cuts in services to improve the balance sheet it is a very difficult message to get across" (*HSJ*, 11 December 1997).

More health bosses were struggling to get across precisely this unpalatable message, with cuts bigger than ever as the centre of their agenda. Many were contemplating a hospital service effectively reduced to little more than emergencies only, with waiting lists continuing their upward path and Patient's Charter targets – which fixed an 18-month maximum wait – increasingly unachievable. Some had begun to cut back on precisely the areas of care which the White Paper had singled out for praise. The threatened closure of "intermediate" and community hospital beds would simply increase the "blockage" of acute beds in the general hospitals.

New Labour had done little more than tinker with the market and inject a minimal additional amount of funding into a system that was seriously under-funded. But this regime of crisis continued largely unchanged until 2000. That was the year in which the announcement of the Blair–Brown plan to boost NHS spending towards European Union average levels, was coupled with the NHS Plan, which set out to introduce more controversial "reforms" that would fragment the NHS, strengthen the elements of the competitive "market", and remodel the NHS along lines of a European-style social health insurance fund, sweeping away many of the features of Bevan's NHS.

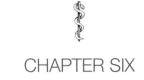

CHAPTER SIX

The NHS Plan – Mr Milburn heads back to market 2000–2005

OF ALL THE HEALTH CARE SYSTEMS in developed countries, not only in Western Europe but throughout the world, the British system has perhaps been the most repeatedly and thoroughly subjected to market-driven and market-style reforms over the last 25 years (Lister 2005a). The process has accelerated in England since 2000 with a rapid succession of reorganisations, structural reforms, and increasing levels of privatisation and use of private sector providers.[16]

The New Labour reforms revolve, perhaps more than those of the Tories, around the New Public Management principle of "steering, not rowing" – to such an extent that the National Health Service could be reduced to little more than a "brand name", a centralised fund that commissions and pays for patient care. The model could be a tax-funded version of the "sickness funds" of European social-insurance-based systems. This would leave the NHS hospitals reduced to providing care for emergencies and the chronic sick, while competing on ever less favourable terms with private sector companies for a share of the budget for elective services, and for the staff they need to sustain basic health care (Pollock 2004). By 2002, as the pace of change began to increase further, a new policy statement from the Secretary of State, *Delivering the NHS Plan*, argued Alan Milburn's view that "the 1948 model is simply inadequate for today's needs":

> We believe it is time to move beyond the 1940s monolithic, top-down centralised NHS towards a devolved health service, offering wider choice and greater diversity bound together by common standards, tough inspection and NHS values.
>
> (DoH 2002a: 3)

By 2004 Tony Blair's former advisor on NHS policy, Simon Stevens, was setting out a full-scale scenario for a mixed economy in health:

> Government is now stimulating a more mixed economy on the supply side, to expand capacity, enhance contestability, and offer choice. Free standing surgical

---

16 Wales and Scotland have been able to take advantage of devolved powers to steer in a substantially different direction, looking towards the reintegration of purchasing and providing care in Scotland, and rejecting increased hospital autonomy in Wales.

centres run by international private operators under contract to the NHS are a first step. Private diagnostics and primary care 'out of hours' services are next.

(Stevens 2004: 41–2)

After three years of minimal change, constrained by Conservative-established cash limits, it was the summer of 2000 before New Labour's contradictory policies for the NHS began to emerge in full view, with the publication of a ten-year NHS Plan – which centred on the promotion of a market in health care, sponsored and underwritten by the taxpayer. And if the notion of a "plan" being used to establish a "market" was not enough of a contradiction, there was the added complication earlier in 2000 of adopting a plan for more hospital beds, while implementing changes to the system that would strip away the financial framework that could support them.

The shortage of beds was also eventually acknowledged in 2000. Frank Dobson had set up an inquiry 18 months earlier into NHS bed numbers – headed by Clive Smee, the Department of Health's chief economist during many years of the rapid bed closure programme. The evidence of long queues for treatment and long delays in A&E departments should have been quick and easy to gather, but the inquiry conducted its investigations at inordinate length and in secret, with no attempt to engage with campaigners, the wider public or health unions. The report was eventually published in February 2000 (DoH 2000a).

It was immediately very obvious that as a consequence of its narrow view and cloistered production the Beds Inquiry was seriously out of touch with the situation taking shape in the NHS. At a point where new hospital projects funded through the Private Finance Initiative were reducing bed numbers by an average of over 25 per cent, and New Labour ministers were explicitly arguing that PFI was "the only show in town", the report made no reference to PFI or its consequences. Instead, it offered a variety of alternative scenarios ranging from calls for an extra 35,000 acute beds over 20 years to a reduction of 12,000 beds and a massive expansion of GP and primary care services: none of the proposals was costed. The inescapable conclusion was that the closures had gone too far: the NHS had too few beds, and needed more. The short term recommendation was for an expansion of acute bed provision, with a target of an extra 2,000 by 2004, along with 2,000 more ill-defined "intermediate" beds (DoH 2000a).

The Beds Inquiry also began the systematic use of what have become stock phrases to describe alternative scenarios for the development of health care and social services. The most long-lived – and cynically misused – of these has been the call for "health care closer to home". This approach was eagerly seized upon by ministers: the Beds Inquiry report was published a few months before the NHS Plan, and just weeks after Alan Milburn as Health Secretary had made a keynote speech at the King's Fund which portrayed a future NHS involving much more emphasis on primary care, and intermediate care in cottage hospitals. Similar phrases and approach were also echoed in the subsequent 2002 report on NHS funding and resources by former NatWest bank boss (and Northern Rock advisor) Sir Derek Wanless.

Mr Smee had given ministers the kind of ambiguous and open report they wanted. Statistics for NHS bed provision show that the overall numbers of acute beds did increase by slightly over 2,000 in the following four years, a rise of around two per cent, as the additional money allocated from 2001 began to flow into the NHS, enabling Mr Milburn and his successors to hit their target.

But the year 2003–4 proved to be the high water mark of bed provision, equalling the level established back in 1993–4: since then economic pressures on NHS Trusts have helped squeeze numbers back down again – by more than 5,700 over two years, to reduce the total to a new historic low of 104,000 in March 2007. This is around three per cent *lower* than when Mr Smee submitted his report.

NHS Plan 2000

The NHS Plan unveiled by Alan Milburn in the summer of 2000 created a framework within which very large increases in funding would be used to reshape and reorganise the NHS, giving a further central role to market mechanisms. And at the centre of the plan for a dramatic expansion of the NHS was Gordon Brown's decision, following Tony Blair's public commitment (in a 16 January TV interview with David Frost) to implement a qualitative and sustained increase in UK health spending. Brown's budget announced plans to allocate an extra £2 billion above inflation to NHS budgets each year for the next four years: this was an increase of 6.1% per year. In 2002, after the Spending Review, Brown went further and upped the rate of increase to 7.5% until March 2008 (DoH 2002b). This meant that the total share of national wealth on health (NHS plus private) was projected to rise from 6.9% in 1999–2000 to 9.4% by 2008, and bring the UK closer to EU and OECD averages. After three years of brutal austerity, the NHS budget was set to rise, from £35 billion in 1997 when Blair was elected, to £92 billion ten years later (Klein 2006).

Milburn's Plan was the first attempt to set out how this extra money was to be spent. It was almost immediately followed up with more radical and forthright documents that began to force the pace (DoH 2001, 2002b). New Labour had kept its foot off the throttle until it had turned the bend, and was now to crank up the pace towards its favoured market-style solution.

The NHS Plan, following on from the Beds Inquiry, declared the aim of expanding capacity, with a commitment to:

- 7,000 more beds in "hospitals and intermediate care"
- 7,500 more consultants
- 20,000 more nurses
- 6,500 more therapists
- and 2,000 more GPs.

The extra staff and beds were intended as the means to deliver a series of pledges for improved services, set out in the NHS Plan:

- Maximum wait of 48 hours to see GP by 2004

- Maximum wait of 3 months for outpatient appointment by 2005
- Maximum wait of 6 months for hospital admission by 2005.

It will have come as some surprise to some of the government's critics in 2000 to discover that most of these targets had either been achieved five years later, or were on course to be achieved. A major study in *Public Finance* magazine incorporated a King's Fund audit which showed that in the five-year period, 68 of the promised 100 new hospitals had either been completed or commenced building (64 of them financed through PFI); 800 new critical care beds and 2,197 additional acute beds had also been opened by 2004 – although we now know that this was the point from which bed numbers would fall sharply away. According to *Public Finance* 4,455 "intermediate" beds had apparently also opened (Whitfield 2005) – although exactly where they could be found in the NHS statistics has never been explained. The closure of NHS elderly care beds had gone so fast that the combined total of "general and acute" beds grew by just over 1,000 – less than one per cent by 2005 – before falling away even more (DoH Hospital Activity Statistics from website, 2007).

Medical school places had expanded by 52 per cent to over 6,000 by 2003–4, and the NHS had hit or exceeded all its targets to recruit consultants, nurses and therapists, although the success of GP recruitment hinged on "headcount" rather than whole-time equivalents.

The additional capacity had also begun to deliver some of the performance targets, although some of these proved to be a little less useful than they at first appeared. On the plus side, waiting times for outpatients were on course to reduce to 13 weeks, and inpatient waiting lists to be no more than six months by the end of 2005 (Whitfield 2005). However, the story is not quite the same on primary care, where, as one survey concluded "Expectations potentially conflict, such that there is a tension between highly accessible care and continuity" (Bower et al. 2003). The 48-hour maximum wait to see a GP proved to be one of those targets that may diminish rather than enhance the quality of the service, since most GP surgeries were able to meet the target only by switching patients to see any available GP rather than their chosen and regular GP, and by restricting the ability of patients with long-term conditions to make bookings well in advance (Royal College of General Practitioners 2004; Bevan and Hood 2006).

The proposed staff numbers were subsequently increased further in *Delivering the NHS Plan* (DoH 2002a), which promised an extra 15,000 "GPs and consultants", 30,000 more "therapists and scientists" and 35,000 more "nurses, midwives and health visitors" by 2008. Once again most of these promises have been fulfilled. The most recent figures available at time of writing (December 2007) flow from the 2006 workforce census, but indicate that ministers had even then overshot the target dramatically on nursing staff (up by over 62,000 – 19% – on 2000 figures, although in many areas these numbers are now static or beginning to decline as spending constraints take effect), and fairly close to the 2008 target on therapists and scientists (up by almost 29,000 – 27%). There had also been a strong growth in numbers of consultants, up by over 8,000 (35%)

since 2000, but not so strong among GPs with 5,000 extra amounting to just 17%.

However, ministers were less eager to trumpet the runaway winner in the rising numbers stakes: managers and senior managers had gone up in number by 11,500 since 2000. This was a staggering 46 per cent increase in this controversial section of the NHS workforce in a period in which ministers had promised to cut bureaucracy and centre on patient care (DoH Information Centre 2007).

No wiser, no cleaner...

Some promises made in 2000 remained unfulfilled at the end of 2007: the promise of clean hospitals, for example. This grew from an obvious point that many health workers, patients and members of the public had been making for around 15 years:

> Patients perceive a major deterioration in the cleanliness of hospitals since the introduction of Compulsory Competitive Tendering and the internal market. Patients expect wards to be clean, furnishings to be tidy. The new resources will allow for a renewed emphasis on clean hospitals.
>
> (DoH 2000b: 46)

But while many people would draw from this the conclusion that New Labour had learned the lesson, and would therefore bring cleaning services back "in-house" and scrap the perverse incentives of the "internal market", the NHS Plan offered no such commitment. Instead it suggested that

> ward sisters and charge nurses will have the authority to ensure that the wards they lead are properly cleaned. Hospital domestics will be fully part of the ward team – and respected for the important work they do.

Yet without bringing the services back in to the NHS neither of these objectives could properly be achieved: private contractors' staff were managed by and accountable to the company paying their wages, not the NHS; and the poor terms and conditions, and inadequate staffing levels had led to a rapid turnover of domestic staff that made any serious team-building impossible. Without a fundamental rethink of the whole process that had undermined hospital cleaning standards – with the downward pressure on staffing levels and resources that had flowed not just from private contracts but from the tendering process where it resulted in cheaper in-house contracts – no real change could be achieved.

Four years later the Department of Health itself explicitly recognised the link between competitive tendering and the falling quality of what remain labour-intensive services. Its document *Revised Guidance on Contracting for Cleaning* noted:

> Following the introduction of compulsory competitive tendering, budgets for non-clinical services such as cleaning came under increasing pressure, and too often the final decision on the selection of the cleaning service provider was made on the basis of cost with insufficient weight being placed on quality outcomes.
>
> Since NHS service providers were in competition with private contractors, they

too were compelled to keep their bids low in order to compete. The net effect of this was that budgets and therefore standards were vulnerable to being driven down over an extended period until, in some cases, they reached unacceptable levels.

Although improvements have been seen in recent years following the introduction of the Clean Hospitals Programme and the investment of an additional £68 million in cleaning, there remains concern that price is still the main determinant in contractor selection.

(NHS Estates 2004)

This echoed the 2002 warning by the Chief Medical Officer that the last 30 years of the twentieth century had brought the return of Hospital Acquired Infection (HAI) as "a major problem for the NHS" (Chief Medical Officer 2002). Two years earlier the National Audit Office had concluded in its 2000 report that, despite the large numbers of patients who suffer as a result of HAI and the dramatic impact this has on the NHS, HAI was still not seen as a priority within the NHS (National Audit Office 2000).

Ministers, too, have increasingly conceded to the consensus view of clinicians, researchers and others that standards of hospital cleanliness have declined. In October 2004, then Health Secretary John Reid argued that one reason for the proliferation of one of the most serious HAIs, methicillin-resistant staphylococcus aureus (MRSA), had been the Tory government's decision to contract out cleaning work, with contracts going to the lowest tender (Carvel and White 2004).

Dr Reid also conceded that cleaners did not always feel part of the NHS health care team: but he did nothing about it, even when the link between privatisation and poor standards of hospital cleaning was further underlined by the national report from the Patient Environment Action Teams (PEATs) at the end of 2004. While just over a third (440 of the 1,184 hospitals surveyed) employed private contractors, 15 of the 24 hospitals deemed "poor" were cleaned by private contractors. This suggested very clearly that the incidence of poor cleaning was twice as common among privatised contracts.

Presenting the figures, Health Minister Lord Warner rejected this implication, but urged Trusts to "spend a bit more of their budget on improving cleaning" (Russell 2004). Unfortunately this welcome suggestion came at the same time as figures showing many Trusts facing extremely large deficits in the final three months of the financial year, with even more uncertainty ahead.

Talking the talk...

Even if more money were spent, how would it be used? Despite Mr Milburn's urgings and Dr Reid's later warm words, few of the initiatives launched by the government to improve cleaning standards made any attempt to include input from the staff who actually do the day-to-day cleaning in our hospitals.

The Clean Hospitals Programme in 2000 promised more money for hospital cleaning, but primarily focused on the role of "Modern Matrons", who were to be given powers to advise that payments should be withheld for cleaning contracts where services persistently failed to achieve local standards: this might close the dirtiest wards, but was not a means to ensure all were clean.

As an additional measure, annual inspections by Patient Environment Action Teams (PEATs) were established, which again managed to draw together a cross section of NHS professional and managerial staff, and service users... but not to involve anyone who actually does the cleaning.

While the unhelpfully titled "Matron's Charter" did include some limited participation by UNISON as the trade union representing cleaning staff, there was no such input into the much more comprehensive and prescriptive DoH document *Revised Guidance on Contracting for Cleaning*, which managed to consult an array of private sector and NHS employers, managers, nurses, and even patients about the work, but not one person who actually cleaned a ward, or any of their representatives. The Revised Guidance took refuge in denial when it failed to address the ongoing problem of under-resourcing of hospital cleaning which has prevailed since the competitive tendering regime in the mid-1980s.

In 2005, UNISON stepped up the pressure for serious new resources to be put in to improve hospital cleaning, and for services to be brought back in-house with improved staffing levels (Lister 2005b). However, the management agenda was dominated by a welter of other "targets" and "priorities" – not least mounting evidence of cash crises – and little of substance has changed in most hospital Trusts, leaving MRSA, C-diff and other hospital-acquired infections as a major issue of public and ministerial concern.

The issue hit the headlines again in 2007 with the shocking revelation that over 90 patients had died unnecessarily from hospital-acquired infection in one outbreak in the chaotically mismanaged and overcrowded Maidstone and Tunbridge Wells hospitals Trust (MTW). This was by no means purely a local issue: while the death toll and the sheer disregard for basic standards of patient care emanating from the most senior management of the Trust may have been exceptional, the underlying circumstances were not. Many other NHS Trusts were facing one or more of the pressures on MTW management:

- cash pressures forcing dangerous cuts in nurse staffing levels

- £3.5 million wasted on management consultants at the expense of frontline staff – with nursing vacancies running at the danger level

- too few beds, too close together, with geriatric beds running in 2006–7 at an AVERAGE occupancy level of over 98 per cent

- cleaning services decimated after two decades of ruthless competitive tendering and the effective casualisation of a workforce that was once a crucial part of the NHS team

- management obsessed with signing a major PFI deal for a new hospital, fending off competition from a new private treatment centre, and meeting government targets on finance and waiting times.

Hardly a district hospital in England, for example, is able to run at the recommended safe 82 per cent bed occupancy level for minimising MRSA and other infections: under the crazy new "Payment by Results" system, which only funds them per patient treated, they cannot afford to do so. All this therefore amounts not just to poor management by one unpleasant sacrificial chief executive and a few blundering consultants, but a system failure: this means that despite the rhetoric, a Maidstone-type crisis could take place again in a variety of places.

(Barely edible) food for thought

The NHS Plan also made a big focus on improving hospital food, promising "a 24-hour NHS catering service with a new NHS menu, designed by leading chefs" (DoH 2000b: 47). But while this got a few friendly headlines at the time, it generated no sustained action, and was not coupled to any readiness to bring services back in-house and provide the necessary increased resources: as a result, surveys have time and again revealed huge public concern at poor or inedible food in hospitals.

Just one year down the line, the Audit Commission published a damning report on the state of hospital catering, warning that patients were running the risk of malnutrition on the wards. But it emerged that the Department of Health had already abandoned its hope of getting hospitals to include at least one "leading-chef-inspired" dish on each daily menu. According to the Whittington Hospital Trust these were potentially the "most expensive part of the programme", since the ingredients would cost more and portion sizes were larger, increasing costs per day by almost 40 per cent from £2.61 to £3.64. Even giving patients the options of two biscuits in the morning and a piece of cake in the afternoon could have cost the Whittington an extra £33,000 a year (*Health Emergency* 54, 2001).

In 2006, a Food Watch survey by Patient and Public Involvement Forums of 2,240 patients at 97 hospitals in England found more than a third had abandoned their food, and 40% had had food brought in by visitors. Around 26% who needed help with eating did not receive any; 18% said they did not always have their choice of meal, and 81% said they had no choice of meals in advance (BBC News 2006).

More than a year later another survey, this time by consumer magazine *Which?*, questioned 1,000 patients in hospital and found only a third of them happy with the food they were served. Well-known food critic Lloyd Grossman, who had been very publicly brought in to work with the "leading chefs" in revamping the NHS hospital menus, now argues that ministers have failed to take hospital nutrition seriously, and have no political commitment to improving food for patients (BBC News 2007a).

Mental health

Several other areas of policy have also run into problems since the NHS Plan, but perhaps none have been as far adrift of the targets as mental health services. The government had published its National Service Framework for mental health in September 1999, outlining seven key standards, Among these:

- Ensure all services are available around the clock
- Patients are to receive care which "prevents or anticipates crisis"
- A hospital bed or "suitable alternative bed" to be available "close to home" for those needing urgent acute admission.

These ambitious plans appeared to be addressed by some of the proposals nine months later in the NHS Plan, which called for:

- Additional teams specialising in care of younger patients
- 335 extra Mental Health crisis-response teams
- 1,000 new "graduate primary care mental health workers"
- 50 extra "assertive outreach" teams on top of the 170 promised by April 2001:

> 14.32 There are a small number of people who are difficult to engage. They are very high users of services, and often suffer from dual diagnosis of substance misuse and serious mental illness. ...*Services to provide assertive outreach and intensive input seven days a week are required to sustain engagement with services and to protect patient and public.*

- By 2003 all 20,000 people estimated to need assertive outreach will be receiving these services.

(DoH 2000b: 120, emphasis added)

A number of these proposals were ambiguous from the outset: the precise role and responsibilities of the 1,000 "graduate primary care" workers, for example, remained undefined: were they to be employed by GPs, by PCTs or by mental health Trusts? Exactly what courses were they to be graduates of? Would they be nurses, health professionals... or something else? What career structure might be open to them?

Even on clearly defined issues such as the "extra" crisis response teams, confused priorities and contradictory pressures have served to hold back the necessary investment in improved mental health services, with many of them singled out as a soft target for cuts as Primary Care Trusts have run into financial trouble: the teams have in some cases been merged with existing teams, or taken the place of day hospital and other services.

The 1999 NSF commitment to improve availability of NHS mental health beds has also been more widely acknowledged in the breach than the observance: in fact numbers of mental health beds increased by just 41 (from 34,173) between 2000 and 2001, but have declined each year since, losing almost 3,000 by 2005, before an even more dramatic reduction in the last two years (DoH Hospital Activity Statistics from website, 2007).

By the autumn of 2003 a survey of 45 mental health Trusts by the Royal College of Psychiatrists revealed that their situation had deteriorated: half of them had been running deficits in 2001 and 2002, with an overall reduction in funding and three Trusts reporting cuts of 5 per cent or more, at a time when their services were supposed to be a priority. RCP research director Paul Lelliott warned that mental health Trusts were facing cuts to help pay for deficits elsewhere in the NHS. This followed a similarly gloomy report by the Sainsbury Centre which examined the finances of 18 mental health Trusts and found two-thirds of them running deficits ranging from just £1,000 to a massive £5 million. Pressure group Rethink warned that a quarter of the £1 billion announced as new spending on mental health in the previous five years appeared to have disappeared into a general NHS pool of money (*Health Emergency* 58, 2003).

Early in 2004 three national mental health charities – Rethink, SANE and The Zito Trust – joined forces with top clinicians to launch a disturbing report on the state of hospital care for people with psychiatric illness. *Behind Closed Doors* talked openly of a "crisis" in mental health services, and revealed that, despite no fewer than 650 national strategies, guidelines, frameworks and protocols issued by the government over the previous five years, much still needed to be done to improve the harrowing conditions under which some of society's most vulnerable people were being treated.

> Too many psychiatric wards remain overcrowded, unhygienic, chaotic and run-down," said Paul Corry of Rethink. "Added to this, serious staff shortages and safety concerns persist, patients are often left for days on end with nothing to do, and abuse of street drugs is commonplace.

SANE's Marjorie Wallace added:

> There can be no freedom of choice or chance of better treatment while the acute wards remain in many places filthy and overcrowded, and staff demoralised. It is no wonder that people who are disturbed or depressed will only stay in hospital if sectioned, and that doctors are forced to take the risk of not admitting people who may urgently need inpatient care.

"To make matters worse," added Jayne Zito of the Zito Trust,

> Too many people with severe mental illness are still being prescribed outdated medicines with intolerable side effects – despite rulings by the government's medicines' watchdog NICE that they should receive improved, modern drugs.

> (Rethink, SANE and Zito Trust 2004)

Free nursing care?

The NHS Plan also saw the long-awaited government response to the Royal Commission on Long Term Care, which had been set up in 1997 and reported in February 1999, triggering a prolonged and constipated silence from ministers. The reason for this was not hard to find: the Commission had recommended not only the abolition of means-tested charges for nursing care for people in nursing homes, but also that social care provided in nursing homes should be funded by the taxpayer – effectively becoming part of the package of care for the individual client.

This would leave those with the means to do so still paying a contribution towards the "hotel" costs arising from their accommodation in the nursing home, even though few would voluntarily have chosen to be living in this accommodation, and fewer would have any genuine choice over which home they were placed in. The additional cost of lifting charges for social care was estimated by its opponents at anything up to £1.2 billion per year at 1995 prices (Pollock 2004: 182).

After lengthy consideration, the NHS Plan sided not with the majority of the Sutherland Commission, but with the two-person "minority report", which took a completely different approach on most issues of substance, and argued that only nursing care should be provided free of charge, since delivering free social care to those with the means to pay towards it would "weaken the incentive for people to provide for themselves privately" (Royal Commission on Long Term Care 1999).

In their "Note of Dissent", Joel Joffe and David Lipsey quote approvingly from Blair's philosophical guru Anthony Giddens as the basis for their alternative approach,[17] before invoking private care homes boss Chai Patel as the inspiration for a cut-price scheme to offer minimal nursing care. Yet even Joffe and Lipsey feel obliged to echo widespread concerns over the chronic underfunding of continuing care services:

> All this is endangered by a lack of resources – there is simply insufficient money in the system to provide adequate long-term care. … In the five year period 1992–3 to 1997–8 the basic amount of the Personal Social Services Standard Spending Assessment has actually decreased by 6.1% in real terms at the same time as the number of elderly people needing such care has progressively increased. We welcome the proposed additional resources Government has decided to make available as a result of the Comprehensive Spending Review for 1999 to 2000–2 but we agree with the Association of Directors of Social Services that "there is still some way to go before the accumulated deficit of the past is eradicated".
>
> (Royal Commission on Long Term Care 1999)

It is worth noting that the Commission did investigate the possibility of a private sector solution. It had carried out an extensive investigation of the possibilities that private insurance cover might be more widely used to guard against the risk of heavy costs for individuals requiring long-term care. But they drew the conclusion that this was not a viable policy: even in the USA where private

---

17 "It is not enough merely to focus on public activity in this field. We believe that there is also dignity that comes from providing for oneself in old age if one can afford to do so. As Professor Anthony Giddens says in his book *The Third Way*, 'old age shouldn't be seen as a time of rights without responsibilities'. Universal welfare provision discourages thrift and self-reliance. The central role of families and friends in caring for elderly people should be recognised. The state should nurture that contribution, not merely because otherwise the burden on the public purse will rise – although it will – but also as a compelling matter of social justice."

insurance is the predominant system, only 4–5 per cent of Americans take out Long Term Care Insurance, while 10–20 per cent of them might be able to afford it, and 80–90 per cent would be either unable to afford it or excluded on health grounds:

> The Commission conclude that private sector solutions do not and in the foreseeable future, will not offer a universal solution. Even schemes for partnership can make only a limited contribution. Inevitably, of course, people may consider one of the many schemes available from the private sector to be worthwhile for them provided they can pay the premiums. Overall however, the funding problem cannot therefore be solved by the private sector.

The NHS Plan in 2000 sided quite clearly with the minority, embracing not the principle of a universal service (from which, inevitably, the wealthiest opt out, making their own arrangements outside the framework of public provision) but of means-tested charges ensuring that those receiving funded care were only those on the lower income levels and possessing no property assets. It argued in identical terms to the Commission dissenters that:

> In fact, personal care has never been free. It has been means tested by social services since 1948 although three-quarters of people in nursing and residential care currently receive help with some or all their personal care costs.

> Actioning the proposal would absorb huge and increasing sums of money without using any of it to increase the range and quality of care available to older people. For that reason it is not supported by the Government.

> Our proposals will involve spending as much money as the majority report recommended but in ways that will bring greater benefits in terms of health and independence for all older people both now and in the future.

The process of assessing elderly people's nursing needs (to be measured against three "bands" of public sector provision, up to a maximum of £110 per person per week), and of trying to disentangle "social care" from nursing in nursing homes, began against the background of a continuing squeeze on nursing home finances. Cash-limited and desperately under-funded social services departments were still setting unrealistic "benchmark" limits on the amount they would pay for nursing home care, while simultaneously tightening their own "eligibility criteria" to exclude all but those with the most serious needs from routine support (*Health Emergency* 55, 2002).

Seamless care? Care Trusts and cross-charging

Another innovation in the NHS Plan was to outline plans for new "Care Trusts" which were supposed to span the historic divide between NHS community services and local government social service departments. All Primary Care Trusts were required to invest in an expansion of "intermediate care" – a consistently vague phrase that has been used in varying contexts ever since – and in particular they were supposed to put in place a basic structure of services:

- rapid response teams: made up of nurses, care workers, social workers, therapists and GPs working to provide emergency care for people at home and helping to prevent unnecessary hospital admissions
- intensive rehabilitation services: to help older patients regain their health and independence after a stroke or major surgery. These will normally be situated in hospitals
- recuperation facilities: many patients do not always need hospital care but may not be quite fit enough to go home. Short-term care in a nursing home or other special accommodation eases the passage
- arrangements at GP practice or social work level to ensure that older people receive a one-stop service: this might involve employing or designating the sort of key workers or link workers used in Somerset or basing case managers in GP surgeries
- integrated home care teams: so that people receive the care they need when they are discharged from hospital to help them live independently at home.

(DoH 2000b: 71–2)

These plans for enhanced care for frail older people ran flatly counter to the dynamic of many NHS services which, since the Griffiths Report of 1988, had been pulling back from any real commitment to care of the elderly, and eagerly handing over to the private sector and social services: geriatric beds had been slashed in number, and day hospital and other services had been among the easiest targets for short-term cuts. The change had not just hit nursing home places: public provision of residential care beds had also plunged from 134,000 in 1980 to just 56,000 20 years later, while the private sector had ballooned from 40,000 to 185,000 beds (*Health Emergency* 55, 2002). By 2002 the Wanless Report was also underlining the fact that the decline in both residential and nursing home places had resumed after a brief respite in 1998 and 1999 (Wanless 2002: 107).

To make matters worse, the increased funding that was to be made available to expand social service provision fell far short of the increases being pumped into the mainstream NHS, and appeared completely unrelated to the scale of the extra responsibilities ministers were dumping on to councils. Central government spending on "Personal Social Services" was sharply increased compared with five years of near standstill in the mid-1990s, but was to rise by just 3.3% a year from 2001–4, and then 6% per year up to 2006 (DoH 2002b: 10): but this compared with increases of 6% and 7.5% for overall NHS spending, and came after years of cutbacks and crisis, and took no account of above-inflation price increases from the private sector providers (Social Policy on Ageing Information Network 2001).

The notion of "rapid response teams" ignored the long-standing problem of securing genuine GP commitment to supporting frail older people at home, and the organizational and managerial effort required to run such a potentially complex service.

Hospitals generally lacked the staff and the commitment to develop intensive rehabilitation services. Recuperation facilities had been among the first elements of elderly care to be axed as cash constraints and internal market pressures drove Trusts in the 1990s towards a greater focus on acute care and day case treatment. Moreover, the call for integrated home care teams ignored the bitter divisions between health and social care that had been widened by the cash limits and constant additional demands placed on social services and the NHS at local level.

In fact, care of the elderly has been another consistent and near-universal example of market failure: the private sector has time and again failed to deliver services where they were most needed, while the public sector has been starved of the resources it would require to put a proper and comprehensive service in place. Indeed, this is one factor that genuinely does link the NHS providers with social services – both are ripped off by, and unable to control, the private sector suppliers. These suppliers have a monopoly over nursing home provision, control the large majority of residential care, and in many areas have also taken over domiciliary services (once the centrepiece of local authority provision but now 70 per cent privatised).

Milburn's NHS Plan failed to address the key issues of this failed market in elderly care. Instead, where health and social care could not deliver in parallel, the Plan called for new types of organizations to be formed, which would bring together health and social care in a single structure – a Care Trust:

> Care Trusts will be able to commission and deliver primary and community healthcare as well as social care for older people and other client groups. Social services would be delivered under delegated authority from local councils.

The idea might make sense in abstract, but in practice there were still really serious problems involved in launching a Care Trust: harnessing together two cash-strapped organisations operating with tight "eligibility criteria" to exclude all but the most desperately frail and vulnerable would not necessarily generate a new, enlightened and well-resourced organisation geared to patients' needs.

In addition there was a profound contradiction in the variant routes towards establishing a Care Trust. It might either flow from a solid and productive working relationship already established between NHS and local government... or from precisely the opposite situation. According to the NHS Plan:

> Care Trusts will usually be established where there is a joint agreement at local level that this model offers the best way to deliver better care services.

But according to the very next paragraph, the opposite situation might also give a pretext for a shotgun wedding between two failing or incompatible organisations:

> Where local health and social care organisations have failed to establish effective joint partnerships – or where inspection or joint reviews have shown that services

are failing – the Government will take powers to establish integrated arrangements through the new Care Trust.

(DoH 2000b: 73)

As this book is completed (December 2007) most local managers of PCTs and social services have managed to steer clear of these proposals in the NHS Plan. There are just eleven Care Trusts across the NHS, and two of these are conspicuously poor role models for the provision of responsive or high-quality care.

Manchester Mental Health and Social Care Trust has been dogged by financial crises and chronic bad management for its whole existence. Recently the Trust has been hitting the headlines as a result of its scandalous decision to sack community mental health nurse and trade union activist Karen Reissmann, on a dubious charge of bringing the Manchester Mental Health and Social Care Trust into disrepute, triggering a solid strike in support of her reinstatement. The victimisation of a leading and outspoken union member seems to have been a desperate device to divert attention from those who have genuinely brought the Trust into disrepute: the managers themselves, whose years of incompetence had reduced the Trust to 173rd out of a league table of 175 mental health Trusts.

Managers had closed vital beds, resulting in bed occupancy rates standing at over 120 per cent by the end of 2007. Changes in community and mental health teams, implemented despite warnings from staff and trade unions that they would fail, left patients without vital key workers and held up the establishment of crisis response teams. Respite services and an elderly care ward have been closed as the Trust struggles with a chronic financial crisis, with another £5 million cuts this year, while its record on human resources management has been a disaster (UNISON MCMH Branch 2007). Many will conclude that the wrong person was sacked: Karen Reissmann has stood up for patients and for quality mental health care, while chief executive Sheila Foley and other senior managers have shown little concern for either, and have allowed the Manchester example to cast doubt on the Care Trust model.

So too, for different reasons, have the managers of the Bexley Care Trust in South East London, who have connived throughout with efforts to solve the financial problems affecting NHS Trusts and PCTs in neighbouring London boroughs by closing down acute hospital services at the only major hospital in their catchment area, Queen Mary's Hospital in Sidcup. The Care Trust has made it clear to local hospital staff that they favour the diversion of patients to hospitals miles outside the Borough, despite the fact that these hospitals lack the capacity to take the additional numbers of emergency admissions that would result. It has ignored the obvious views of the public, the local press and public expressions of concern by elected representatives, and opted instead to join with managers of bankrupt Trusts and other PCTs rather than meet the needs and wishes of its own catchment population (Lister 2007d).

If Care Trusts like Bexley and Manchester are the model, many people would draw the conclusion that most of the rest of the country is better off without them.

There seem to be few if any stories of improved working or genuine synergies in the Care Trusts that have been established, while the crisis in social services has sharpened in recent years making any real convergence less likely than ever.

Even if PCTs were to link up successfully with social services, it would still leave one of the central contradictions unresolved: hospitals seeking to discharge patients even more rapidly as a result of the perverse incentives of the Payment by Results system run time and again into the restrictions, complexities and inadequacies of the social care system, which in many areas functions with far too few nursing home beds and extremely limited provision of domiciliary care. NHS budgets and financial pressures remain separated from social service budgets and pressures – and in conditions of cash limits, each organisation is obliged to act as best it can in its own self defence.

Another question mark still hangs over the hybrid bodies: while deals have been done to establish whether groups of staff are paid on NHS or local government terms and conditions, it still seems open to doubt whether Care Trust patients might be subjected to social services-style means-tested charges for some forms of care, or whether the NHS principle of treatment free at point of use would always apply.

Money has raised its head as ministers have tried to square the circle of health and social care by creating financial incentives where appeals for collaboration and cooperation had clearly failed. In 2002, *Delivering the NHS Plan* outlined plans to allow hospital Trusts to levy charges on local authority social services which failed to provide adequate nursing home and other support to facilitate rapid hospital discharge, resulting in "bed blocking". The policy was based on the experience in Sweden – but with a significant difference in the case of the UK. While Sweden's 1992 Adel reform was designed to place pressure on municipal authorities which own and run Swedish nursing homes, in Britain social service departments have always purchased this type of care from the private sector – and the private sector takes its investment decisions not on the basis of local health needs but the possibility of coining a profit. Even in Sweden the reforms put a severe strain on the municipal authorities, and effectively forced higher costs onto older patients who pay higher out-of-pocket charges for nursing homes than for hospital care (Dixon and Mossialos 2002; Lister 2005a).

As the new system of fines – which began in 2004 at £100 per day (£120 in London) – was introduced, social services departments were braced for hefty bills that would further undermine their ability to deliver services to frail older people outside the hospital system. In the autumn of 2003 it was estimated that some 3,500 frail people aged over 75 were marooned in hospital beds for lack of alternative accommodation or supporting systems to care for them. Councils had been given a puny £50 million nationally to allow them to expand preventive services and secure additional accommodation (Health Emergency 58, 2003).

But there is no way, within the current system of fixing benchmark fees for nursing home care, to enable local authorities to ensure sufficient places are available for all those frail older people who need them. Instead it seems that some other complexities of the discharge process are being exploited to delay the NHS Trusts' decisions to discharge and thus avoid excessive liability to pay the "fines" when councils cannot find spaces. The government seems to have made this relatively easy for evasive local authorities by bringing in the Mental Capacity Act and the Independent Mental Capacity Advocate (IMCA) service from April 2007, which adds new complexities and dimensions to patient discharge and puts fresh obstacles in the way of hospitals seeking a speedy solution (DoH 2007d).

Private intentions

The consolidation of the private sector role in the provision of continuing care for the elderly was not the only concession made to private sector involvement in the NHS Plan. It also pledged a further major expansion of hospital building under the Private Finance Initiative, with 100 new hospitals by 2010 – virtually all of them to be financed through PFI – see Chapter nine.

The private sector was also to be brought in as a "partner" to the NHS in the provision of a new network of "Diagnostic & Treatment Centres", which would be new units offering diagnostic tests and elective surgical treatment. Although this concept was already being pioneered by the NHS, and some more were to be built as NHS units, the focus soon shifted towards private sector provision, which soon became referred to as "Independent Sector Treatment Centres" – see Chapter nine.

The most immediate impact of the NHS Plan's turn towards the private sector centred on the "Concordat" outlined in the Plan, and signed in the autumn of 2000 by Alan Milburn with the main providers of private hospitals – to boost NHS use of private hospital beds to relieve pressure on acute services and avoid what had become an annual "winter crisis". The Concordat aimed at closer working links between the NHS on three distinct levels:

- elective care: this could take the form of NHS doctors and nurses using the operating theatres and facilities in private hospitals or it could mean the NHS buying certain services

- critical care: this will provide for the NHS and the private sector to be able to transfer patients to and from each other whenever clinically appropriate

- intermediate care: this will involve the private and voluntary sector developing and making available facilities to support the Government's strategy for better preventive and rehabilitation services.

(DoH 2000b: 97)

It was immediately obvious to NHS staff that flows of patients would be in different directions for each of these categories of care. While the private sector would happily cream off a profitable slice of the less-complex NHS elective operations, and some new facilities may be developed for "intermediate care" if the price was right, allowing NHS hospitals to discharge older patients more swiftly from frontline beds, the story was very different on critical care.

Private hospitals are geared purely around the least complex elective operations: they are too small and mostly lack the resources to deliver full-scale critical care, as well as lacking full-time consultant and medical staff. Far more likely, then, was that this new "partnership" would be invoked as a basis for more of the private sector's medical mistakes and unexpected emergencies to be transferred rapidly to the nearest NHS emergency department, which would have the skills and the resources lacking in the private hospitals.

New bureaucracy, reduced accountability

The final key aspect of the NHS Plan that will be discussed here was the extraordinary process described in *Health Emergency* as the "March of the quangos": half a dozen new organisations were to be created and take their place in the increasingly complex and fragmented management of the NHS, alongside the Trusts, PCTs, NICE, CHI, Health Action Zones (since axed) and others. They included:

- A new Modernisation Agency, complete with regional teams, charged with "rolling out" the NHS Plan – this once employed as many as 760 staff but has since been axed, with little sign of any ill effects on the NHS

- A Leadership Centre for Health – this appears to have suffered a similar fate: web links from this now lead to a new NHS Institution for Innovation and Improvement

- Patient Environmental Action Teams (PEAT) to check on hospital hygiene

- A national clinical assessment authority to investigate the performance of doctors subject to complaints

- A UK council of health regulators to coordinate disciplinary matters for NHS professional staff

- An Appointments Commission – effectively a quango tasked with choosing non-executive board members for Trusts and PCTs

- An "independent reconfiguration panel" to advise ministers when controversial plans for hospital closures are referred back for ministerial review: in practice this panel has acted as a rubber stamp for closures

- A new citizen's council to advise NICE

- And a complex and ineffective new system of Patient Advocacy and Liaison Services (operating at Trust level), local Patient and Public Involvement Forums and council Oversight and Scrutiny Committees to replace the established and often very effective Community Health Councils, which had enjoyed statutory powers since 1974. The abolition of CHCs (in England: they have remained in place in Wales, although generally much more subservient to local NHS managers) was clearly a move to remove a thorn in the side of ministers, and cynically exploited the passivity and servility of many of the worst CHCs in order to shut down the best ones. This legislation, which cost a staggering £200 million (*Health Emergency* 55, 2002), did not take effect until December 2003. Now in turn the PPIFs are to be abolished, and replaced in the spring of 2008 with the even less effective "Local Involvement Networks (LINks)".

(DoH 2007b)

The NHS Plan boasted the signatures of large numbers of top professionals and senior managers: but as the policies were rolled out and put into practice much of this consensus proved illusory. Nonetheless ministers have driven a relentless and accelerating pace of "reform", with repeated reorganisations in England's NHS since 2000. One strongly critical *BMJ* Editorial on the issue notes that:

> Reorganisations are a clumsy reform tool, and research shows that they seldom deliver the promised benefits. Every reorganisation produces a transient drop in performance, and it takes a new organisation at least two or three years to become established and start to perform as well as its predecessor. Yet the NHS is reorganised every two years or so, which probably means it sees all the costs of each reorganisation and few of the benefits.

(Walshe et al. 2004)

In the period 2000–5 the Regional offices, last remnants of Regional Health Authorities, were scrapped, along with 100 health authorities: in their place 28 Strategic Health Authorities were established (subsequently merged into ten) (Klein 2006).

Primary Care Trusts

Primary Care Groups were also replaced with 300 Primary Care Trusts (PCTs) – local commissioning bodies established in 2002, which within a few years were in control of upwards of 75 per cent of the total NHS budget for primary, community and hospital services (Stevens 2004).

The early promise that PCTs would exercise substantial local autonomy was thrown into question by the Department of Health's insistence that PCTs in Oxfordshire had no choice but to agree to the establishment of a controversial private sector treatment centre delivering cataract treatment, despite PCT concerns that it would undermine the financial viability of Oxford's existing NHS Eye Hospital (Hanna 2006).

The widely held view that PCTs had failed adequately to establish themselves as effective purchasing bodies forcing maximum value from hospital Trusts soon led to fears among some observers that these organisations would themselves be effectively broken up, and see some or all of their commissioning functions and some – though probably not all – of their provider functions privatised: *Guardian* correspondent Tash Shifrin perceptively warned, well ahead of the moves that were to take shape the following year, that:

> There is speculation that, in the long term, under-performing PCTs may be "taken over" under NHS franchising arrangements, by private commissioning

organisations from the US and elsewhere.

(Shifrin 2004)

By the summer of 2004, as Shifrin reported, the perceived failures of PCTs had led to a round of PCT mergers, including Hampshire, where PCTs began by combining their management teams, and Cambridgeshire and Derby which both opted for joint chief executives. In Newcastle and North Tyneside, three PCTs had been bullied by the Strategic Health Authority into a "mega merger" to form a single consortium (Shifrin 2004). Each time, the process of reforming PCTs involved a further step away from local accountability, towards more remote organisations – entities more willing to take a tough line in forcing concessions from the hospital Trusts, which were now firmly outside the loop of decision-making.

Foundations for a new health market

One of the centrepieces of New Labour's structural "reforms" to the NHS was the establishment of Foundation Trusts, with the linked changes to the financial system that pays providers for the services they deliver.

Under the Thatcher reforms, NHS Trusts were launched from 1991 as "public corporations", each governed by a Trust board of directors composed of executive directors and direct and indirect government appointees, conducting most business behind closed doors. Their main income would come from contracts with purchasing health authorities, for which they would be required to compete on the basis of price and quality. New Labour took this concept and added a further twist: from 2003 onwards "three star" Trusts, already shown to be performing best against the government's targets and star ratings system, were urged to apply to become "Foundation Trusts", on the model of similar hospitals in Sweden and Spain and Portugal's "hospital companies" (Lister 2005a).

The plan was denounced by health unions and by the BMA as a return to the type of market-style methods wheeled in by Margaret Thatcher's government in the early 1990s, and which Labour ministers claimed to have swept away after 1997. Former Health Secretary Frank Dobson and other former ministers also attacked the plan for precisely these reasons, pointing out that the new "freedoms" to be granted to Foundation Trusts could only be at the expense of other NHS Trusts that have been excluded from the elite status.

Foundations were to be non-profit public companies (sometimes even described as "mutuals" – Blears et al. 2002; Lea and Mayo 2002), controlled by local boards and accountable not to the Secretary of State but to a new independent regulator (known as Monitor). Some of Milburn's colleagues, such as Ian McCartney, took the rhetoric of democracy seriously and went even further over the top, claiming that Foundation Trusts – supported as they were by the Tory Party, and Thatcherite organisations such as the Institute of Directors and the Adam Smith Institute – represent "popular socialism" and hark back to the "old Labour", "socialist" values of the cooperative movement (McCartney 2002).

But the Foundations were to be run as businesses, and were encouraged to show entrepreneurial spirit: they would have to pay commercial interest on any loans they took out with the private sector. They may not have become "for-profit" bodies distributing their surplus to shareholders, but they would have to break even. They would seek to retain a growing surplus year on year: so they would inevitably seek to strengthen their market share by competing against other Trusts for contracts to treat more NHS patients, as another aspect of Milburn's reforms – the re-establishment of a full-scale market system through a new system of Payment by Results – took effect.

Foundation Trusts might even use their "freedoms" in order to pick and choose which specialities and services they saw as economic to offer to local Primary Care Trusts – and which they saw as less attractive, and to be left for non-Foundation Trusts.

As Mohan (2003a, b) argued, the claims made by New Labour ministers to be treading in the footsteps of pre-NHS voluntary hospitals represented both a distortion of the actual events and organisations which operated in British health care prior to 1948, and a substantially retouched version of the level of democracy and involvement that actually occurred, in which large-scale participation fund-raising was met by "tokenistic" representation on governing bodies:

> With few exceptions democracy and consumer control were not strong features of these hospitals… Moreover any serious assessment of the pre-NHS era would have to acknowledge the enormous variations in provision and finance, such that there were five-fold variations in patients' chances of obtaining treatment in a voluntary hospital, depending on where they lived.
>
> (Mohan 2003a, b)

In other words, the increase in "localism" came with a heavy cost in terms of rising inequality, on a level that could not be tolerated in a twenty-first century NHS. Foundation Trusts would begin as elite, top-rated hospitals, and would have no obligation to share their surpluses and resources with any other part of the NHS. And the objective of entrepreneurialism meant that the initial inequalities would not narrow, but would rather tend to widen, as Foundations were promised new freedoms over and above those available to non-Foundation Trusts.

Foundation Trusts were to have extra freedoms to borrow, including from the private sector – but their borrowing would count against the total cash limits on the NHS, and so any extra borrowing by them would mean less capital for maintenance or new building in other Trusts. They would be free to retain any cash raised from the sale of Trust property assets, prompting fears that some may embark on a new round of asset-stripping – a fear borne out by the sale by London's University College Hospital Trust of the old Middlesex Hospital building for a cool £175 million (Gadelrab 2006), none of which has been shared with other organisations delivering health care in the area.

They would be free to set up private companies that could offer managerial and other services inside or outside the NHS and which could bid to take over neighbouring "failing" Trusts under the government's franchising scheme: a version of this has already occurred in Birmingham with the takeover of Good Hope Hospital Trust by Birmingham Heartlands Foundation Trust (Timmins 2007a).

Ministers were eventually forced to retreat from early promises that Foundation Trusts would be free to borrow on the money markets: borrowing would be strictly limited, and policed by Monitor. By 2004, Health Minister Lord Warner revealed in the House of Lords the borrowing limits for the first ten Foundation Trusts – which ranged from just £3.3 million to a maximum of £17.1 million – well short of the borrowing required for any major schemes, and the expected freedoms when Foundations were first proposed (*Lords Hansard*, 19 April 2004).

Foundations would also have freedoms to vary the pay of their staff, giving scope in some areas to offer more to recruit staff with particular skills – subject only to vague restrictions on "poaching" staff from other Trusts. Although Alan Milburn said that Foundation Trusts would be covered by the new NHS "Agenda for Change" pay structure, it was clear that they would be effectively free to vary from the new, laboriously negotiated national pay scales. Indeed, if Milburn's plan that ALL Trusts should eventually become Foundations were ever to bear fruit, it could potentially demolish any coherent national pay structure, taking unions right back to the chaos of local pay rates unleashed by Thatcher in the early 1990s.

Foundation Trusts were also given a guarantee of independence from legal direction by the Secretary of State – raising serious questions as to whether they could be prevented from using these other freedoms in ways which might threaten the survival of other Trusts: they would be accountable only to Monitor, the independent regulator.

Mr Milburn insisted that the Foundation Trusts would be non-profit-making bodies, with their assets "locked" to prevent Foundations being privatised at a later stage (Milburn 2002). But what of a Foundation Hospital whose main buildings were already owned by a private consortium through PFI? What protection would there be against it being converted into a straightforward business, selling care to the NHS, with profits bolstered by its local monopoly position? The government ignored the grim warning from the experience of the first Foundation-style experiment in Sweden, where St Goran's, a major hospital in Stockholm was privatised by its board – sold to private operator Capio – against the wishes of the local health authority and the government: St Goran's is now described as "Sweden's largest private emergency hospital". In 2001, the government legislated to prevent further public hospitals being privatised (Dixon and Mossialos 2002; Lister 2005a).

However, Milburn did retreat in front of those warning that Foundations would (like the first-wave NHS Trusts in the Tory reforms) seek to expand their treatment of private patients and numbers of private beds. He insisted that they would be prevented from doing so, and that applications would be preferred if they proposed to switch existing pay beds back to treat NHS patients: it was not clear if any such plans existed.

Milburn also argued that Foundations would remain "part of the NHS", and that they would be controlled by elected "stakeholder" members from the local community, who would elect representatives to comprise a majority of a board of governors.

However, it was obvious from the outset that the real power would remain in the hands of an unelected management board, and the extent to which local "stakeholders" would actually influence the day-to-day running of the Trusts – if at all – was never clear. There were also big questions to be answered over the extent to which such "stakeholders" groups would be representative of anybody, let alone the ethnic and social mix of the communities the Trusts are supposed to cover.

The legislation eventually passed through the Commons in December 2003 with a majority of just 17. The reality was that while New Labour still had enough of a majority and a parliamentary machine to force through the law, Foundation Trusts remained almost completely bereft of popular support. The policy that struggled to get airborne when the first dozen or so Foundations launched on April Fool's Day 2004 was anything but popular, democratic or socialist.

So puny was the base of public support on which even monster Trusts had based their Foundation bids that consultation meetings during the application process frequently drew attendances in low single figures: one joint meeting in South East London, called jointly by Guy's and St Thomas's and King's College Trusts to promote their parallel Foundation bids, drew a total attendance of five people, including a chief executive with a powerpoint presentation!

The striking absence of bums on seats was predictably matched by a lack of punters signing up to "join" the Foundations. In autumn 2003 a Department of Health spokesperson announced that Foundations would be expected to establish a minimum "membership" of 7,000–10,000 people. In practice, according to a *Guardian* survey in January 2004, only two of the first-wave Foundation Trusts (King's College Hospital and University Hospital Birmingham) even topped the 3,000 mark, with many languishing in the low hundreds (Carvel 2004).

The flagship University College London Hospital – with its gleaming white £420 million PFI hospital taking shape at the top of Gower Street – had so far mustered only 600 members, and was the first to voice fears that with so few people interested, they could fall prey to "entryism", and be captured by "an interest group or a Trot element". UCLH's Foundation project director told the *Guardian* that the progress so far had been a "fiasco" (Carvel 2004). The UCLH warning was taken to heart by other Foundation hopefuls, including Hackney's Homerton hospital, where Trust bosses echoed fears that the election of a governing council could be hijacked by "single interest groups". Elsewhere,

Foundation applicants promised that would-be candidates for the new governing councils, to be elected from the limited ranks of "members", would be required to sign a pledge – a latter-day McCarthyite promise that they were not now, nor ever had been, proponents of a "single interest".

But how democratic was this new procedure to gerrymander elections and filter out the feared "Trots" and the (apparently less-seriously feared) fascists of the BNP et al.? Why should it be necessary for Foundations – supposedly designed to make NHS Trusts more responsive to local people – to begin life by drawing up a list of local people whose opinions were to be excluded a priori from consideration at all costs? How tightly defined was the notion of a "single interest group"? Would it potentially mean the exclusion of pensioners' groups, kidney patients, rheumatic patients or diabetics? Conversely, how many apolitical, disinterested and ignorant citizens were likely to be found who would willingly involve themselves in the potentially complex process of policy-making for an NHS Foundation Trust?

By making a lack of interest or commitment a precondition for allowing punters to become involved, the Trusts were excluding precisely those concerned and motivated local movers and shakers who might genuinely make Foundations accountable and democratic. As the Bill reached its final phase, ministers had a bright idea to make up the numbers: simply draft in the existing staff... and patients... of the Foundation applicants. The amended Act included a provision that Foundations may count as "members" any past or present patients and staff members who have not specifically written to "opt out" of membership.

This brought a double threat:

- potential harassment of any staff members who resisted this unequal and unrewarding "partnership" with management

- and a potentially vast "membership" of thousands of unwitting patients, who for one reason or another had not understood, or not got around to writing back to the Trust to decline the offer of membership.

From a Trust point of view, the entire procedure involved maintaining a data base of the passive and unresponsive: the ideal membership base from the point of view of maintaining control would include thousands of elderly patients too polite, too confused or too immobile to send back forms declining to join.

Such large numbers might impress the regulator, but few if any of these members would vote, or put themselves forward for the governing council: the risk of capture by a small, active, organised minority would remain. But in the real world, existing Trust chairs and non-execs who wished to stay on had been guaranteed at least a year of tenure after Foundations were launched, and existing chairs would become chairs of the new governing councils. Who would expect the first round of elections to generate any visible change in the Trusts?

The extent of the autonomy on offer to Foundations was thrown into question the following autumn (2004), when one of the first wave, Bradford Hospitals, found itself facing a substantial deficit (predicting a £4 million deficit after just six months) in place of the modest surplus it had predicted in its business plan.

Despite the fact that this level of deficit was modest compared with the crisis situation then developing in many NHS Trusts, Monitor immediately intervened, and called in a firm of New York-based business trouble-shooters to sort out the growing financial crisis. The company, Alvarez & Marsal, was chosen and called in by Monitor: but the costs of flying in the team of "turnaround management consultants" (who had to be told that British health care is priced in pounds and not dollars) had to be paid by the Bradford Trust. Their recipe for turning around included axing sandwich snacks for elderly patients and security guards on the hospital car park (Revill 2005).

Yet even after the regulator had seen fit to intervene so publicly and dramatically, Ministers predictably washed their hands of the whole business. In the House of Commons, Health Secretary John Reid issued a statement refusing to answer parliamentary questions on any Foundation Trusts, declaring that:

> Ministers are no longer in a position to comment on, or provide information about, the detail of operational management within such Trusts. Any such questions will be referred to the relevant Trust chairman.

Only a limited number of Foundations had been established before the 2005 General Election. However, this did not stop the Blair government making it clear very early in the process that if they were re-elected then all hospitals would be pressed to become Foundations.

Provider payment reform

As a vital part of its new, wider-reaching marketising reform, New Labour began to introduce a much more complex system for financing health care providers. There were two main strands in the new system ushered in from 2001: the first was a brainchild of Gordon Brown's Treasury team, a system known as Resource Allocation Budgeting (RAB). RAB was introduced in April 2001, and took full effect from 2004, with two important effects on NHS Trusts: it halted the long-established device of fudging revenue deficits by transferring capital to revenue, and it brought in the "double deficit effect" (Commons Health Committee 2006: 26). This meant that Trusts were effectively penalised in the following financial year by a cut in allocation equivalent to any deficit incurred the previous year. The combination of RAB with the many other financial pressures and rising demand on frontline NHS care was a succession of the largest deficits ever recorded by NHS Trusts, until the scheme was eventually axed in 2007 (Mooney 2007a; Edwards 2007).

The second change was originally described in the NHS Plan as "reforming financial flows", but has become known (misleadingly) as "Payment by Results" (PBR). In fact the payments have nothing to do with the "results" of the treatment: the hospital secures the same fee whether the patient jogs out in a tracksuit or is carried out in a box. PBR is a cost-per-case system, linked to a fixed national tariff of "reference costs" for each item of treatment they deliver –

the old system of block contracts is being scrapped. PBR has been introduced firstly for Foundation Trusts (beginning in 2004) while its roll-out across other acute hospital Trusts is being phased in.

The official explanation of Payment by Results is that it is "fair", "transparent" and "rules-based":

> The aim of the new financial reforms being introduced across the NHS is to create a fair transparent system for paying NHS Hospitals and other NHS service providers. Payment by Results will end relying on historical budgets and locally negotiated settlements as payments for services will be directly linked to activity and results. Payment by Results will therefore reward efficiency and quality and encourage the better management of demand and risk.
>
> (DoH 2007a)

However it is no coincidence that the introduction of PBR came simultaneously with the roll-out of Foundation Trusts and the move towards ISTCs. Indeed as the DoH statement makes quite clear, the new scheme is a "system for paying NHS Hospitals *and other NHS service providers*". Elsewhere, the DoH argues that:

> It will reward efficiency, support patient choice and diversity and encourage activity for sustainable waiting time reductions.
>
> (DoH 2007d)

Reading between the lines, therefore, the new structure was designed with two prime objectives:

- to create a new framework within which Foundation Trusts could secure a wider share of the available contract revenue in a competitive health "market", while Trusts less well resourced (or whose costs for whatever reason are higher than the reference price) could lose out

- and to open up a portal through which NHS funds could be extracted to purchase care from private providers ("patient choice").

By effectively commodifying health care at such a basic level, the PBR system facilitates the New Labour objective of breaking down the barriers between the public and private sectors, and ensuring that every patient who chooses or is persuaded to accept treatment in a private treatment centre or hospital takes the money with them out of the NHS. To use Thatcher's famous phrase, "the money follows the patient" – and the crisis and cash shortfalls remain within the NHS while the private sector collects a guaranteed margin. NHS Trusts have therefore increasingly had to compete not only against other NHS Trusts, but also against private hospitals which have a much more selective, purely elective, and thus much less complex and costly caseload. But of course the competition is even more unfair than this suggests: treatment centre contracts are ring-fenced so that only private sector providers are allowed to bid for them.

One down-side of PBR is that a fixed tariff of cost-per-case fees can act as a perverse incentive for NHS Trusts to discharge patients swiftly, regardless of their individual needs and pace of recovery.

Ministers have attempted to create the illusion that the situation is driven not by them but by patients: through PBR they appear to have have put the responsibility for spending decisions and the reallocation of funds and resources not on to Primary Care Trusts, but on to individual patients, who are being offered a progressively wider "choice" of where they want to have their treatment. Of course, few patients will have any awareness of the potentially far-reaching impact of their "choices" – and few would willingly choose an option that might undermine their future access to a properly resourced local district hospital. Ministers have consciously destabilised NHS Trusts in what former advisor Chris Ham has called "creative destruction" (Carvel 2006).

By the end of 2005, Primary Care Trusts were obliged to offer almost all patients a "choice" of providers – including at least one private hospital – from the time they were first referred. By 2008, the NHS's sixtieth year, any patient will be allowed to choose any hospital which can deliver treatment at the NHS reference cost (Stevens 2004).

Irrespective of what patients may choose, ministers have consistently made clear that they want at least 10 per cent of NHS elective operations to be carried out by the private sector in 2006, rising to 15 per cent by 2008. This policy has been strongly criticised, not least by the BMA, but also by studies produced by London NHS managers for Health Secretary John Reid, which warned that the plans were "problematic, unaffordable" and of "no benefit" in London, since they would have serious impact on the financial stability and viability of NHS Trusts. The Commons Public Accounts Committee has warned that the policy could result in private sector providers "cream skimming" the most straightforward and lucrative cases, leaving NHS hospitals with reduced resources to cope with the chronic, the complex and the costly patients: it could also give GPs perverse incentives to refer patients to hospitals which did not have adequate facilities or medical support (Coombes 2005; McGauran 2004).

There has been growing concern that hospitals which lose out when patients choose to go elsewhere could be forced to close departments – or close down altogether: ministers and senior NHS officials have said that they are willing to see this happen, arguing that it would not be their policy, but patients who made the decision (Carvel 2006b, c). However, it is not only this factor that could push hospitals into difficulties, but also the problems faced by hospitals – especially specialist hospitals where for whatever reason operations are currently costing above the NHS reference cost. These Trusts face a substantial cut in revenue under PBR which could force them out of business. A number of "specialist" Foundation Trusts were promised a share of a Department of Health "sink fund" to bail out some of the biggest losers in this new market: other Foundations were to get nothing, while non-Foundation Trusts – many of them already facing massive multi-million deficits – would be left to their own devices, and have to fight through yet more obstacles to survival in a new, even more unequal, two-tier NHS. In fact it has become clear that ministers aim to use the tariff system as a means to squeeze specialist services out of district general hospitals and carry though the controversial "rationalisation" process (Vize 2007).

Even where hospitals have been charging less than the new reference cost, and would stand to make windfall gains under the new system, the Primary Care Trusts which buy services from them would find their budgets cut. Estimates of the mismatch in funding in 2004 were as high as £1 billion a year across the NHS, with some Trusts set to lose very heavily (*Health Emergency* 59, 2004). This new market-style system makes no reference to social and other inequalities, and runs the risk of funnelling an ever-larger share of the NHS budget to the best-resourced and largest Trusts and GP practices at the expense of those struggling to cope in more deprived areas.

But the new system also represents the end of 30 years of efforts to equalise allocations of NHS spending on the basis of population and local health needs.

Now PCTs in areas where Trusts have been delivering services below the new NHS reference costs will require extra cash to pay an increased fee – which will become a "surplus" for the Trust. Conversely, PCTs whose Trusts currently deliver relatively high-cost treatment will see their cash allocations for other services reduced.

None of this bears any relation to social deprivation, the age profile or relative health of the population: the new market system emerges as the enemy of equality. The prospect of widespread financial instability seems to have been the key factor in forcing a delay, and then a phased introduction of the new payment system, which was to have applied to 70 per cent of treatments by April 2005, but which by the time of the General Election had already been postponed by 12 months.

Where does all the money go?

Like the Tory reforms, the market-style policies introduced since 2000 have been strongly criticised both by doctors and by health unions for their negative impact on equity of access and treatment – while New Labour ministers have argued that the reforms were necessary precisely to secure these objectives.

While the underlying principle of a public-sector, tax-funded service has been generally upheld, and the New Labour reforms have been accompanied by a substantial increase in government spending on health, partly funded through tax increases, the British reforms are in general on the most radical end of the European spectrum.

Ideological reinforcement for the proposal to increase sharply the share of UK GDP to be spent on health care came in two reports commissioned by Gordon Brown through the Treasury, one by former NatWest boss Derek Wanless (2002), and another – an overview of the (largely economic) trends and challenges facing health care systems in eight high-income countries – commissioned from the European Observatory on Health Care Systems (Dixon and Mossialos 2002). Both reports flagged up the very low comparative level of spending on health care in Britain, while the European Observatory collection raised critical points on some of the "reforms" implemented in other high-income countries.

Wanless went in much greater detail into the resources required to improve the British health care system, but his Interim Report in November 2001 was widely welcomed for revealing the extent of the gap that had opened up in health care resources between Britain and other comparable countries, which was variously estimated at £200 to £267 billion in the 25 years from 1972:

> The cumulative underspend (relative to the unweighted average of EU spending) between 1972 and 1998 has been calculated as £220 billion in 1998 prices. Relative to EU average spending on an income-weighted basis, the cumulative underspend is £267 billion. Not surprisingly, with such significantly lower spending, UK health service outcomes have lagged behind continental European performance... The surprise may be that the gap in many measured outcomes is not bigger, given the size of the cumulative spending gap.
>
> (Wanless 2001: 37)

But increasing the flow of funds to the NHS raises the question of how best to spend the money, and which policies can deliver most beneficial results. Labour ministers seeking vindication point to the sharp reduction in waiting lists and waiting times that have been achieved across much of the NHS since the NHS Plan: but since most of these improvements pre-date many of the more controversial marketising reforms and the establishment of most of the independent sector treatment centres, the most fundamental reason for this increase in volume and pace of treatment has been the increased spending and increased numbers of frontline staff (nurses, doctors and support staff). Staff productivity has increased, while overhead costs of goods and services bought in from the private sector have spiralled upwards.

A report by the Office of National Statistics in 2004 revealed that between 1995 and 2003 – a period in which the NHS workforce, according to the ONS, increased by 22 per cent – spending on labour went up just 44 per cent (from £22 billion to £32 billion). This suggests an actual rise in staff pay of just 22 per cent over eight years, a far from over-generous level of increase: by contrast spending on "intermediate procurement" rose by a massive 133 per cent – from £16 billion to £37 billion. In other words for every £1 spent on staff in 1995, just 71p was spent on goods and services from the private sector and outside the NHS, but by 2003, for every £1 spent on staff £1.14 was spent on procurement – an increase of over 50 per cent. Over this same period NHS output (ignoring factors which might be argued as improving the quality of care) increased by 28 per cent according to the ONS (ONS 2004; *Health Emergency* 60, 2004; Lister 2005a). With this constant drain of resources to more costly private sector providers, leaving the NHS to cope with the most complex and high-cost treatments, New Labour was recreating a market-style system more wasteful and wider in scope than the "internal market" that Thatcher began in 1989–90.

The extra cash in the system had brought a pause (from 1994 to 2004) in the rapid rundown in numbers of acute hospital beds which had characterised the 1980s and early 1990s – driven by the expansion of day surgery and new anaesthetics and surgical techniques – and government guidance began to underline the need for additional hospital and "intermediate" capacity to deal with a rising proportion of older patients. In theory, all new hospital schemes after 2000 were supposed to contain at least as many beds as the facilities they replaced: however, many plans for costly new hospitals to be funded through the Private Finance Initiative began again to look to reducing numbers of acute hospital beds, to hold down the size (and rising cost) of the project (see Chapter nine). The new onset of financial pressures after 2004 served to intensify this process, and numbers of acute beds began to fall rapidly. And there had been little if any pause in the very heavy cutbacks in beds for older patients and mental health beds, which continued after 1997, although at a slower pace than the early 1990s (DoH Statistics, 2007).

Countdown to crisis

By 2004–5 the NHS budget, at £67 billion, was double the 1996–7 figure. Billions of this extra spending, however, were increasingly being funnelled into contracts with private health providers, making profits for the private companies, whilst many NHS hospitals faced bigger than ever cash deficits and were forced to close beds and cut jobs. There were increasing concerns that the NHS was not getting sufficient value for money and that the extra cash was being wasted.

During 2000, the year of the NHS Plan, ministers still waiting for the first tranche of additional funding to flow from Gordon Brown's budget the following year managed to secure an extra £150 million to help the NHS in England deal with the coming "winter pressures". But half of the 85 health authorities surveyed by the Press Association believed their local social services would not be able to cope with the rising demand for care packages to support older people discharged from hospital (*Health Emergency* 52, 2000).

In 2001 as the extra cash began to flow, a rising tide of "unavoidable cash pressures" on health authorities, along with tough new government targets, began to swallow up much of the new money. In East London and City Health Authority, covering three of Britain's most deprived boroughs (Hackney, Tower Hamlets and Newham) an eight per cent increase in funding (£45 million) was almost matched by a massive £342 million of unavoidable cost pressures. In Lambeth, Southwark and Lewisham Health Authority a first draft of its business plan looked to extra spending of £57 million, only to discover than just £12.6 million was available to fund new developments. A second draft still left a spending gap of £35 million, before managers resorted to a further effort to scale down expectations:

> "Further down-sizing was undertaken on the basis of a pragmatic assessment that LSL would not be in a position to fund anything other than the minimum 'must do' targets and non-discretionary pressures": even this, which excluded any national targets, or priorities not specifically required in 2001–2, and any locally decided priorities, left a £14 million gap.
>
> (*Health Emergency* 53, 2001)

By early 2002 the Commons Health Committee was hearing evidence that the government's cash increases for the NHS had lagged way behind the list of "priorities" and targets it had imposed upon Trusts and health authorities. Croydon HA told the committee that just to implement the top 20 priorities would cost it an extra £70 million a year – ten times the increase it was to receive. In SE London, Lambeth, Southwark and Lewisham HA warned that simply to implement the recommendations from the National Institute for Clinical Excellence (NICE) on new drugs would cost an extra £15 million a year: as a result LSL had ignored much of NICE's guidance. In West London, Ealing, Hammersmith and Hounslow's Local Modernisation review found that meeting revised access targets in elective and emergency care could cost around £15 million (2.5 per cent of turnover), while mental health targets could cost another £3.6 million: all of the plans together would stack up to an extra £40 million. Even Kensington, Chelsea and Westminster, the health authority with the largest cash increase in the country, warned that it could not afford to deliver all of the targets, and it would have to make savings to balance the books (*Health Emergency* 55, 2002).

The continued increase in the flow of NHS funds brought no reprieve from the rising tide of deficits: by early 2003 a *Health Emergency* snapshot survey of Trust and health authority board papers showed eleven London Trusts in the red to the tune of £33 million, with several Trusts facing £4 million-plus shortfalls. Problems were mounting in Worcester (where the PFI hospital had immediately run out of beds), the Oxford Radcliffe Hospitals (£13.6 million deficit), Manchester (where PCTs were facing a £27 million total shortfall), Bristol and Cornwall.

The final months of 2004, with an election approaching, saw deficits projected to reach unprecedented levels across the country. A snapshot survey of England's Strategic Health Authority websites by London Health Emergency revealed combined deficits in excess of £500 million by November – but the very patchy and late publication of figures meant that this figure was likely to be a serious underestimate, as Trusts grappled with ever-more ambitious government targets and slammed on the brakes in a last ditch effort to balance the books.

A *Daily Mail* telephone survey of 72 NHS Trusts in late November showed that two-thirds of them were in deficit, and some were implementing major cutbacks.

- Leeds Teaching Hospitals Trust, facing a £16 million shortfall had closed eight wards (250 beds) and four operating theatres
- Southampton University Hospitals Trust, £11 million in the red, had axed 85 beds, merged two wards, cut out 400 jobs and imposed 100 redundancies
- Hammersmith Hospitals, £6 million in the red, had closed 90 beds and limited staff recruitment
- Oxford Radcliffe Hospitals Trust, seeking to address an underlying £42 million deficit, had made specialist nursing staff redundant – while spending £20 million a year on agency staff

- Bradford Teaching Hospitals Trust, the Foundation Trust whose deficit had rocketed from a projected £4 million to £11.3 million, had axed five wards and four operating theatres

- St George's Hospital, South London, facing a deficit of between £20 million and £35 million, had barely scratched the surface with the closure of 24 beds and axing 100 mainly vacant posts.

As Trusts contemplated their options for saving money with just four months of the financial year to go, an extra pressure compelling them into action was the new Resource Allocation Budgeting (RAB) set of rules, which for the first time prevented them spending money from their capital funds to bail out the revenue account. The stock response from the Department of Health was that Trusts could borrow their way out of trouble by approaching the NHS Bank for a loan. Health Secretary John Reid insisted that ministers would not bail out Trusts in financial crisis. Replying to the Commons Health Committee in November, he argued that pumping extra cash into Trusts facing deficits just meant that somewhere else a patient would have to wait longer in pain. "If necessary Trusts facing financial problems should change their management," suggested Dr Reid (*Health Emergency* 60, 2004).

By the summer of 2005, when Patricia Hewitt took over as Secretary of State after New Labour's historic third election victory, the *Health Service Journal* was warning that 8,000 jobs were likely to be axed in English Trusts and PCTs as SHAs battled to clear deficits which totalled more than £750 million (*HSJ*, 14 July 2005). Strategic Health Authority chiefs had even hatched out a bizarre plan by which 11 of the SHAs with the smallest overall financial shortfall would lend money to bail out the six SHAs regarded as financial basket-cases with "no hope" of clearing debts in 2005–6. A middle group of 11 SHAs would need to make "significant savings" to balance their books by March 2006, when the Payment by Results regime would begin to throw the system back into the melting pot.

The Department of Health had reportedly brokered the scheme, under which SHAs which were still in the black would offer loans totalling £200 million on terms which ensured interest payments of at least 10 per cent per year – more than the level then charged by many credit cards.

The six hopeless cases that would need to borrow the cash were NW London, Norfolk, Suffolk and Cambridgeshire, Bedfordshire and Hertfordshire, Surrey and Sussex, Hampshire and Isle of Wight, and Cheshire and Merseyside. This left some of the SHAs with the biggest individual problem Trusts in the middle group, where cutbacks were the order of the day, with up to 8,000 jobs predicted to go.

Obviously, Trusts within the other 14 SHAs would also be adding their contribution to the cuts, closures and redundancies that were set to be a feature of the NHS into the autumn and winter. What was clear to many health workers and campaigners was that for a lot less than the £3 billion she had controversially just allocated to purchasing more elective treatment from the private sector, Patricia Hewitt could have wiped out the cumulative debts that were dragging down Trusts and services across England, and expanded NHS services to meet the government's targets.

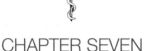

CHAPTER SEVEN

Hewitt and Blair crank up the pace 2005–2008

Two faces of Patricia Hewitt MP

1) The "listening" Secretary of State:

Over the next three months I will be doing a lot of listening and learning from the real experts – patients and staff. I intend to get around all parts of the NHS, finding out for myself what patients feel about the care they are receiving and shadowing staff as they carry out their duties. I will listen to everyone, whether medics or midwives, cleaners, porters or physiotherapists, stop-smoking teams or our new breed of personal health advisors.

(Department of Health, Tuesday 10 May 2005, 17:22)

2) Three days later, the relentless Blairite moderniser:

While I am Health Secretary there will be no let-up in the pace of reform and no change in the direction of our modernisation. That's why I have announced today that the NHS will purchase an extra 1.7 million operations from the independent sector over the next five years.

(*The Scotsman*, Friday 13 May 2005)

BY ELECTION DAY 2005, on the face of it, the NHS was looking pretty good. Spending on the NHS, at £67 billion, was running at twice the level that Gordon Brown inherited from the Tories in 1997. More than 2,000 extra acute hospital beds had opened up, waiting lists had been drastically reduced, along with waiting times, and the equivalent of more than 270,000 additional doctors, nurses and support staff had been added to the payroll. But despite all these positive changes, the coming autumn and winter already threatened headlines of cuts, closures and a large wave of redundancies across English hospitals and PCTs. Questions were beginning to be raised over where all the extra money had gone and how wisely it had been spent.

The strangely relaxed attitude of the Department of Health at the beginning of the year to the spectacle of dozens of Trusts and many Primary Care Trusts (PCTs) failing by miles to hit their financial targets, could be directly explained by the imminence of the general election: nobody had wanted to trigger a round of pre-poll closures. But some NHS finance chiefs were soon complaining that their earlier warnings of problems getting worse had been downplayed or dismissed in the months up to 5 May, resulting in even bigger problems to be confronted afterwards.

For exactly the same reason ministers had staged a tactical withdrawal on their plans to force through the new 'Payment by Results' (PBR) system, which had been planned to be the method of financing 70 per cent of NHS treatment from 1 April – but which also threatened to push dozens of hospital Trusts and even more specialist departments over the edge, triggering wholesale cuts and closures. Roll-out had been held back to April 2006. Some even began to doubt whether the full PBR policy would ever be implemented, for fear of the consequences in terms of the closure of busy local hospitals.

However, the PBR system helped New Labour turn health care back into a marketable commodity, and break down the post-1948 barriers between the public and private sectors: this in turn would enable them to switch more work to private sector providers. Ministers clearly wanted to build up sufficient capacity in the private sector to generate a real fear that failing NHS Trusts would be allowed close down, with services delivered from alternative private providers. Early in 2005 the government had invited private tenders to deliver a further 250,000 operations a year, worth an estimated £500 million annually: in addition another £400 million worth of X-rays, scans, blood tests and pathology tests were to be hived off to the private sector. These moves would almost double the number of private sector operations to be purchased by the NHS, pushing the government's total spend in the 'independent sector' up towards £1.5 billion – two-thirds of the total £2.3 billion turnover of the private medical industry in 2003.

Their plan was no longer for an 'internal' market – but simply a market system, in which NHS Trusts would have to compete not only against other NHS Trusts, but also against private hospitals which have a much more selective – and thus much less complex and costly – caseload, with no emergencies to deal with. So, bizarrely, NHS hospitals, under the cosh to deliver endless year-on-year 'efficiency' savings were now told they would be allowed to spend taxpayers' money on advertising to attract patients. The pace of the competition was to be forced by putting the responsibility not on to Primary Care Trusts, but on to individual patients, who would be offered a progressively wider 'choice' of where to have their treatment, but not made aware that the potential consequences of their decisions could include forcing the closure of their own local NHS hospital.

By the end of 2005, Primary Care Trusts would be obliged to offer almost all elective patients a 'choice' of providers – including at least one private hospital – from the time they were first referred: but eventually (from 2008) Blair had pledged that any patient would be allowed to choose any hospital which could deliver treatment at the NHS reference cost. Ministers began to insist that 'patient choice' was a more fundamental principle than maintaining local access to NHS hospital services, following a line from Tony Blair:

> Choice is not a betrayal of our principles. It IS our principles.
>
> (Knight 2004; Eaglesham 2003)

What the New Labour scenario did not address was the wide range of emergency and other services which have only ever been available from NHS hospitals, and which the private sector has shown no interest in providing. NHS Trusts would have to close services which attracted too few patients, and the NHS Bank was told to stand by and offer "support to services in transition, where exit or recovery is needed."

Almost as soon as the votes had been counted in the 2005 General Election the real scale of the financial crisis facing England's NHS Trusts and Primary Care Trusts began to emerge. Within days of the 5 May General Election the first cuts in hospital services began to hit the headlines locally and nationally: Lewisham Hospital in SE London was among the first, revealing an £8.5 million deficit and plans for ward closures (Ebrey and Revel 2005).

The new Health Secretary, Patricia Hewitt, was reportedly astonished at the size of some of the deficits, but instead of listening to the reasons for them, immediately ordered Trusts to take whatever action was necessary to balance the books – and not to expect any additional injection of government funding.

Health workers may have been groaning under the non-stop barrage of reforms, but Ms Hewitt clearly believed that the instability her government's policies had created was good for the NHS. In a 14 June interview with the *Financial Times* correspondent Nick Timmins, she admitted that too many NHS staff feel that "change upon change has been done to them, rather than with them", but spelled out the scenario:

> It's not only inevitable, but essential that payment by results and these other elements create instability and change for the NHS. That is precisely what they are designed to do.
>
> Yes there is a real risk of a unit closing because it simply can't deliver the quality of care and the value for money that all of us as patients and taxpayers want.

The changes would be rammed through in the next two or three years, in the hope that voters would have forgotten by the next big polling day:

> It's much better to take the pain and change now – in the first year or two after a general election, than to do it in the year or two running up to the next election.

Hewitt appeared to be firmly in denial, telling the *Health Service Journal* that while she had her foot "flat down on the accelerator" of reform, it would be "ridiculous" to imagine that hospitals would close all over the country as a result of her policies (*HSJ*, 16 June 2005). And she argued on BBC radio's *Today* programme a week later that there was "no question" of putting hospitals delivering A&E services in jeopardy "because the A&E service is absolutely essential." (*Today*, BBC Radio 4, 24 June 2005)

Not everyone agreed with her: some calls for a change of line came from unexpected quarters. The *HSJ* reported appeals from a health authority chief executive and from Bill Moyes, the chair of Monitor, the Foundation Trust regulator, for the government to write off the debts of some of the struggling

Trusts. Many had debts so large that Moyes would not have been able to rubber stamp their applications for Foundation status by the target date of 2008. He went on to point out that many Trusts which appeared to have broken even had in fact concealed deficits by in-year borrowing ("brokerage") which simply stores up long-term problems.

A survey of top NHS managers by the NHS Confederation found that two-thirds of them did not believe their organisations could meet all of the government's targets for improving services with their current levels of funding. Four out of five believed that unless funding levels continued to increase at the rate they have been in the last few years, patient care would decline after 2008, when the NHS Plan allocations came to an end. A third of the managers responding felt that the quality of care would not be improved by offering patients more choice on where to get their non-emergency surgery.

As the NHS braced itself to publish figures showing more Trusts running bigger debts than ever before, Hewitt told managers at the NHS Confederation's conference in Birmingham that more reform to the already massively "reformed" system was not an optional extra, but "your highest priority". Managers were failing to tap in to "major productivity gains to be had from the extra investment already in the system", insisted Hewitt. She went on to demonstrate how little she had learned in just over a month in the job when she argued that the key to improved productivity was reducing average length of stay for hospital inpatients, ignoring the fact that many hospitals were struggling to discharge patients because of a lack of adequate support from other agencies – PCTs, community services and social services, all of which were also faced by heavy financial pressures (Hewitt 2005).

Among the many soaring deficits that came to light, one of the biggest appeared to be the £30-million-plus hole in the finances of the Surrey and Sussex Healthcare Trust. Auditors warned that without an additional injection of government funding the Trust would effectively be bankrupt, failing its statutory duty to break even over the three years to March 2006. So desperate was the financial plight at the end of the 2004–5 financial year that the Trust board considered delaying March staff salaries to April and withholding PAYE tax and national insurance payments to make the deficit seem smaller: a full payment of debts outstanding would have left it £36 million in the red (PricewaterhouseCoopers 2005).

Another straw in the wind was the combined deficits of Oxfordshire Trusts and PCTs, which totalled over £50 million, with South Oxfordshire PCT topping the list with a staggering £25 million deficit. Across six of its community hospitals, 37 beds were to close. North Oxfordshire PCT had been offered a £4 million handout towards its shortfall of £10 million, and was looking at handing over community hospitals in Bicester and Chipping Norton, complete with staff, to private management. The third PCT, Oxford City, was planning to cut the skill mix of its nursing staff, and hoping to cut emergency admissions by 15 per cent to cut costs by £3 million. Oxford Radcliffe Hospitals Trust, which claimed to have cut £20 million from spending in the previous year faced another £11.7 million cuts which "may require the Trust to reduce service capacity" (*Health Emergency* 61, 2005).

The logic of Hewitt's position was simple: any hospital that failed to balance its books must also have failed to attract sufficient patients – and patients had therefore exercised their choice. Since patient choice was the main mantra of New Labour's NHS policy, those hospitals which were not chosen would be allowed to close. "I am not going to force patients to choose services they don't want", she told NHS employers (Timmins 2005a).

But she had made no equivalent promise to patients whose first choice would be to use services at their local NHS hospital, but who faced being dispatched for private sector treatment to meet new privatisation targets for Primary Care Trusts.

Crisp provokes a crunch

Normally the middle of a sleepy holiday period, 28 July 2005 marked the launch of a round of restructuring and "reforms", unveiled in a circular to NHS managers by NHS chief executive Sir Nigel Crisp. While Crisp purported to be re-shaping the way services were commissioned "to reflect patient choices", it was all too obvious that the very last people to have been consulted – or have their views taken into consideration – were patients. Even though Crisp and ministers insisted that the reforms were reshaping "from the bottom upwards", it was clear that the opposite was the case: the reforms were being relentlessly driven from the top, allowing no time to hear or heed critical views from professionals or the public.

In fact opinion polls and surveys confirmed that the first choice of NHS patients was the opposite of government policy: people wanted continued access to comprehensive local NHS services in the hospitals they knew and loved. In a BMA-commissioned YouGov poll of June 2005, "Choice" came bottom of a list headed by clean hospitals and improved A&E (BMA 2005). Most of the public had been bemused and disorientated by the constant rounds of 'reform' that had stripped away the old local health authorities and the recognisable Regional Health Authorities, only to bring in a confusing and constantly changing system involving varying permutations of Trusts, Primary Care Trusts and Strategic Health Authorities (SHAs); and scrapped the Community Health Councils that once had a brief to stand up for local people, replacing them with a baffling array of toothless and pointless bodies that few people heard about or understood.

Meanwhile, many news editors on newspapers and in the broadcast media had also succumbed to confusion and change fatigue, and simply stopped covering health policies. Indeed, there had been so little press coverage or public debate on the various rounds of NHS 'reform' since the public debates over Foundation Trusts that few people, even among NHS staff, would have been able to make head or tail of Sir Nigel's latest far-reaching proposals. Nevertheless, the policies set out in Crisp's circular of 28 July, 'Commissioning a Patient Led NHS', were important: they set out to drive another critical nail into the coffin of an NHS based on principles of planning and social justice. This would open the door still wider to a health care "market" in which health care would be reduced to a commodity, and NHS providers forced to compete at every level with the private sector and rival NHS providers, with the losers going to the wall.

In 2005 PCTs, which held the purse strings for most health care services, employed upwards of 250,000 health workers, many of them delivering community and mental health care. Crisp's plan would have meant the PCTs would have to be broken up, and reduced to commissioning only, with their role in provision of services "reduced to a minimum". It was never made clear how this would be done: services may have been hived off to existing Trusts, privatised, or handed to the voluntary sector.

PCTs also faced the prospect of more mergers, on the basis of plans to be drawn up not by patients or health workers but by SHAs. Sir Nigel's 28 July circular gave the SHAs until 15 October to submit proposals – which would then be vetted by the Department of Health, and in some cases then put out to "consultation" at the end of November. SHAs themselves were also to face mergers, even though there were only 25 of them in England, already covering large areas and populations. Mergers would inevitably make them less local and even less accountable: one of the targets of the new reforms was to cut management and administrative spending by a minimum of 15 per cent (£250 million).

Meanwhile in the same circular Crisp tried to pressurise PCTs to ensure that the commissioning of all contracts for services was transferred to groups of GP practices "no later than the end of 2006" – although it was by no means clear that many GPs wanted this additional responsibility. This new policy was the direct opposite of the Department of Health's own guidance just seven months earlier that "There are no targets: we simply have the aspiration that all practices will be involved in Practice based Commissioning by 2008" (NHS Confederation 2004).

There were problems too for hospital Trusts, many of which were facing huge problems as a result of long-term deficits, to be compounded by a new system of "Payment by Results" to be introduced next spring. The 28 July circular insisted that Trusts had to be press-ganged by SHAs down the road of Foundation Trust status, despite the fact that many were carrying deficits which would rule out any serious application to the regulator.

The focus of the circular – and the flurry of activity which followed – was purely on "commissioning", emphasising the purchaser–provider split and the new market-style system emerging under the NHS Plan, and strengthening up the "commissioners". Proposals emerged almost immediately in Oxfordshire to merge the county's PCTs and privatise the commissioning role bringing in a large corporation – universally believed to be UnitedHealth – to use its alleged expertise in helping to carve up the £600 million annual budget for health services (Lloyd and Donnelly 2005).

Even where privatisation was not part of the proposal, the process of restructuring was designed to cut spending on NHS hospital care, diverting more patients to private providers, and encouraging GPs and PCTs to "free up" cash by developing alternative forms of "care outside of hospital".

Exactly how this could result in a "patient-centred NHS" remained a mystery to all but Sir Nigel, Hewitt's ministerial team, and their backroom band of pro-market advisors. Angry trade unionists joined with frustrated and befuddled Labour backbenchers to protest at the scheme, which had been hatched up by a few back-room mandarins and health ministers without any wider discussion. After months of protests and pressure some of the more outlandish proposals were toned down, postponed or dropped: Patricia Hewitt even came to a UNISON seminar and a conference of chief nurses and apologised for having got it wrong (Mulholland 2005).

The proposal to hand over responsibility for commissioning and control of Oxfordshire's health budget to a private company generated such a unanimous tide of local protest, linking all parties in condemnatory votes on the County Council, inflaming the anger of GPs, winding up trade unionists and galvanising MPs in opposition, that ministers were eventually obliged to step in and call a halt to the experiment. The SHA was told to drop – or at least postpone – its plans, and it seemed that the issue of privatised commissioning had been put on the back burner.

Autumn query: where has the money gone?

If spending had doubled since 1997, why were so many Trusts and PCTs in such deep trouble? September 2005 saw the first serious attempt to provide answers, in the form of a major report from the NHS employers' body, the NHS Confederation, entitled *Money in the NHS: The Facts* (NHS Confederation 2005). It cited the 2002 Wanless report into NHS funding, which had calculated the cumulative under-spend between 1972 and 1998 at up to £267 billion, to explain why almost three-quarters (73 per cent) of the additional money in 2004–5 was allocated to services that had previously been "chronically underfunded". This increased spending included 30 per cent on employing new staff, and 20 per cent on increased pay.

When the Labour government had taken over in 1997, many Trusts were already facing deficits which had been "managed" by one-off financial measures year by year. And for the first three years of the new government, in which Gordon Brown upheld Tory cash limits, and NHS spending only rose marginally against inflation, the deficits continued unresolved. Some Trusts had carried forward deficits in one form or another ever since: others had been better resourced. When the new government policy of substantial real terms increases in NHS spending year on year was introduced from 2001, every additional £1 million pumped in to the NHS came with NHS Plan strings attached – in the form of at least an additional £1 million worth of new targets, including reduced waiting lists and waiting times, and improved performance in A&E.

The NHS Confederation reported that just 20 per cent of the extra money had been spent on providing additional services, which had delivered a dramatic cut in waiting times, and noted a substantial increase in the numbers of staff across the health service, with an extra 230,000 staff in post by 2005. But staff cost money: pay settlements for GPs and consultants and the European Working Time Directive had substantially increased costs for PCTs and NHS Trusts, while the new Agenda for Change pay reforms had also increased the overall pay bill across all sections of staff: the Commons Health Committee in 2006 blamed the rising deficits in part on "poor central management", noting the "hopelessly unrealistic" government estimates of the costs of these contracts, while targets such as the four-hour maximum wait in A&E had imposed extra costs (Commons Health Committee 2006: 42).

External supplies and services from the private sector had gone up in price even more rapidly than the pay bill. The NHS Confederation pointed out that the drug bill had increased by 46 per cent in five years, to £8 billion, pushed upwards by costly new drugs (like the cancer drug Herceptin) and increased use of drugs like statins (up six-fold to £720 million a year), while PFI schemes were forcing up overhead costs and taking an increased share of NHS Trusts' income, averaging 11 per cent of the total budgets of 60 Trusts. Costs of the new IT systems needed to implement the government's controversial "choice" agenda were also rocketing upwards, even though the introduction of the new system had been postponed yet again (NHS Confederation 2005).

There were other upward pressures on spending. The constant national-level reorganisation of the NHS had consumed management time and resources and confused and demoralised staff: the 2005–6 shake-up, involving the merger and restructuring of SHAs and Primary Care Trusts, was the fifth major change since 1997. Preparation for the new, competitive system of "Payment by Results" in April had further increased administrative costs for Trusts, and left some sections of NHS departments under-used and less efficient.

New rules introduced by the Treasury from 2004 had prevented NHS Trusts and PCTs from resorting to the age-old trick of switching money from their capital accounts (to pay for new buildings, repairs and new equipment) to revenue to avert larger deficits, and begun to "double" deficits by penalising overspending Trusts: the result had been ever-larger deficits showing up on balance sheets. Throughout much of the previous financial year (2004–5) it had been clear that many Trusts and PCTs were running up large and unbridgeable deficits, with National Audit Office figures (a relatively conservative estimate) showing 28 per cent of Trusts in the red in 2004–5,[18] sharing an estimated underlying deficit of £328 million (Commons Health Committee 2006: 9): but this was the run-in towards the 2005 General Election, when there was little if any government pressure to balance the books at the expense of politically embarrassing cuts in services.

---

18 This number was up from 8 per cent in 2001–2, rising to 31 per cent in 2005–6 (Commons Health Committee 2006).

As a result, much larger debts than usual were rolled over into the 2005–6 financial year, and this was the background to the paradoxical cash crisis: the NHS was receiving more money than ever, but facing much bigger cuts than at any time in its history. By February 2006, the King's Fund analysis of new data from the Department of Health suggested that nearly 40 per cent of the £4.5 billion cash increase for Hospital and Community Health Services (HCHS) would be absorbed by pay rises, with higher prices and increases in costs associated with NICE recommendations, clinical negligence and increased costs for capital estimated to absorb a further 32 per cent of the increase.

Damaging as they were, the first round of cuts, job losses and "efficiencies" proposed by Trusts fell far short of the sums needed convincingly to balance the books or secure recurrent balance for future years. That's why a round of limited cutbacks in the summer and autumn of 2005 was followed early in 2006 by a fresh round of real, painful cuts in jobs and services, affecting not only Trusts with large carried over debts but also other Trusts seeking savings to balance the books in the financial year 2006–7.

On 16 February 2006, Tony Blair himself staged a formal "welcome" into the "NHS family" for eleven profit-hungry private companies. This spectacle followed the shambolic hand-over of the supply of bottled oxygen to vulnerable patients at home to four profit-seeking companies – with predictably disastrous consequences (Norfolk and Lister 2006; Cressey 2006). Blair signalled an even bigger bonanza on the way for the private sector, predicting that the NHS would soon be purchasing up to 40 per cent of private operations, meaning a huge expansion programme for private providers… at the expense of widespread crisis and closures in the NHS (Mulholland 2006). In some areas and specialties this would mean private providers creaming off a majority of routine surgical cases from NHS Trusts: this would not only have a financial impact, but would strike a body blow at the training of junior doctors, and at medical research which is only carried out in major NHS University hospitals.

Shortly after her appointment as Health Secretary, Patricia Hewitt had announced a second round of "Independent Sector Treatment Centres" in England, to share out the additional £3 billion to be spent on NHS-commissioned private treatment (Johnston 2005). However, NHS hospitals – even Foundation Trusts – were excluded from the bidding process: the "competition" would be between Blair's 11 greedy private sector "partners" to carve up the available contract income between them. The Department of Health document proposing the second wave of ISTCs no longer claimed that the private sector was being brought in to create additional capacity. It admitted that under DoH direction waiting list operations would be *transferred* from NHS hospitals to private providers (leaving under-used departments with inflated costs and a caseload of complex, chronic and costly patients the private sector does not want). Indeed, *because* the services were being transferred, the DoH argued that it should also allow the transfer of NHS staff to carry out the work – permitting them to be seconded from NHS hospitals: publicly funded NHS treatment centres and facilities were also likely to be handed over to private operators.

As if all this was not a big enough bonanza for the private sector, there was even more to come. PCTs were still required to hive off their directly provided services, some of which could be an attractive proposition for private companies: but there was also a chance to get in on a new primary care market. The first GP practices were already being privatised, and giant US corporation UnitedHealth had set up a European subsidiary with a long-term plan to grab control of the multi-billion budget for commissioning primary and community health care and hospital care for local populations.

To cap it all, the ostensibly bland new NHS White Paper contained a provision for local service users to be able to petition to force their local Primary Care Trust to put any public sector NHS service out to competitive tender from "any willing provider". All this had always been a one-way process: New Labour ministers had never suggested any corresponding right for patients or local people aggrieved at the abysmal quality of privatised services to force them to be brought back in-house.

Every aspect of this new policy agenda centred on New Labour's bizarre and baseless ideological conviction that the private sector is always somehow superior in quality to public services.

Payment by Results

The PBR scheme, which had begun on a relatively small scale, was due to be rolled out on a generalised basis to cover 60 per cent of hospital Trusts' budgets from April 2006 – but it was already deep in crisis. The final weeks of Sir Nigel's tenure as chief executive were marked by a shambolic decision by the Department of Health: the basic tariff of reference costs, which stipulate how much Trusts will be paid for each item of treatment, had to be withdrawn and rewritten at the last minute – leaving Trusts, PCTs and would-be Foundation Trusts completely in the dark. The situation was aptly summed up in a *Health Service Journal* cover headline "It's a total cock up" (2 March 2006).

Many campaigners and union activists saw the PBR system as part of the same process of fragmentation that underpinned the reorganisation proposals. As Hewitt had said right at the beginning, the destabilisation – and enforced rationalisation – of existing NHS units was another important part of the government plan. It was clear that from the chaos and downsizing of the NHS they aimed to create space for a growing and sustainable private sector, delivering care commissioned and funded from NHS budgets.

To cap it all, it was becoming increasingly obvious that the promised savings of £250 million across England from the reorganisation of PCTs and SHAs would not be achieved. The Commons Health Committee estimated likely savings of, at most, between £60 million and £130 million – between a quarter and a half of the projected total. The West Midlands plan to close 66 per cent of existing SHAs was predicted to save just 53 per cent of the current core budget of just over £14 million.

Crisp becomes toast

Sir Nigel Crisp abruptly resigned as NHS chief executive on 7 March: he took early retirement at the age of just 54, standing down from his £200,000-plus annual salary with the consolation of a £100,000 early retirement package and a reported overall pension package worth £3.2 million (Helm and Hall 2006; *Daily Express*, 8 March 2006).

Although it was hotly denied by Tony Blair and by other government spokespeople, it was widely believed that Crisp was being forced out, effectively carrying the can for a succession of policy failures. These included his 28 July circular launching the first abortive move to divest PCTs of their direct services; hopelessly inaccurate projections of NHS deficits; a reorganisation of Strategic Health Authorities that he himself had established just three years earlier; a catastrophic blunder in calculating Payment by Results tariffs; and a ludicrous suggestion in the midst of a rising tide of shortfalls and crisis cutbacks that the NHS should be starting not just to balance the books but to run with a surplus. He had visibly fallen out with his Health Secretary, Patricia Hewitt, and with her team of marketising advisors (Timmins 2006a).

Beyond any dispute was the fact that NHS deficits were still rising rapidly despite frantic injunctions from Crisp himself and leading DoH bureaucrat Duncan Selbie. Four days before the end of month 11 of the 2005–6 financial year, Selbie issued a diktat to NHS finance chiefs instructing them to take "immediate action" to tackle the worsening NHS financial situation and to sign off plans to "materially improve the position for months 11 and 12." Local managers were warned that Crisp himself would personally be checking on their progress. At the same time, bungling DoH apparatchiks were recalling the tariff of fees they had sent out for the roll-out of Payment by Results because errors had been detected at the last minute. At the end of February, Trusts and PCTs were left in the dark on how much they would receive or pay for treatment beginning in April.

Days later Sir Nigel had "retired".

Another reorganisation: another phoney consultation

The proposal for the mergers of Strategic Health Authorities across much of England, and the accompanying proposals to merge many of the existing PCTs to form county-wide or rural-plus-urban PCTs were set out in a series of consultation documents early in 2006. Each of the documents carried as an introduction a letter from Sir Nigel Crisp, to make it quite clear that the proposals flowed from his controversial circular to all NHS managers the previous July – 'Commissioning a Patient Led NHS' – which pressed for the separation of PCTs' commissioning role from their direct provision of services. This was curious, since by the time the consultation process began, Sir Nigel had already been forced out of his position as chief executive.

All of the consultation documents were desperately lacking in detail, ignoring the underlying context and framework within which this further reorganisation of the NHS was taking place. Campaigners argued that the process towards mergers of PCTs was being driven by an accelerating national drive towards the fragmentation, privatisation and marketisation of the NHS.

Crisp questions

Sir Nigel's call for PCTs to divest themselves of their directly provided services had not by any means been withdrawn: it still left unanswered the question of who should take over these services. Did he mean it to be the private sector? The voluntary sector? Or other sections of the NHS – perhaps local hospital Trusts would be encouraged to move back in to an expanding community and primary care sector?

Who did Sir Nigel expect would be employing up to 250,000 hard-working PCT staff once his full proposals had come into effect, reducing the PCTs to a role of commissioners by 2008, delivering no further services themselves? And, since he was now an ex-chief executive, why did his views matter anymore anyway?

Strikingly, Crisp himself, right up to the point of his enforced "early retirement", never offered any clarification or assurances despite the wave of anger which during the autumn of 2005 forced many Labour MPs to make strong representations to ministers, and ministers reluctantly to step in and insist that there was no actual instruction for all PCTs to divest themselves of all services immediately.

Despite these assurances it was clear in 2006 that many PCTs were continuing to work towards precisely the separation of services that ministers had disavowed. The Commons Health Committee, in a hard-hitting report of December 2005 expressed itself "appalled" at the lack of clarity over the future of services provided by PCTs, and unconvinced by ministerial assurances.

The MPs concluded that:

> As far as we can see the overall direction of travel in fact remains unchanged, and PCTs will ultimately divest themselves of provider services.
>
> (Changes to Primary Care Trusts, 15 December 2005, para.35, p.16)

Largely indifferent to the Committee, making no secret of her agenda, and defending the line of privatisation, Health Secretary Patricia Hewitt went as far as to claim at a press briefing on 17 February that PCT staff were eager to be privatised:

> there was "widespread enthusiasm" from staff to move out of the NHS and work for the social enterprises invited to bid for primary care provision.
>
> She called for "unions and professional bodies to start to see it as something which their own members are very interested in, and that there is a need out there to which they should be responding".
>
> (*HSJ*, 23 February 2006: 7)

However, there is no evidence at all that market-based health care could deliver a comprehensive health service, address issues of equity and health inequalities, or improve the quality of care. Nor, of course would more private-sector services save money: evidence from around the world confirms that far from reducing costs, competitive systems in health care increase transaction costs, requiring more bureaucracy and administration, while private-sector providers will also always cream off an additional profit from any payments they receive.

It was this underlying background of marketisation and fragmentation that made it impossible to endorse the proposed reorganisation of SHAs and PCTs. The NHS needed some form of mechanism to make local services accountable to local people, and while the pre-Crisp PCTs and SHAs were far from perfect in this regard, the new, larger, and more remote PCTs threatened to make matters even worse, while offering no compensating improvements.

Fewer, larger, and less accountable PCTs were always going to be more vulnerable to future pressures from above to privatise, hive off or close down services. Even during the consultation process itself steps were taken towards the privatisation of GP services in Derby and in North Derbyshire – with rumours in the medical press that up to 15 per cent of GP practices across the country could be hived off in similar fashion to private companies such as UnitedHealth Europe or for-profit groups of GPs.

There was no reassurance in the consultation documents on SHA mergers, which said little or nothing about the proposed new bodies that would control billions in NHS budgets and in some cases span areas of thousands of square miles with millions of residents.

They said nothing about:

- How many members would sit on the new SHAs
- How they would be selected
- On what basis, for how long, or by whom
- Whether or not there would be any attempt to ensure geographical areas are represented
- Any means by which these new super-quangos might be held to account by any of the local people whose health care services would be under their control.

Staff cuts in Staffs

One of the first hospital Trusts to announce really large-scale redundancies was the University Hospitals of North Staffordshire Trust, which hit the financial skids in the final few months of 2005. In March 2006 it unveiled a plan to axe 1,000 jobs, almost 15 per cent of its workforce – including 370 nurses and midwives – as the cumulative financial shortfall hit £18 million. Health Secretary Patricia Hewitt named it as one of the 18 worst Trusts in England, and the financial melt-down had already brought the departure of two chief executives, a finance director, the Trust chair and all of its non-executive directors. A hard-hitting response from UNISON to the UHNS situation argued that – after six previous years in which the Trust had achieved balanced budgets – the crisis was not so much the result of individual management incompetence, but rather evidence of a systems failure within the NHS as a whole.

A lethal combination of ambitious targets to reduce waiting times, under-funded pay settlements, contradictory guidelines on prescribing, and soaraway inflation from the pharmaceutical industry and private sector providers had a forced busy, successful Trust into crisis (Lister 2006a).

In the period prior to the 2005 election, when NHS managers around the country were being tacitly urged to avoid making cuts to balance their books, UHNS managers had in addition been preparing their case to win support for a £400 million project for a new hospital, to be funded under the Private Finance Initiative (PFI). In seeking to minimise the apparent financial difficulties of the Trust, Trust managers had been doing exactly what ministers wanted them to do (Lister 2006a). The UNISON report concluded that there were no grounds to believe that the new replacement directors, or the government-appointed 'hit squads' of management consultants who were being wheeled in by the Strategic Health Authority and the Department of Health, would be any more successful at delivering the necessary level of services within an inadequate budget.

Flying in the face of opinion

The North Staffordshire announcement effectively breached the dyke, opening the way for a flood of similar job losses and cutbacks as NHS Trusts and Primary Care Trusts across the length and breadth of England wrestled with massive deficits. There was no relief in the form of a Budget hand-out from Gordon Brown: his speech made no mention of the NHS, effectively forcing the pace of painful changes and cutbacks. But in the midst of the chaos which grabbed many local and national headlines came an obscure report which helped to explain the scale and cope of the problems in the NHS.

The report had been commissioned by ministers from the so-called 'National Leadership Network', comprising a number of prominent NHS bosses, academics and top figures in NHS-related quangos. It was misleadingly entitled *Strengthening Local Services: The Future of the Acute Hospital*, although its proposals would have been viewed with dismay by most of those actively campaigning to protect their local hospitals and health care services from cutbacks. It focused on problems in sustaining services, and pressures towards a far-reaching new rationalisation of hospital services, and claimed that unchanged hospital services would "risk becoming unpopular, unstaffable, unsafe, unsustainable, resulting in service failure" (NHS National Leadership Network 2006).

In fact local NHS hospitals have remained among the most popular of all British public institutions: any threat to cut or close local NHS hospital services is the one thing most likely to provoke thousands of angry people of all ages and political persuasions into active protests and campaigning – while active, amateur supporters of the government's market-style reforms (which have been swallowed whole and without question by the "Leadership Network") have remained pathetically few and far between. It was also clear in the spring of 2006 that government policies – including the new spending squeeze that was forcing job losses, and also the promotion of a new private sector in health care that was eagerly poaching key sections of NHS staff and siphoning tens of millions from NHS Trust budgets – were the key factors collapsing morale and making NHS hospitals "unstaffable"; while the imposition "Payment by Results" threatened to render many existing NHS departments and whole hospitals unsustainable.

The Leadership Network proposals represented an attempt not to criticise or challenge these policies, but to accommodate the chaotic new system being ushered in as Tony Blair's legacy of "modernisation" and "reform". Hospital services were being remodelled not to meet patients' needs or wishes, but to meet the new economic pressures of a market system that was being artificially created – at enormous expense – to make room for a new, heavily protected private sector. So in place of what the "Leadership Network" derisively referred to as a "one size fits all" model of district general hospitals, it proposed 'networks' of hospitals and community services – and even a separation of emergency services from many of the surgical and other specialist services which are currently regarded as essential support for an A&E department. The end result of these proposals would be the downgrading and downsizing of many existing general hospitals, leaving many people who need emergency treatment facing much longer journeys or delays in accessing care.

The "Leadership Network" also suggested that A&E units could be managed without the on-site 24-hour access to services normally seen as vital – including emergency and specialised surgery, trauma and orthopaedics, paediatrics, obstetrics and gynaecology, and mental health. One of the driving forces pushing them to these outlandish conclusions was the acknowledged loss of a growing share of waiting list (elective) treatment from the NHS to new contracts with private sector hospitals and treatment centres.

In January, in an uncanny pre-echo of the Leadership Network's report two months later, Patricia Hewitt had told the *Financial Times* that her reforms would mean "reorganising services, reconfiguring hospitals, doing more treatment and diagnostics in the community, in primary care centres and community hospitals" because the NHS cannot "do everything, or as much as we are currently doing, in acute hospitals." The *FT* pointed out that this policy would mean the closure of some hospitals, with many more losing A&E departments and the full range of procedures (Timmins 2006b).

This proved the keynote for later reports. By the summer the NHS Confederation had jumped aboard the sinking ship, endorsing the NHS Leadership Network's call for a fresh round of rationalisation and bed closures. Dragging out a pathetically tired and inappropriate set of statistics, the NHS Confederation claimed that a third of NHS beds had closed over the 20 years to 2004 – without troubling to point out that the closures of acute hospital beds (which treat emergencies and waiting list cases) had effectively ground to a halt over ten years earlier, when hospitals recognised they could not cope with peaks in demand if any more beds closed. To confuse matters further, a large share of the beds closed over the two decades cited by the NHS bosses had not been acute hospital beds, but beds for mental health, learning difficulties and specialist long-stay beds for older people (Carvel 2006b).

Hewitt rouses the unions

April 2006 brought a rude awakening for Patricia Hewitt and her New Labour team, in a bruising encounter with reality at conferences of UNISON and the Royal College of Nursing. The staunchly pro-Labour UNISON health conference in Gateshead hung Hewitt out to dry, greeting her speech and statements with stony silence, and went on to adopt not just one but two emergency resolutions cranking up the union's resistance to the job cuts, hospital closures and privatisation she was trying to justify, promising to ballot for industrial action wherever cutbacks threatened members with compulsory redundancies. The non-affiliated RCN dropped even the trappings of politeness: whereas UNISON stewards had ordered delegates to take off campaigning T-shirts before the TV cameras came on to cover Hewitt's humiliation, dozens of normally staid and conservative RCN delegates sported T-shirts with the RCN's campaign slogan 'Keep nurses working: Keep patients safe' – and noisily gave the Health Secretary the bum's rush with cat-calls and booing that forced her to scrap half of her patronising speech. Afterwards, the RCN awoke from decades of inaction, and issued a call for resistance to cuts in nursing posts, publicly calling on its members to stop working unpaid overtime.

But while normal politics would dictate that ministers who find themselves in a hole should at least consider stopping digging, urged on by a speech from Tony Blair himself, they opted instead to press ahead with what a former government advisor, Professor Chris Ham, described as "creative destruction". Ham warned that if ministers stuck to their guns "the changes to the NHS so far will look like minor skirmishes compared with the bigger battles that lie ahead" (Ham 2006).

Instead, health minister Lord Warner stepped up a gear, and revealed the underlying strategy as he warned that local NHS hospitals would have to "face up to the need to reconfigure services" as a result of reforms which were aimed to enable new "independent sector providers" to enter the NHS market. The logic was simple enough: in order to make room for the development of a brand new private sector, Hewitt, Warner and Blair had to slash back existing NHS services. In other words, the NHS situation hitting daily headlines is not chaos but a cynical plan: busy, popular local hospitals were being deliberately driven into crisis, to force local management into rationalisation and closures. That was why deficits amounting to around £1 billion – just a few day's NHS spending – many of them historic deficits and the result of long-term under-funding were being used to force the pace and drive forward the closures.

The meaningless mantra of "health care closer to home" was also being wheeled out as a pretext to axe hospital care, regardless of whether any alternative community-based services were available, and oblivious to the parallel cutbacks in provision of social services and domiciliary support. But while ministers could get away with this among servile layers of NHS managers, they had not managed to convince any serious numbers of the wider public – nor the frontline health workers who now found themselves under the hammer. While ministers appeared to shut their eyes and ears to the evidence that their plans lacked even the most rudimentary public support, just one faint glimmer of reality appeared to have percolated through.

At the end of April, ministers were forced to announce a substantial retreat in the scale of their controversial second wave of Independent Sector Treatment Centres, due to be announced in the summer. Seven of the original 24 local schemes were axed, while the rest were postponed by up to a year, after a number of Strategic Health Authorities succeeded in persuading Department of Health bureaucrats that the new capacity was not required in their areas (*HSJ*, 27 April 2006).

Slamming the gate on patients

The summer of 2006 saw panic measures in London to ration numbers of patients referred by GPs to hospital consultants. News of the cash-led rationing scheme, which would process each GP referral through a team of bureaucrats in "referral management centres", broke with the publication of a leaked document. The London-wide clampdown on GP referrals and consultant-to-consultant referrals was imposed by top civil servant John Bacon (Davies and Elwyn 2006; Hawkes 2006a). In another covert measure to impose rationing irrespective of health needs, the Department of Health early in 2006 announced a bizarre new formula designed to reduce demand for emergency care, which would mean that hospital Trusts would be paid only half the standard rate for treating any "extra" patients admitted as emergencies above the previous year's levels. PCTs were also urged to limit elective referrals to a maximum of 3 per cent above 2005–6 levels (*HSJ*, 26 January 2006). Both these instructions from the Department of Health clearly rode roughshod over the notion of patient choice, and placed financial concerns above patient care.

Profiteers wanted

Ministers once again triggered a summer of controversy, this time by advertising to invite private insurance companies to take over control of a large slice of the £64 billion NHS commissioning budget. The first inkling of this proposal came in a front page article in the *Financial Times* (18 June), headlined 'Insurers invited into NHS economy'. *FT* correspondent Nick Timmins concluded that:

> The move is likely to attract interest from the big US insurers such as UnitedHealth and Kaiser Permanente, Discovery of South Africa, BUPA, PPP and Norwich Union in the UK, and possibly German and Dutch insurance funds.

At first sight the very notion was a sick and silly joke: putting these companies in charge of the NHS budget was like putting Dracula in charge of a blood bank. No wonder ministers had kept these plans close to their chest: with New Labour candidates already as popular with voters as a dose of herpes, which backbenchers would fancy their chances of persuading their constituency to welcome the arrival of Kaiser Permanente or UnitedHealth as the stewards of billions of taxpayers' money for health care?

To make matters worse, there was of course not the slightest shred of evidence that these insurance companies – which specialise in screening out and excluding potential subscribers with pre-existing illnesses, chronic conditions, and of course the low-paid and unemployed who cannot afford their premiums – have any relevant expertise that could inform the commissioning of a comprehensive health care service for a whole resident population of a PCT. The US companies in particular come from a system which consumes one dollar in six of the US national wealth, while leaving one American in six (51 million at the latest count) uninsured. They spend only around 70 cents of every health dollar on health care, carrying huge overhead costs including inflated salaries to chief executives whose pay and bonuses are dependent on holding down risks by excluding the poor – precisely those in most need of health care. US health care corporations have become collectively notorious for apparently defrauding the Federal government, and their own patients, to the tune of tens or hundreds of millions of dollars. What expertise could they offer to PCTs or other NHS managers seeking to deliver comprehensive and cost-effective care?

So while campaigners began to flag up the danger that was developing, it still seemed possible that the whole story was a kite-flying exercise to test out public response… until it was revealed that an advert had indeed been placed that week in the Official Journal of the EU, inviting companies to bid for framework contracts to deliver commissioning and management services to PCTs. The terms of this invitation made it quite clear that virtually all aspects of the PCTs' role were to be offered out to private bidders:

> This will include, but not be limited to, responsibility for population health improvement, the purchasing of hospital and community care, supporting local GPs develop practice-based commissioning [sic], the management and development of community health services for the PCT resident population, and other services.
>
> (Carvel 2006e; Lister S. 2006; *OJEU* 2006)

The new arrangement would leave the PCTs with next to nothing to do other than brew the tea and open the biscuits for occasional board meetings. So handing over these services to a multinational, multi-billion-dollar corporation would clearly sound the death knell for Primary Care Trusts, which had only been established in 2002, and which had just been extensively and expensively reorganised. However, once again, as it had been the previous autumn, the adventure was brought to a premature halt: the advert was suddenly withdrawn as a result of unexplained "drafting errors", and a letter from Hewitt was hastily published, attempting once again to assure an even more confused and sceptical public that there was no plan to privatise the NHS, leaving us with more proof of the old adage: never believe a rumour until it is officially denied (Fleming 2006).

Big business as usual

But in July it was back to privatisation as usual – not creeping, but galloping through the NHS. Ministers stamped the foot back on the accelerator, arrogantly stuck up two fingers to the wide cross section of union leaders, professional organisations and Labour MPs who had expressed concern over the advert – and gave the go-ahead to a fresh advert, which was identical in all essentials.

Nor were ministers the slightest bit deterred by the unexpectedly critical report by the Commons Health Committee on the way private sector treatment centres had been allowed to cherry pick a growing share of the least complicated NHS "elective" (waiting list) operations. Ministers casually brushed aside the MPs' evidence-based critique with a cosmetic sound-bite, and continued with plans for an ever-widening use of these costly units, whose benefits the MPs found questionable and unproven.

While first-wave treatment centres were already coining in guaranteed contracts and profits, many of them shamelessly milking the funds from local NHS Trusts while falling massively short of their contracted levels of work, BUPA was in pole position to win two more lucrative treatment centre contracts in Cheshire and Merseyside, involving some 6,000 operations a year (*HSJ*, 31 August 2006). Meanwhile, the prospect of a new treatment centre in Essex grabbing up to 20 per cent of the NHS Trust's elective income (£7.8 million a year) had been cited as a major factor in forcing Essex Rivers Healthcare Trust to scrap plans for a new £160 million PFI-funded hospital in Colchester (Bennett 2006).

While the NHS suffered painful cutbacks, the private sector was on a roll: the floodgates of privatisation were being wrenched open in other areas, too. Five commercial companies had been selected as "preferred providers" for a new £1 billion package of diagnostic procedures (X-rays and ultrasounds, etc.) over the next five years – yet another contract which had excluded any NHS providers from bidding (Timmins 2006c).

And after a high court judge rejected local appeals and rubber-stamped the bizarre tendering process which had allowed UnitedHealth Europe, a subsidiary of a major for-profit US health corporation, to secure a contract to deliver primary care services in rural Derbyshire despite having no staff, track record, expertise, or local links, the private carve-up of primary care services was beginning to accelerate. The primary care market was already estimated to be worth upwards of £150 million a year to the independent sector, and almost a third of Primary Care Trusts were already involved or beginning to put services out to tender (Marsh 2006).

There was also a bonanza in management consultancy work for city slickers such as PricewaterhouseCoopers and McKinsey, with hundreds of highly paid "experts" being brought in by local NHS Trusts and Primary Care Trusts to draw up "recovery" and "turnaround" plans – dressed up as "independent" advice. The Private Finance Initiative, along with the primary care equivalent, NHS LIFT, was back in business, too, despite evidence of its inflated costs: in Birmingham the long-delayed new hospitals project, the £553 million PFI-funded university hospital and psychiatric hospital, which was once promised to be a 'building-only' PFI, was signed, and turned out to include the full privatisation of support services – promising a long-term income stream of £300 million for the Balfour Beatty subsidiary.

To cap it all ministers were forcing through the biggest and what many critics regarded as one of the craziest privatisations of the lot, the carve-up of the award-winning (and profitable) NHS Logistics, the public sector organisation then in charge of more than £4 billion of NHS procurement budgets – handing the contract over to the Texas-based Novation, a company still under investigation for overcharging the US federal government for health supplies (Hawkes 2006b).

This lurch towards privatisation brought a welcome if unusual initiative from the TUC, which brought together a dozen or so organisations including the main health unions, professional bodies and the Royal College of Nursing to mount a major autumn campaign to defend the NHS against cutbacks and privatisation.

Given the mounting frustration and feeling of isolation that had haunted many local campaigns, a coordinated programme of action was very much what campaigners had been calling for. Even before this new action plan a UNISON regional protest in Cheltenham showed the potential, mobilising upwards of 5,000 protestors from the South West to challenge cutbacks and privatisation (BBC News online 2006a).

In a world of their own

Despite the evidence of opinion polls showing New Labour's health reforms had become an electoral liability (lagging in popularity behind even David Cameron's nebulous and largely identical policies on privatisation of the NHS) Hewitt and her team of kamikaze ministers closed their eyes and ears to the mass protests which were now an increasingly common occurrence in many of England's towns and cities. They were egged on by a Labour Conference in which it seemed almost every constituency delegate was from Fantasy Island. With speakers from the floor urging Hewitt to press on regardless, only the insistence and block votes of the trade unions ensured that a resolution calling for a slower pace of privatisation was eventually carried: almost two thirds of the hand-picked delegates from constituencies voted to support the government. Patricia Hewitt seemed a little disorientated when her headmistress-like speech was not heckled but even lamely applauded at New Labour's Manchester conference (Toynbee 2006).

Outside in the real world, New Labour's health policies had radicalised unlikely towns such as Hastings (5,000 marching), Chichester (4,000), Eastbourne (3,000), Worthing (4,000), Banbury (4,000), Epsom (5,000),

Cheltenham and Ludlow, along with much of Cornwall (27,000 on the march), with too many more local campaigns to list here (Keep Our NHS Public 2006). Many of the protests centred on cutbacks in local services. As if to whip up even more public hostility, Hewitt joined with NHS chief executive David Nicholson to support calls for the rationalisation of services in at least 60 hospitals across England, claiming that services would somehow be "improved" for patients through a process of closing down A&E units and replacing them with fewer, bigger A&E units and alternative, community-based models of care (Carvel 2006b; Wintour and Carvel 2006).

But her claims were devoid of supporting evidence. The arguments, echoing the theme kicked off by Hewitt at the beginning of the year, were endorsed in a provocative "Briefing" by the Blairite "think tank" IPPR, which in September revealed the results of a crude number-crunching exercise calculating the catchment populations of different hospitals. This led them to conclude that up to 58 A&E units should be closed in England – including nine in London (five of them in NW London) (IPPR 2006).

There was an immediate outcry. The BMA and the Royal College of Surgeons had initially (Revill 2006) been reported as endorsing the IPPR report (which had actually been part-funded by the BMA and the Royal College of Nursing) but were swift to issue denials and take their distance from findings which would threaten frontline emergency services in many parts of England (*HSJ*, 5 October 2006). Indeed far from there being any evidence to support a plan for fewer A&E units and any further reduction in hospital care, the most recent government statistics showed a continued and significant increase in numbers of patients attending A&E units, and an increase in numbers admitted as emergencies as a result. Across England the increase in attendances had been over 6 per cent. In other words, despite 15 years of rhetoric from successive Health Secretaries since Virginia Bottomley promising that a "primary care-led" policy would reduce the need for hospitals and unleash a new model of patient care, the reality was that more and more patients every year were still requiring hospital services, and there was little or no sign in most areas of community services developing to take their place (NHS Hospital Episode Statistics (HES), 2007).

In London – where many Primary Care Trusts faced major cash gaps, compounded by the "top slicing" of 3 per cent of their budgets to build a reserve to cover deficits – the increase in A&E attenders was far higher than the national average – 10 per cent overall, with some units notching up double digit increases. And with one in six London A&E patients requiring admission to hospital, any suggestion of closing even one of the smaller surviving A&E units in the capital raised serious knock-on implications for surrounding hospital Trusts – as well as threatening the future survival of the scaled-down hospital (Lister 2007b).

So while New Labour seemed deliberately to have destabilised hospitals and triggered high-profile and unpopular cuts, there was little to suggest that the system that would emerge out of this baptism of fire would be adequate to the actual pressures of patient needs. Worse, they had effectively dismantled any system for planning the allocation of health care resources to match local needs. Having laboriously forced down waiting lists and waiting times through expanding the NHS workforce, opening more beds and injecting some of the necessary resources, Hewitt and co. seemed set to force them back up again in many areas, as PCTs and Trusts struggled to balance their books by slashing back on patient care (Hall 2006).

As news leaked out that Labour chair Hazel Blears was working on a "heat map" to respond to local political pressure and minimise hospital closures in Labour marginal seats, ministers argued that the Department of Health had simply been tracking those areas where active campaigns were challenging their "rationalisation" of care. Either way the message was clear: if you wanted to save your hospital you had to keep the heat on ministers, MPs, and councillors (Carvel and Mostrous 2006).

The health unions responded by calling a lobby of Parliament for 1 November.

Third way to NHS privatisation

The White Paper *Our Health, Our Say…* was published in January 2006. Despite an overtly bland content it soon emerged as a significant new element driving Primary Care Trusts towards further and faster privatisation and "outsourcing" of services, reducing their own role to one of commissioning. In October 2006 the Department of Health implementation document *Making it Happen* stressed the need for "better partnership working with third and independent sectors".

The so-called "third" sector is a woolly category which ranges from voluntary sector organisations and charities (with their uneven record on accountability, employment practices, trade union recognition and quality of services) through to "social enterprise" and not-for-profit companies which run to all intents and purposes like a normal private business. Public schools, the Royal Opera House and even BUPA, Britain's largest private medical insurer, apparently all fit the model of "social enterprises". Apparently over 26,000 organisations described as "third sector" are currently involved in delivering health and social care services in England, with a combined annual income in excess of £13 billion (Lister 2007e, i; Amicus 2007).

In July 2006 a policy paper from the "Third Sector Commissioning Taskforce" had been published by the Department of Health, entitled *No excuses. Embrace partnership now*. It emphasised the government's relentless drive towards privatisation:

> delivering health and social care services is no longer the preserve of the public sector, and… third sector as well as private providers have a valuable role to play in shifting the balance of provision closer to where people live, and the type of responsive services people want.
>
> (DoH 2006a: i)

Indeed, local PCT bosses were urged to develop "partnerships" which would not only privatise the living, but also hive off the dying to various outsourced forms of care, with a brief to:

explore current and potential community resources, including workforce, community hospitals, third sector, independent and social enterprise provision; and create End of Life networks.

(DoH 2006a: 16)

Meanwhile newly reorganised PCTs were being pressurised into putting more and more of their directly provided services as well as more GP services out to competitive tender. To make matters worse, government hard-man Lord Warner insisted that there was "no excuse" for PCTs not pressing further ahead with the establishment of "Practice Based Commissioning" that would devolve a much greater share of NHS budgets to the level of GP practices – despite the clear evidence that very few GPs actually wanted to be lumbered with this level of managerial responsibility (Greener and Mannion 2006).

GP practices operating Practice Based Commissioning (PBC) are encouraged to address the needs only of the patients on their list, with an eye to balancing their books and retaining a surplus, but with no wider responsibilities for accessible services to the surrounding community. But some GP practices were also already being privatised, and PBC also meant that in those areas where private companies such as UnitedHealth Europe and others succeeded with bids to take over GP practice contracts they would also gain immediate access to a tasty slice of the NHS purchasing budget (Barrett 2006).

However, the whole rush towards privatisation has remained entirely a one-way process: while patients were to be encouraged to petition PCTs to press for services to be put out to competitive tender, with PCTs obliged to respond to as few as 1 per cent of their local population, there is still no corresponding mechanism through which patients angry at poor standards from private providers can insist they be brought back in-house.

Not much care in the community

New Year 2007 revealed the hidden crisis in care services for frail older people that had been taking shape behind the scenes of the high-profile debates over hospital care and the "reforms" in the NHS. The crisis stemmed from the far-reaching process of privatisation that began in the early 1980s but continued under Blair and Brown, and now leaves little public-sector provision for a crucial area of health and social care where the market has palpably failed.

A New Year report by the Local Government Association pointed out that if current trends continued, by 2009 no councils would be offering any preventative social care or packages of social services support for clients whose needs are classified as less than "critical" or "substantial" (Public Finance 2007a, b). Almost three-quarters of local authorities in England had already withdrawn domiciliary support from those judged to have low or moderate need for care – applying increasingly stringent "eligibility criteria" to escape the costs and responsibilities of sustaining a more comprehensive service. And the services that remain have been increasingly privatised – or, like the old home help services in many areas, effectively abolished. Well over 70 per cent of home care services are now privatised, with staff paid on minimal terms and conditions which often do not cover travel time between clients. The network of residential homes once run by social services has also been largely hived off to a burgeoning private sector (Lister 2002), while other private companies also control the vast majority of nursing home places – and remain free to pick and choose where they wish to provide services and where (such as in large areas of Greater London) they choose not to do so, thus leaving chronic shortages.

With many Primary Care Trusts also facing massive cash crises, the scope for expanding and improving support for patients discharged from hospital or needing help with living at home is increasingly limited: some services, especially in rural areas, are closing down, leaving new gaps in care and offering ever fewer options for frail older people and their families. Even where social services are available, they are subject to means-tested charges which still result in tens of thousands of people having to sell their homes and empty out savings accounts to pay for their continuing care in old age (Mandelstam 2007).

The landmark 1988 report by Sainsbury boss and Thatcher favourite Sir Roy Griffiths triggered a rapid rundown of NHS geriatric beds. Bed numbers plunged by 43 per cent in ten years, from 53,000 in 1987 to just 30,000 when Tony Blair took office in 1997. But the rapid rundown continued under New Labour: another 23 per cent closed to leave just under 23,000 specialist elderly care beds available, many running at near 100 per cent occupancy levels (DoH statistics, 2007). Many of the 3,000 beds that closed in the cash squeeze of 2006 were beds for older patients.

The disappearance of public sector and NHS provision has run alongside the expansion of long-stay beds in private sector nursing and residential homes, most of them for-profit, which now account for 89 per cent of care home places, providing over 373,000 places – almost three times the number of NHS general and acute beds. Increasing numbers of care home places are funded by the NHS – which only pays for nursing care: analysts Laing and Buisson estimate that 37,000 people (23 per cent of all independent sector nursing home residents) were NHS funded (Laing and Buisson 2007).

The numbers needing care are expected to increase: Gordon Brown's own figures in the pre-budget report pointed out that over the next decade the number of over 85-year-olds will increase by 38 per cent. NHS Trusts are being urged by accountants and Blairite "think tanks" to discharge older patients faster than ever to "care closer to home". But in reality the statistics show repeated year-on-year increases in numbers of emergency admissions to hospital – many of these frail older patients with medical rather than surgical problems, who have not been properly supported by primary care, community services or social services. Far from recognising or responding to the problem, and allocating increased resources to plug the gaps that have widened even in years of increased NHS spending, Gordon Brown as Chancellor demanded that social care make savings of 3 per cent on its already over-stretched budgets (Public Finance 2007b).

The inevitable result will be more frail older people left high and dry, discharged by the NHS to a non-existent system of care. It's hard to remember that these are the same ministers who came to office in 1997 blathering on about the need for "joined up government".

Mental health under attack

On 31 January, an angry one-day strike against job losses, downgrading, cuts in patient care and possible privatisation was staged by 250 Manchester nurses, therapists and support staff working in mental health. By the end of 2007, they were obliged to strike again, this time in defence of their victimised branch chair, Karen Reissmann, sacked by Manchester Community and Mental Health Trust for standing up in defence of services and patient care (MEN 2007a, b; Crook 2007).

More people with the courage of Karen Reissmann and her colleagues have been desperately needed in 2006 and 2007 as mental health services have been singled out around the country for some of the most devastating cuts.

Early in 2007 Patricia Hewitt's constituency patch of Leicestershire faced a double dose of mental health bed closures, confirmed as permanent in March (*Leicester Mercury* 2007a, b), and drastic cuts in consultant staffing were threatened in Oxfordshire's already battered mental health services, as well as cuts in Sheffield. More cuts were threatened in London, with drastic reductions in Brent PCT, and the threatened closure of two specialist services for older people in Lambeth and Southwark (Lister 2007a).

Meanwhile the Sainsbury Centre for Mental Health published a report arguing that if the government really wanted to implement its National Service Framework for mental health it would need to increase spending on services by 50 per cent in real terms, with a 40 per cent increase in staff. By contrast, at least one university that trained nurses for mental health and learning disability was announcing a fall-off in recruitment – arguing that the spectacle of redundancies among nurses had not helped attract able young applicants to join what were already shortage specialty courses (Boardman and Parsonage 2007).

It is impossible to avoid the conclusion that mental health and care of the elderly have been singled out as soft targets for cuts because they have little day to day media profile. This means that when campaigns are waged which force the cuts in mental health into the media, they can be very influential: the campaign to save the unique 24-hour mental health emergency clinic based at the Maudsley Hospital secured an extremely wide base of support from service users, relatives, community groups, most political parties and of course the UNISON health branch, which has for years been consistently challenging the mental health cuts in South East London. The opposition became so intense that the local "scrutiny committee" covering Lambeth and Southwark councils was even persuaded to refer the emergency clinic closure back to Patricia Hewitt, while her cabinet colleagues Harriet Harman and Tessa Jowell were among the MPs lobbying against closure. However, Hewitt was unmoved on the Emergency clinic, rubber stamping the closure and forcing the councils to consider a possible legal challenge. But already another UNISON-led campaign was under way to save the trail-blazing services at the Felix Post unit and the Eamon Fottrell unit in Lambeth, which deliver vital support to older patients, but faced closure to make savings of just £300,000 from a directorate budget of £26 million (Lister 2007a).

Even Ms Hewitt was not above seeking a cheap round of applause for a few trite phrases on mental health. In April 2007 she responded to campaigners by telling the Mind conference in Bournemouth that mental health Trusts would no longer be required to "bail out" other NHS organisations that overspend. It was "completely unfair" that mental health should face cuts on this basis, she argued (*HSJ* 2007). Who could disagree? Except of course those who noticed that unless Hewitt was planning to ring-fence mental health budgets, her "reforms" had set up a market-style system that drives in precisely the opposite direction. It allows each local Primary Care Trust, and increasingly GPs involved in "practice-based commissioning", to allocate funds as they wish – but it also imposes stringent targets for performance in acute services which drive PCTs to prioritise them above less high profile and less tightly monitored areas of care such as mental health.

Meanwhile, the Camden and Islington Mental Health and Social Care Trust was being forced into swingeing cuts as a result of reduced allocations from Camden PCT. Again the cuts target was £8 million, and one of three day hospitals was to close, with the loss of a quarter of the total places, along with all three remaining wards at St Luke's Hospital. The Trust was aiming to slash the average inpatient length of stay from six months to just three, despite devastating cuts to community-based services. To make matters even worse, a psychiatric intensive care unit at St Pancras Hospital also faced the axe, and there were fears for the future of a walk-in centre at Tottenham Mews which was to be "reconfigured", with staff redeployed. A grimly familiar blame game was being played out in which the Trust blamed the PCT for the cuts while slashing vital services, and none of the management appeared to pay any attention to the needs or views of the clients using the services. Camden and Islington Trust Chair David Taylor claimed that "mental health care is a national priority" – before reverting to the more sober view that "we have to do the best we can with the resources available" (Gadelrab 2007).

A real straw in the wind was a conference on 12 September that underlined the incongruity of lumping mental health into a market-style NHS: Mental Health Forum 2007 had attempted to move with the Brownite times by adopting the incongruous title of: "Modernising mental health to embrace business challenges and achieve service transformation". Day one was to focus on "mental health corporate development":

> As the NHS moves towards a more commercial and competitive environment, mental health services must rise to the challenge. However behaving as a business and maintaining a focus on 'customer' care [sic!] is no easy task. This is a unique day to put this new NHS world into context within mental health.
>
> (Mental Health Forum 2007)

But elsewhere too the grim reality of mental health as the poor relation of the NHS, and the first in line for financial cutbacks was still making itself felt. A new round of cuts had come in North Essex. Despite the fact that according to NHS figures all three PCTs covering the area were set to break even or make a small surplus, a consultation document showed that between them they were seeking cuts in services aimed at saving over £6 million. On a combined budget totalling over £1 billion this might not seem too serious – two-thirds of the cuts (£4 million) were to land on mental health services, which accounted for just 8 per cent of the PCTs' combined turnover: the remaining £2 million was to be cut from the "other" 92 per cent. Mental health had been blatantly singled out as the easiest soft target for cuts, one attracting few headlines and relatively little public involvement. The result was a plan for a brutal package of cuts, slashing back on beds and services for older patients, adults and those currently being cared for in supported schemes in the community (Lister 2007f).

The three PCTs didn't even bother to pretend that the axed beds would be replaced by alternative services: and only a fraction of the projected savings was to be reinvested in mental health. Even as these plans were being pushed through, mental health "Tsar" Louis Appleby was claiming that huge progress was being made, and stressing only the increase in resources that had taken place over the previous seven years, ignoring the developing problems taking shape (Appleby 2007). Somebody else was living in denial.

Foundations and market forces

Spring 2007 brought official confirmation that New Labour's new competitive market system could kill off local NHS services, in the form of recent statements by Bill Moyes, chair of Monitor, the regulatory body supposed to keep track of Foundation Trusts. He and Monitor were urging Foundations to act more like any other business, and to re-examine the financial situation of each of the services they provide, regarding each service as a "profit centre", and ruthlessly discarding those services which do not offer sufficient return on investment.

The aim, Moyes told the *Financial Times* correspondent Nick Timmins, was to "understand profitability, efficiency and quality – and to strike the right balance between the three" (12 March 2007). Hospitals should in his view be "behaving like any other business". As a result, said Mr Moyes:

> The time may come when foundation trusts may be able to walk away from a service, provided we are confident that the primary care trust has alternative suppliers.
>
> (Timmins 2007b)

And of course, if this is the logic behind services continuing or closing, there can be no guarantee any unprofitable – or less profitable – service could be maintained whether or not a local Primary Care Trust has an alternative provider to turn to. By the autumn there was information to confirm the emergence of a two-tier NHS: figures from Monitor showed that while many NHS Trusts had been desperately slashing back staff numbers, services and beds to tackle runaway deficits, Foundation Trusts had been piling up fat surpluses and unspent reserves which totalled almost £1 billion. Profit margins of FTs had now increased to an average 6.7 per cent a year: many had supplemented this by flogging off some of the land and property assets they inherited from the taxpayer, and stashing the cash in reserves (Timmins 2007c).

The giant Addenbrooke's Hospital, now the Cambridge University Hospitals NHS Foundation Trust, had notched up a net surplus of £6 million on a turnover of almost £340 million, and made clear that it intended to build up a war-chest of surplus cash to avoid any future reliance on the costly Private Finance Initiative for future capital investment. Meanwhile its main purchaser, the newly merged Cambridgeshire PCT, was facing a deficit of £51 million, and proposing to make savings by running down services at the modern and popular Hinchingbrooke Hospital in Huntingdon, which was also facing a hefty £13 million deficit. A UNISON Eastern region report argued that Hinchingbrooke was another classic example of a Trust which had done as required by government but found itself "caught in the crossfire" of government reforms and the new marketised, competitive NHS – which in their case included two Foundation Trusts, Peterborough and Addenbrooke's (Lister 2007h).

As a low-cost provider, Hinchingbrooke should have been making a surplus under the controversial "Payment by Results" system: that alone should have been enough to turn around the Trust from heavy deficit to surplus. But instead of being able to charge the new, higher NHS tariff for treatment, Hinchingbrooke would not even be entering the PBR system until 2008 – while Addenbrooke's and Peterborough as FTs had been able to hoover up extra cash. But by 2008, the PCT cash crisis would mean that instead of collecting extra cash for its work, Hinchingbrooke would have to reduce the amount of treatment provided to match the limited cash available (Lister 2007h).

No opportunity was offered for Hinchingbrooke to work its way out of this problem. The Trust signed up for a new state of the art £22 million treatment centre, which had to be built through PFI – at a cost of at least £93 million. The business case for this NHS-run treatment centre hinged on promises from Cambridgeshire's PCTs to refer additional patients: the promises were broken. The expected extra patients never arrived in Hinchingbrooke, but it seems some were lured instead to rival projects in Cambridge and Peterborough – leaving Hinchingbrooke stuck with an under-used facility and a hefty bill for years to come: worse, the new PCT plan wanted to cut Hinchingbrooke's caseload (and budget) further by diverting £2.3 million worth of patient care to private sector units... 20 or more miles away in Peterborough or Cambridge (Lister 2007h).

The switch from Blair to Brown brought no slowing of the relentless pace of "reform" in the National Health Service. As Brown's juggernaut squashed any serious opposition, he and his key supporters went out of their way to stress their commitment to more of the privatisation and marketisation they had begun under Blair. Brown's coronation came just after with the decision – clearly sanctioned by both Blair and Brown – to appoint a senior executive from a subsidiary of the US health insurance giant UnitedHealth to one of the top positions in the NHS management, commissioning services from private and NHS providers. R. Channing Wheeler was to bring us his years of experience running a profit-seeking, exclusive insurance company in the world's least efficient and most bureaucratic health care system. Exactly how that equipped him to commission universal and comprehensive services in the NHS was never explained (Timmins et al. 2007).

On the same day as Brown's guaranteed succession to the premiership, Work and Pensions Secretary John Hutton made a speech to a CBI forum, emphasising that Blair's public sector "reforms" – including the "marketisation" of public services and "an open minded approach to who provides" – had now been "built into the DNA" of public services. However, Hutton was later forced to admit that these policies have yet to win the acceptance of the large majority of the NHS workforce (Hutton 2007).

Cabinet Secretary Gus O'Donnell, appropriately speaking to a forum convened by ubiquitous city slickers PricewaterhouseCoopers on the eve of Brown's coronation also joined the chorus praising the role of market-style policies, and insisting that "we need market incentives to improve efficiency". Yet at the same time O'Donnell admitted that an essential element to usher in the level of "choice" that Blair and Brown have promised is that "you have to have some spare capacity" (Timmins 2007d). But the existence of unused spare capacity – especially if some of it is additional capacity provided by the private sector at increased cost above NHS rates – is by definition LESS efficient than making full use of the appropriate amount of capacity. In fact the new system of "Payment by Results" ensures that the NHS cannot afford to maintain spare, unused capacity: Trusts are forced into contemplating cutbacks and closures when patients are diverted to private treatment centres.

Small wonder that with contradictory thinking and double standards like this at the very heart of government policy there is still no evidence to show that the costly introduction of "contestability" in the NHS with the establishment of a new, expanding private sector in elective (waiting list) treatment has done anything to improve efficiency or deliver value for money. Brown had been easily as big a culprit as Blair in the rapid and continuing expansion of private sector provision in the NHS: in the view of these two architects of New Labour, even the sharpest-toothed sector of private enterprise is preferable to public-sector provision.

Brown has also been a key figure in the implementation and expansion of the ruinously expensive Private Finance Initiative – described even by Tory MP Edward Leigh as "the unacceptable face of capitalism" – as the only means of financing most new hospital developments (Timmins 2006e). Brown's last budget outlined plans for even more PFI-funded projects in health and elsewhere, even while NHS Trusts were ruefully counting the escalating cost of schemes already operational.

Building magazine has revealed that at least five early PFI projects had involved the Department of Health handing over leases as long as 125 years to PFI consortia, giving private firms control over the land new hospitals have been built on (Leftly 2007). And it was increasingly clear that PFI – far more than the pattern of patient needs – was shaping the next round of "reconfiguration" of hospital services. South East London was one of several areas in which NHS Trusts faced a process of mergers and rationalisation: three of the SE London Trusts (Bromley, Lewisham, Queen Elizabeth Woolwich), had substantial PFI contracts to pay off for 30 years or more – leaving the fourth, Queen Mary's Hospital Sidcup, firmly in the frame as the cheapest one to close (Lister 2007d).

However, not everything was going exactly the way the private sector wanted. In early summer 2007 it suffered two substantial setbacks:

- Plans for a new network of "Independent Sector Treatment Centres" (ISTCs) in South London had been shelved. The £35 million a year contract had been expected to skim off some of the simplest and least risky elective operations – but threatened to undermine almost every NHS and Foundation Trust south of the river, and this seems belatedly to have been recognised by the new London Strategic Health Authority.

- Plans for a new ISTC in Hertfordshire, based in Hemel Hempstead had also been scrapped, after county PCTs and Trusts had concluded that an NHS unit would offer better value (Herts PCTs 2007).

But ministers were reluctant to retreat from their objective of establishing new private units and what the Department of Health has called a "sustainable Independent Sector market". In the North West, plans were being laid by the Strategic Health Authority to police the numbers referred by Primary Care Trusts to the new "clinical assessment and treatment services" which were to be run by South African multinational Netcare and Partnership Health Group. There was an implicit threat that PCTs that sent insufficient numbers would face some form of penalty – regardless of whether patients chose the new units in preference to NHS facilities. However, the public resistance to the new services, which seemed certain to result in embarrassingly low numbers of patients being treated, and poor value for money has now resulted in this experimental plan being axed at national level in late 2007 by ministers and eventually by the Primary Care Trusts, which had tried to carry on regardless (Lancashire PCTs 2008).

Now you see them, now you don't

There were plenty of riddles in the figures proudly unveiled by Patricia Hewitt in June 2007, which purported to show the NHS in England running a £500 million surplus in place of the previous year's deficit – especially after her previous projections of an overall surplus of just £13 million.

A closer look at the figures showed that a number of chronic and massive deficits appeared to have been miraculously expunged, with little if any explanation as to how such large sums could be made to disappear. Lewisham

Hospital Trust, for example, had been projecting a hefty £12 million deficit at month 9, but wound up claiming a £2 million surplus three months later. The nearby Queen Elizabeth Hospital Trust, a notorious casualty of the Private Finance Initiative, projected a £36 million deficit at month 9, but reported a year-end shortfall of just over £7 million (DoH 2007e). It soon became clear that many of these deficits had been made to disappear through large-scale longer-term borrowing, leaving Trusts with substantial amounts top-sliced from their revenue for years to come.

But another key factor in London, and in other areas too, was the extent to which the apparent financial health of the area has been hugely distorted by surpluses run up by the Strategic Health Authority: in London, this surplus amounted to a staggering £180 million – enough to make it appear that the whole London health economy was in surplus to the tune of £92 million, while in fact Trusts' and PCTs' debts exceeded surpluses by almost £90 million, with eleven hospitals headed for really large shortfalls. 19 of those reporting a balance or surplus were expecting to hold on to less than 0.5 per cent – far less than the margin for error. Teams of trained masseurs had clearly worked long hours trying to pummel the NHS figures into shape: but with services up and down the country still in turmoil as another year of cash squeeze takes effect, a £500 million surplus suggested that much needless agony has been imposed on NHS staff, managers and patients, who in many areas have seen new "minimum" waiting times imposed to hold down spending (Mandelstam 2007).

Coupled with the £1 billion held by unaccountable Foundation Trusts, and the £2 billion a year now being funnelled out to private sector providers, plus the ever-increasing £500-million-plus pocketed each year by PFI consortia and their shareholders, these figures help explain why so many health workers and service users feel ministers have not spent the extra cash wisely, and they have not secured the results that should have been achieved.

July 2007 saw the publication of the Darzi Report on London's NHS (Darzi 2007a).[19] Professor Darzi, a high-flying surgeon who had dabbled in health care planning issues in Wakefield and Teesside, was a surprise appointment as junior health minister in Gordon Brown's reshuffle, picking up a peerage in the process. His report on London, drafted before his governmental appointment, grabbed headlines, but generated remarkably little response to NHS London when it became clear that it lacked any specific proposals on the allocation of services (Lister 2007b).

Almost all responses seized upon the progressive language, Darzi's focus on health inequalities and the talk about "partnership", while only including those who adopted the most superficial approach saw this as a signal that the whole report should be uncritically welcomed. However constructive the approach, a serious analysis has to begin with the old fashioned method of reading the whole

---

19 For a more detailed discussion of the Darzi Report's implications for primary care, see Chapter twelve below.

document and the accompanying technical paper, and analysing the proposals and their impact.

As Londoners know full well, not all plans are progressive and helpful: there are bitter memories of the wretched King's Fund report, followed by the 1992 Tomlinson Report proposing wholesale hospital and bed closures to shape up the NHS for Thatcher's "internal market".

One fact is clear from the outset: any substantial reorganisation is also going to involve a shake-up in ways of working that in many cases go back to 1948 and beyond. This will inevitably annoy some groups of professionals who prefer things just as they are. It may be a tough challenge to win over those affected. But this is not necessarily an immediate reason to reject any change: that would give a total veto over health policy to relatively small groups of professionals.

However, Darzi's report does display a number of problems and weaknesses.

Even though it was written in the midst of an ongoing financial squeeze on Trusts and PCTs in the capital, it makes no reference at all to the financial context and takes no position on the various processes towards rationalisation already taking place around London. The words "closure" and "downgrade" do not appear despite the fact that they are at the centre of debates which have continued in the North, North East, South West and South East of London.

The report also ignores the dreadful and inadequate state of social care services in the capital, and the problems posed for any reorganisation of services by inadequate public transport and chronic traffic congestion. It proposes improvements in midwifery services, mental health, palliative and terminal care – but again fails to identify the funding, the staff or the locations for these new services.

Although widely trailed as proposing the downsizing of up to a third of London's district general hospitals, and proposing a new division of clinical responsibility between "local hospitals", "elective units", "major acute" and "specialist hospitals", Darzi gives no idea of how many of each should be provided, or where they should be located. Despite the fact that jobs and working conditions for the capital's 200,000-plus health workers are at stake, Darzi's list of "partners" in the process of reform significantly omits the trade unions and professional bodies – such as the BMA – and any involvement of the wider public through pensioners' groups or other means.

The report is almost entirely devoid of specifics: the only precise proposals are for a network of 150 polyclinics (although there is no discussion on where they should be located), and for seven "hyper-acute" hospitals to gear up with enhanced technical resources to improve stroke care, and two new Trauma Centres. The polyclinics proposal (establishing a network of large-scale hybrids between health centres and outpatient units, each with a staff of over 100 including 35 GPs) appears to be set out and costed in detail: but on closer examination it is clear that many costs have been omitted or seriously under-stated, and the clinical case for switching some of the services from hospitals to polyclinics is very weak. The immediate hostile reaction to these plans from

London's GPs, and the obvious lack of any prior attempt to win support for the proposals must throw doubt on the short-term prospect of establishing more than one pilot polyclinic.

Despite fears that the plan is simply a framework for privatisation, Darzi makes little reference to the private sector, and none to private sector treatment centres: all of his examples of good practice are in NHS units, including the NHS-run SW London Elective Orthopaedic Centre – which remains in the public sector thanks to the intervention of local campaigners. Darzi's report appears oblivious to the financial consequences of his proposals for NHS Trusts under the "Payment by Results" system.

His proposal to switch 40 per cent of outpatient appointments and 50 per cent of A&E attendances to Polyclinics would – on the basis of the figures contained in his own Technical Report – siphon around £500 million a year from hospital budgets, and leave the NHS stuck with all the more expensive and complex cases. The consequences would be a haphazard pattern of service cuts and closures – potentially undermining services that Darzi's plan would want to see operational. All these and other inconsistencies and errors suggest that the plan as it stands will not, as Darzi claims, save up to £1.5 billion a year from health budgets by 2016, and cannot be implemented as it stands.

There is another problem: while the plan itself identified no specific hospitals for run-down and closure, it is vague enough for local managers with their eyes on cash-driven cuts to begin to invoke the Darzi Report and its talk of "local hospitals" as a basis to ram through closures. This is already happening in SE London, where four hospital Trusts (Bromley, Lewisham, Queen Mary's Sidcup and Queen Elizabeth Woolwich) are contemplating possible mergers and proposing three "options" – all of which mean downgrading services (to a "local hospital") and closing the A&E at Queen Mary's (Lister 2007d). Elsewhere in London PCT and Trust bosses are also looking to drive forward their local rationalisation of service regardless of Darzi's attempt to establish an overall plan.

Closures endorsed

September saw a resumption of New Labour's relentless drive for "reforms", and more evidence of the cash pressures which are forcing NHS Trusts and PCTs to contemplate ever more unpopular "centralisation" of services and cutbacks in local access to care. The zealotry of reform was back with a vengeance as Health Secretary Alan Johnson rubber-stamped his first raft of hospital closures – brushing aside local protests including those of ministerial colleagues to sign the death warrant for a series of maternity units in Greater Manchester (Hencke 2007a).

The ink was barely dry on Johnson's signature when a damning new report from the Academy of Medical Royal Colleges was published, which concluded that there was no evidence to show centralisation of emergency services into bigger units brought a benefit to any but a small minority of patients, and sharply criticised government policies including "Payment by Results" (AoMRC 2007).

A section from the Royal College of Surgeons, previously cited as major supporters of the call to rationalise services into fewer bigger hospital units, concludes:

> There is some hard evidence that outcome for a select group of patients is improved in specialist centres where surgeons can maintain their specialist skills by treating a greater number of people. People who have experienced major trauma and those requiring specialist neurosurgery and vascular care do fare better if they are treated in specialist units.
>
> **However, there is conflicting evidence that specialist centres are beneficial for other kinds of surgery. At this stage, any decision to withdraw 24-hour surgical cover from some hospitals in favour of centralisation is not supported by current clinical evidence.**
>
> [...]
>
> The Royal College of Surgeons considers that care must be delivered as locally as possible providing there is no compromise on the safety and quality of that care. Our March 2006 report Delivering High Quality Surgical Services for the Future outlined what we believe to be the three main drivers for reconfiguration:
>
> * clinical need (for example, the need to reconfigure specialised services such as paediatric cardiac surgery, or the need to reconfigure services in smaller hospitals);
> * the introduction of contestability and competition in the health service; and
> * the cost of providing services.
>
> **The RCS insists that any reorganisation of health services has a sound clinical and evidence base. Financial, political and managerial expediency must not be primary drivers for service reorganisation.**
>
> (AoMRC 2007, 3.11, A71, emphasis added)

As Gordon Brown scrapped plans for an early election it seemed that even more impetus was put in to boost privatisation in the NHS. This was the only real content in the otherwise inconclusive and insubstantial findings of the interim report of Lord Darzi's much-heralded "review" of health services in England. Darzi tried once again to play the inequalities card, revealing the far from earth-shattering fact that health inequalities continue to widen in Brown's increasingly unequal Britain – the poorest, sickest areas still have the lousiest health care. Darzi's findings confirmed that patterns of provision of GP services continue to fit the Inverse Care Law first identified in the early 1970s – the availability of good quality and well-resourced primary care services tends to be inversely proportional to the need for it. But what was Darzi's solution? Wheel in the private sector to plug the gaps left by GPs who prefer to practise in leafy and prosperous areas. Exactly how the private sector could recruit the extra GPs that would be needed – and how much of a premium payment they would require – was not discussed (Darzi 2007b).

Darzi also ducked the hard questions on another main theme: hospital hygiene. He called for tougher regulation, for nurses to have greater powers to impose standards and for a "deep clean" of filthy wards – but the interim report shirked once again, like ministers have before, the vital call to clear out the cowboy private firms whose cheapskate methods have brought a slump in standards since they were introduced in the mid-1980s.

Unlike his London report, which praised NHS services and offered few encouragements to the private sector, Darzi's report on the rest of England's NHS carried a number of New Labour-style plugs for the (unproven) merits of "Independent Sector Treatment Centres".

The day after Darzi's interim report was published, in a massive new lurch towards privatisation, ministers unveiled a list of 14 giant private companies, four of them major US health care insurers, who are now "approved" to bid for lucrative contracts "advising" Primary Care Trusts how to spend their £70 billion-plus budgets for "commissioning". Four of the approved forms are giant US-based health care companies – Aetna, Humana, UnitedHealth and Health Dialog Services, three of them famous from Michael Moore's recent film *Sicko* – and two of them were currently embroiled in a fresh scandal over their role in the US Medicare system (health care for older people). One thing all 14 companies have in common is that not one of them has any experience of commissioning or providing a comprehensive and universal health care system like the NHS (Milne 2007).

As the NHS came to the end of its 59th calendar year, London's health care faced a fresh shake-up: a consultation based loosely on Lord Darzi's July document *A Framework for Action* was launched on 30 November, to run until mid-March 2008. The consultation will not be cheap: NHS London, the Strategic Health Authority covering the capital's 7.5 million population, has agreed to spend £15 million on "consultation and implementation" of Darzi's proposals (NHS London 2007a, b). But it looks as if the money, and the time and energy involved in the consultation process, could be completely wasted. The consultation document itself, drafted by PR spin-doctors, lacks any of the concrete proposals that might interest or excite the London public, and as a result neither the press nor the TV and radio in the capital have shown any interest in covering the debate or publicising the issue. So almost nobody knows a consultation is taking place. The publication of the original report in July, amid a relative fanfare of press publicity resulted in a miserable 30 responses by post and email to NHS London, a remarkable 0.0004 per cent of the capital's population. With no continuing publicity the response rate to the consultation is likely to be even lower.

To make matters worse, there are question marks over the process itself – and even over the real intentions of the report's author. The situation is a little reminiscent of Robert Louis Stevenson's story of Dr Jekyll and Mr Hyde: are Londoners really dealing with Professor Darzi, the kindly maverick hospital consultant... or are they up against the hard-faced Lord Darzi, the privatising minister in a New Labour government? Are they to respond to the apparent concerns voiced in Darzi's London report over inequalities in health and the need to improve treatment for stroke patients and others whose care has been under-resourced? Or should they instead be alarmed at the subsequent statements by Lord Darzi the junior minister, whose interim report on the NHS in England explicitly welcomed the controversial "Independent Sector Treatment Centres" and called for the private sector to play a larger role in plugging gaps in primary care services?

NHS London representatives have on occasion tried to divert discussion away from allegations of privatisation and the fears that a number of London's District General Hospitals would be downgraded alongside any expansion of specialist services in selected hospitals. But they have been unwilling to respond directly to the concerns people have raised. On several occasions NHS London have been publicly challenged to give a guarantee to Londoners that the Darzi Plan would not result in a massive new privatisation of GP and hospital services. No such guarantee has been given.

Meanwhile, a series of further revelations have linked Lord Darzi and his proposals – both in London and nationally – with the private sector:

- Kingston Hospital Trust is pressing ahead with plans to hand over its entire elective surgical operation to the private sector, arguing that this policy is in line with the Darzi proposals. NHS London has not officially denied the Trust's claim, nor has it used its powers to intervene to prevent this new escalation of privatisation in the NHS (Mooney 2007b).

- One of the senior US managers of UnitedHealth, the biggest and most profitable of the US health insurers, is Simon Stevens, a former health advisor to Tony Blair – who told the Observer on 11 November he had met Lord Darzi, who was "one of his big admirers". UnitedHealth has been included among the 14 corporations approved by ministers to bid for contracts advising Primary Care Trusts on "commissioning" services: the statement listing the approved companies to share in this potential bonanza was issued by none other than NHS Commissioning Director Channing Wheeler – himself a former senior executive with UnitedHealth in the US (Revill 2007).

- Heart of Birmingham Primary Care Trust has drawn up a "bold and ambitious" plan to franchise its primary care services to companies including Virgin, Asda and Tesco. These proposals follow meetings between Lord Darzi and retail chains aimed at forging a new provider role in primary care (Nowottny 2007).

- Discussions on possible developments of new polyclinics have increasingly focused on the involvement of the private sector in building and running the new centres and delivering many of the services they will provide. London Health Emergency wrote in July to NHS London chief executive Ruth Carnall to demand the SHA step in and call the Trusts and PCTs to order, and impose an official moratorium on any decisions and consultations that would undermine services while a debate is supposedly taking place on general principles: but the eventual reply proved evasive.

So, all the signs so far point in one direction. It is beginning to look as if the positive and progressive proposals in Darzi's London report are simply a smokescreen for an agenda of service cuts and privatisation, and his report is effectively a Trojan horse, drawing the public into a false and irrelevant discussion on various issues of genuine concern – while behind the scenes the plans for a new wave of privatisation and for the axing of local hospital services take shape.

Department of Health figures published at the end of 2007 show that a massive 5,500 acute (short stay) beds closed in England over the last two years – 5 per cent of the total. These are the first real reductions in acute beds since 1993, when even the Tory government was forced to concede that a basic provision of beds was vital to cope with peaks of demand and large numbers of medical emergencies. The situation is even more desperate because a massive 3,744 elderly care beds were also closed in the same two-year time frame – 14 per cent of the total (DoH statistics, 2007).

That helps to explain why even before the real onset of winter large hospitals were closing their doors in new "black alerts" – like Addenbrooke's in Cambridge, and the Norfolk and Norwich (BBC News 2007b, c). Both hospitals are many miles from any alternative hospital beds. Addenbrookes' nearest hospital to the east, West Suffolk, was also full to the rafters.

More shocking figures from the Treasury at the end of November confirmed that the Private Finance Initiative (PFI) was a ridiculously expensive way to finance new hospitals, schools and prisons. A few months earlier it had been revealed that the NHS is set to fork out a staggering £53 billion for new hospitals with a capital value of £8 billion. But a Treasury letter replying to the Commons Public Accounts Committee has conceded that the total costs of hospital school and prison PFIs will stack up to a staggering £170 billion to be paid to private sector banks, investors and entrepreneurs by 2032 (Hencke 2007b).

Even the most positive spin from the Treasury, arguing that the value of payments in future years will be less than the present value, admits that the total cost will be £91 billion in today's money. Meanwhile many PFI hospitals are still struggling to pay exorbitant rents to private landlords: Bromley Hospitals Trust has admitted a colossal £99 million historic deficit which has arisen after its PFI hospital lost the "smoothing" payments promised by the Department of Health to make the project appear more affordable (Iggulden 2007).

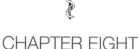

CHAPTER EIGHT

National Health Services?
The changing model in Scotland, Wales
and Northern Ireland

FOR ITS FIRST 50 YEARS IT WAS SUFFICIENT to talk of one National Health Service for the whole of the UK, although clearly there were distinct social, cultural and logistical issues to be addressed in Wales, Scotland and Northern Ireland. However, the implementation of promised legislation to devolve powers to an elected Scottish Parliament and National Assembly of Wales from 1998, and more recently the devolution of powers to the power-sharing administration of the Northern Ireland Assembly in May 2007, have opened up space for increasingly distinctive policies in each of these three UK nations. It is clearly no longer simply one UK NHS, but a composite of four health services (Plumridge 2007).

The increasingly market-based model, and the continued rapid succession of organisational and structural reforms which have marked the last ten years in England, have for the most part not been copied and reproduced in the other UK nations, which in general have stayed much closer to the original centralised model of Bevan's 1948 NHS. Interestingly, however, since this involves services being run through elected and accountable institutions in each country, it offers a greater degree of democratic control for the Welsh, Scottish and Northern Irish people than is available to the English population. There is no equivalent possibility, for example, for English MPs to turn up at decision-making sessions of the Scottish Parliament or Welsh Assembly to force through a proposal such as Foundation Trusts – even though Welsh and Scottish Labour MPs played a conspicuous role in securing Tony Blair's wafer-thin House of Commons majority of just 17 votes to impose this policy in England.

In Wales, First Minister Rhodri Morgan has long proclaimed his determination to maintain "clear red water" between Welsh Labour and their Westminster equivalents, resulting in a more mainstream "old Labour" policy, based on collaboration rather than competition (Williams and Ham 2006). Similarly, Scotland has a distinct political culture and a much stronger legacy of militant trade unionism. This helps to explain the distinctive approach of each of these governments. The establishment of the Assembly in Northern Ireland is still too recent to allow us to detect many long-term political tendencies.

This chapter will examine the process of change taking shape in each of these three nations, beginning with the most recently devolved assembly, which got into action in May 2007.

Northern Ireland

Although very different from each other politically, the four main parties in the 2007 elections had put forward manifestos promising health policies that revolved around two consensus issues which are quite different from the current English model – moving towards free personal care (the two Unionist Parties), and free prescriptions (the Ulster Unionists and Sinn Fein) (Jervis 2008).

Prior to the devolution to Stormont, health services had been included as part of the 2005 Review of Public Administration promoted by Northern Ireland Secretary Peter Hain, although the health proposals also made use of the detailed and extensive review commissioned by Northern Ireland Minister Angela Smith and carried out by the King's Fund's Professor John Appleby in 2005. The health changes were to be the first of the bunch of RPA proposals to be implemented. As a result of this combined process, 47 previous health and social care bodies were to be squeezed together to leave just 18, although only part of this process has been completed, and many of the restructuring changes have now been postponed until 2009 (Kirby 2007).

The Department of Health, Social Services and Public Safety (DHSSPS) was to be slimmed down, and manage a new, unified Health and Social Services Authority, which was supposed to replace the previous four health and social service boards: this is the level at which the health minister Michael McGimpsey has intervened to halt the proposed changes. In theory the HSSA in turn was to oversee seven new "local commissioning groups" comprising GPs, other health professionals and HSSA nominees, which would commission services from a drastically reduced number of merged provider Trusts. This is the level at which the changes have been forced through, and 18 health and social care Trusts were in April 2007 merged into just five new integrated Trusts linking hospitals with community services, with the ambulance Trust retaining its independent organisation (Carlisle 2007a).

One prime objective in the whole package of changes, "the most fundamental change to the health and social services system for decades" (RPA 2006) was to reduce management overhead costs – with 1,700 jobs to be eliminated (Plumridge 2007): another factor likely to raise its head with more ferocity in the future is the drive towards rationalisation of hospital services, or as Plumridge aptly sums up "unpopular hospital consolidation" – which is proving so difficult to sell to the electorate in any of the UK nations.

A major concern in Appleby's report had been the relatively high cost and low productivity of the system, with no obvious driving mechanism to promote the performance of the providers: he told the *Health Service Journal*'s Daloni Carlisle:

> Performance management was pretty poor. There was notionally a sort of split between those organisations with money and those with services. But it seemed to me... that the split was more in name than anything else.
>
> (Carlisle 2007a)

As a result, in an attempt to "sharpen up" the performance management, but not, he has made clear, with any intention of replicating the English NHS market, Appleby recommended the introduction of a "purchaser–provider split":

> This Review would suggest that some form of separation between the providers of services and the funders/commissioners of services would be an important factor in sharpening up incentives in the system. Given the particular circumstances of Northern Ireland, its population size and distribution, the political governance structures, etc., there needs to be further investigation of the most appropriate form of separation, however. …It may be that a single pan-Northern Ireland commissioner would be more appropriate. This arrangement would not preclude some devolution of commissioning to GPs…
>
> (Appleby 2005: 11)

The proposed new structure for the commissioning organisations therefore incorporates the purchaser–provider split, operating a form of Payment by Results – but firmly rejects practice-based commissioning and Foundation Trusts. Northern Ireland's population is considered too small at 1.7 million, with half of this number too scattered in the rural areas to justify any New Labour-style attempt to create "contestability" or meaningful competition and a market structure.

Appleby has made it clear that he is not enthusiastic about further plans to set up another level of "community commissioning organisations" within each of the seven local commissioning groups, covering around 30,000 people each – leaving each organisation very small and unequal to any trial of strength with the new "super-trusts". The Belfast HSC Trust is the largest in the UK, with a budget of £1.1 billion – almost 30 per cent of the total Northern Ireland Health budget – and 22,500 staff (Carlisle 2007b).

The DHSSPS had earlier brought in the expertise of Greater Manchester SHA to help set up a new Integrated Clinical Assessment and Treatment Service (ICATS). By the spring of 2007 this had helped cut the numbers waiting to an all-time low of around 40,000 waiting for inpatient treatment (with a maximum wait of 6 months) – and some 180,000 outpatients waiting to see a consultant, along with nearly 7,000 waiting for scans (*Belfast Telegraph* 2007).

Plans for rationalization of hospitals, however, have been much harder to force through, with Health Minister McGimpsey having firmly nailed his colours to the mast of opening new hospitals soon after the Assembly launched into action, and indignantly rejecting speculation that the hugely expensive programme of PFI-funded hospital building was to be cut back:

> One of my first decisions on taking up office was to confirm Enniskillen as the location for the acute hospital and a £190 million enhanced local hospital for Omagh. The suggestion that acute services should not be provided in Enniskillen is particularly unhelpful given the very advanced stage of procurement on the new £279 million acute hospital. In addition such a suggestion would leave a large proportion of the population west of the Bann some considerable distance from acute services.
>
> (McGimpsey 2007a)

Also nearing completion is a new £60 million hospital in Downe. The combined investment of £529 million for these three projects is staggering in proportion to the Northern Ireland health budget of £3.9 billion in 2008–9 (Northern Ireland Executive 2007), and the financing through PFI ensures that the final bill will be four or five times higher, with the money top-sliced from the Trust revenue budgets. This is likely to become an even more serious issue in the next few years as rapid growth in health spending comes to an end: after growing by 55% in the five years from 2001 (£2.3 billion to £3.6 billion) the health budget is set to grow in real terms by just over 1% in 2008, less in 2009, and by around 2% in 2010 (HM Treasury 2000; Northern Ireland Executive 2007). Spending levels, historically much higher in Northern Ireland than in England, are being squeezed closer to the English level, although health and social care have steadily risen as a share of Northern Ireland government spending, to consume almost half (46%) of the total in 2006–7.

With a tighter budget, the burgeoning costs of the PFI projects will hang like an albatross on the NHS. UNISON had warned that the financial viability of the Enniskillen and Omagh hospitals appeared to hinge on the loss of up to 25 per cent of hospital staff, but in evidence to the Assembly's Health Committee officials have claimed this reduction has subsequently been scaled down to 9 per cent (39 posts). However they refused to comment on UNISON's warning that the Omagh project could face an affordability gap of £20 million, arguing that the figures were "commercial in confidence" (Northern Ireland Assembly 2007).

This investment in new hospitals is linked with a rationalisation that will reduce the overall number of hospitals slightly (from three in Fermanagh to two), but the overall policy runs counter to Royal College suggestions that the whole of Northern Ireland should have only three acute hospitals (Jervis 2008: 30). Although the province has for many years had more beds per head of population than England (Alvarez-Rosete et al. 2005), rationalisation – especially on the sort of level proposed by the Royal Colleges – will be difficult to sell to a sceptical public with all four main parties looking to expand and improve NHS coverage.

But while appearing to follow the English example by immersing themselves in an enormous PFI project, the Northern Irish politicians also began, almost immediately after the handover to the devolved Assembly, to seek ways of lifting charges for personal care and following the Welsh and Scots in moving towards free prescriptions (Jervis 2008: 117). While the apparent integration between the NHS and social services in the new super-Trusts ought to make it much easier to translate these aspirations into a coherent, genuinely seamless service, services are up against another legacy reminiscent of England: the nursing homes, including the latest "state of the art" home opened recently by the minister, remain in private hands (McGimpsey 2007b; *Mid Ulster Mail* 2007).

Northern Ireland seems set to remain for some time a hybrid system, based on the historic base of the NHS with a few isolated features of the market-style system established in England – but amidst a political consensus located much more around the pre-1990 values of the NHS, rather than its twenty-first century English incarnation.

Wales

The Welsh Assembly Government has forged an independent line on health care since devolution in 1999, based far more consistently on notions of public health, prevention and primary care than the English policy. The deliberate creation of "clear red water" between Cardiff and Westminster resulted in policies based explicitly on universalism and equality. Following this logic, the Welsh Assembly have been the trail-blazers in scrapping prescription charges – which are the most unequal of charges, having most impact in deterring the lowest-paid workers – moving first to free prescriptions for people aged 16–25, and then to abolish the charge for the whole population from April 2007. Also free is swimming for those aged under 16 and over 60, and bus passes for residents aged over 60 (Williams and Ham 2006).

The 2001 policy document *Improving Health in Wales, a plan for the NHS and its partners* focused both on health improvement and reshaping the health care system: health improvement policies included healthy schools initiatives, health alliances and community food projects (National Assembly for Wales 2001).

However, the report by Sir Derek Wanless in 2003 found that Wales was not getting full value for its investment in health and social care, and that this was a factor driving pressures on acute hospital Trusts:

> The current configuration of health services places an insupportable burden on the acute sector and its workforce. This is the most expensive part of the system. More acute beds are not a viable or effective long-term response. Actions to reconfigure provision, release acute capacity and raise productivity are needed alongside a rebalancing of the system to meet need earlier in the 'care pathway' and improvements in the way in which the parts of the system work together. Supply is involuntarily rationed by long hospital waiting lists and times and assessments without subsequent social services.
>
> (Wanless 2003)

Wanless went on to call for the Assembly to stop funding Trust deficits – a policy which the Assembly has tried rather ineffectually to implement in the teeth of massive deficits in some of the largest Welsh Trusts – and to seek to develop a seamless provision of health and local care, although he did not propose organisational or structural changes to achieve this. In addition Wanless called on the Assembly to adopt a realistic and achievable programme of change.

However instead of a realistic and achievable programme, Wanless' criticisms resulted in a fresh idealistic response in the 2005 policy statement *Designed for Life: a world class health service for Wales* – a document apparently shaped around a succession of PR consultants' clichés, which sets out a long series of complex milestone targets for the next three years, as well as proposals for the following three, and three more up to 2015. The document was notable for its immense lists of targets and objectives, set out in Appendix 4: a staggering 54 "milestones" were to be achieved by March 2006, among which were:

• Work will commence on the remodelling of social services and social care

- Health communities will work together to ensure medical emergency admissions are reduced by 5% against the 2003–4 baseline, through the development and implementation of needs-based Chronic Disease Pathways
- A review of health and social care policies will be completed
- A review of commissioning covering the strategic context, information needs, responsibilities, and skill development will be completed *and the identified changes implemented* [emphasis added]
- Demand management programmes will be implemented
- Existing NHS deficits will be eliminated or recovery plans agreed.

(NHS Wales 2005)

Such a dauntingly long list of tasks, some of which are clearly beyond the scope of the NHS locally or nationally (remodelling social services is a responsibility of local councils), and some of which are contradictory or competing "priorities", must have been seriously disorientating for Welsh NHS managers – almost akin to the relentless and rapid-fire pressures piled on to English NHS managers in the period since 2000. The list also appears to be seriously incoherent: how does the proposal for "demand management" (normally perceived as attempting to hold down demand for, and use of, hospital beds) fit in with the review of commissioning – if commissioning is seen as identifying and meeting local health needs? And how does the review of commissioning help in the elimination of deficits, if Trusts are already struggling to make ends meet?

Managers who successfully negotiated the barrage of targets in 2005–6 would no doubt have been relieved to find just 25 targets for the following 12 months, although some of these – such as a 10 per cent reduction in emergency hospital admissions – were extremely ambitious given the pressures on NHS services in Wales. Others were so vague and jargon-ridden it would have been hard to determine what outcome was required, such as the document's commitment that:

> Effective but minimalist systems will be developed for the ongoing monitoring and analysis of the impact of the major chronic diseases pathway on the individual and on bed usage.

Other targets were clearly self-serving ambitions for the politicians. Nothing beats a good logo on a bedpan:

> All relevant LHB and NHS Trust materials will carry Health Challenge Wales branding to demonstrate to the public the contribution that services are making to the national effort to improve health in Wales.

For the year 2007–8, there were another 30 assorted targets. So complex is the whole list, covering such a wide range of issues, that monitoring its implementation would be a mammoth task in itself.

Another difficulty with such a diffuse and all-consuming approach as *Designed for Life* is that it tends to eclipse genuine priorities, some of which, such as mental health, have been sorely neglected and under-resourced. *Under Pressure*, a critical report in 2005 from the Wales Collaboration for Mental Health, was based on two-day visits to each of the ten Trusts and the Local Health Board responsible for mental health services. Its findings were "remarkably consistent across Wales." The researchers found services under great pressure despite the efforts of staff, with over-occupancy of inpatient units – "at times exceeding 100%" and high workload on community mental health staff (WCMH 2005). The report warned that there was a risk to the quality of patient care, an increased risk of "high profile incidents where public safety is compromised" and a danger of "a further reduction in staff morale". It outlined a 24-point programme for action over the following year, covering issues such as monitoring units where the occupancy levels exceeded 90 per cent, action to remedy the shortage of supported housing for people with mental health problems, strengthened community mental health teams to enable them to offer 24/7 crisis response services, and many aspects of staff training.

Designed for Life was also remarkable in carrying only indicative costs for the various projects it proposed, and offering little indication of where the money (some £1.6 billion in capital) was to come from – especially given the consistent principled rejection by Welsh health ministers of PFI as a funding mechanism ever since the costly scheme to build the Neath Port Talbot hospital (Lister 2003a). The follow-up document *Spending By Design* was not an explanation of the financial plans, but a new system for improving financial information (Plumridge 2007).

Progress on the new hospital projects has been halting, complicated also by the financial problems faced by the Trusts, and the well-established complexities of capital programmes: plans for the new hospital for Caerphilly, promised for years and now listed as a £97 million project, are still being finalised. Many of the proposals in *Designed for Life* also appear more convincing in abstract than they do in real life. When the first major detailed proposals for restructuring health care provision in South Wales along the lines of *Designed for Life* were outlined in the document *Gwent Clinical Futures*, UNISON, the main health union, raised serious concerns over the practicality and viability of the planned network of hospitals and services (Lister 2006d). Gwent Healthcare Trust was at that time attempting to balance the books in the face of a massive £47 million shortfall in 2006–7, and UNISON warned that the plan itself did not even discuss the related issue of financial viability, or the availability of sufficient revenue funding to sustain the proposed pattern of service.

Gwent has 552,000 residents – 19 per cent of the total Wales population of 2.9 million (2001), and Gwent Healthcare Trust had 1,672 acute beds (the largest total of any Trust in Wales), in addition to 101 Maternity beds, 146 "geriatric" beds and 389 mental health beds (2004–5 figures from National Assembly of Wales). The Trust therefore had the equivalent of 18 per cent of the acute beds in Wales, and a third of the acute beds in South Wales.

Gwent Clinical Futures argued strongly for a new pattern of care, to include six new Local General Hospitals and one much smaller Specialist and Critical Care Centre to cover the county's population. However, the plan required that the local general hospitals should each offer only a limited range of services, raising questions over whether there would be adequate and accessible provision for the clinical needs of the population.

There was little sign of spare capacity: the Trust's average length of stay for acute inpatients was right on the Wales average, while its occupancy level of acute beds, at 85 per cent, was slightly higher than the Wales average, and the fifth highest in Wales. The most recent figures from the National Assembly showed over 62 per cent of Gwent's hospital caseload, and more than three-quarters of the inpatient admissions were emergencies.

Its beds for older patients were even more heavily used: the Trust came after Cardiff and just after Swansea as the busiest beds in Wales, with an occupancy level of 93 per cent. But while Gwent almost matched the Welsh average for numbers of acute patients treated per bed, it achieved just over 40 per cent of the Welsh average of patients per geriatric bed, the lowest in Wales, while its average length of stay for older patients, at 57 days (two months) was by far the longest of any Trust in Wales.

In other words, Gwent has a system that is relatively weak on discharging vulnerable patients to alternative forms of care, and which therefore relies heavily on the availability of sufficient hospital beds. As figures from the National Assembly Government demonstrate, the trend in Wales as a whole since 1999 has if anything been towards an increase or no change in average length of stay. Acute inpatients averaged 6.3 days in hospital in 1999, but this has now edged up by 10 per cent, to reach 7.0 by 2004–5.

Just 17 per cent of Gwent Healthcare's total hospital caseload, and less than half of the total elective caseload, were day cases – very low compared with many Trusts in England. Indeed in Wales as a whole numbers of day cases have actually been falling, after a massive drop in 2002–3, and are still well below the figures from 1999–2000. UNISON argued that:

> Finding ways to increase the use of day surgery seems to be a key issue in improving the performance of Gwent Healthcare and other Welsh Trusts on waiting lists and waiting times.

> (Lister 2006d)

In the context of ongoing cash constraints on the Trust and Local Health Boards, and the lack of a concrete plan to expand primary care and community services to fill in the gaps in hospital care, UNISON was far from convinced that the new plans were financially or organisationally viable.

> The entire infrastructure of community health services and primary care, which are absolutely vital to the plans outlined in the consultation document, is referred to only in passing in this consultation: but it is clear that any attempt to reconfigure services will require detailed and continuing attention to the recruitment, training and retention of an expanded workforce of staff delivering a range of services in community and local hospital settings which until now

have taken place in the large hospitals. There is as yet little sign that this preparation has been thoroughly thought through. Yet a failure of community services to deliver the expected improvements would leave the new network of hospitals facing an immediate crisis.

Since the need for the most specialised treatments is relatively rare, UNISON had no objection to centralising them in a single major hospital, as was largely the case already. The potential problem would arise from a reduced local ability to deliver prompt routine and emergency treatment, obliging more patients to travel to the specialist centre, where the reduced number of beds and facilities would come under pressure.

UNISON's response rejected the piecemeal approach to planning represented by the Clinical Futures consultation document, which did not properly address the mix of enhanced community and primary care services vital to sustain even the level of hospital beds provision it proposes. A viable plan required adequate investment in the whole of the health care system across Gwent: if any sector was under-resourced it would have adverse consequences on the other sectors of care. The union was also unconvinced that – in the absence of any identified costings or guarantees of capital funding – all six of the proposed new hospitals would actually be constructed. It seemed much more likely that a more limited number of new-build hospitals would be obliged to work in tandem with refurbished or even unrefurbished facilities at, say, Nevill Hall in Abergavenny or Newport's Royal Gwent. There was also doubt over the future of many of the Trust's 12 existing community and cottage hospitals; it was not clear whether endorsing this scheme would also be interpreted as agreeing to closure of these facilities – despite the fact that no case had been made to justify closures.

Unfortunately, despite using the language of partnership and collaboration, the consultation process in Gwent on these issues of long-term public concern was run more along the lines of the "consultations" in England, with little attempt by the authors of the plan to respond to difficult questions, clarify areas of doubt or to fill in the missing details sufficiently to win the confidence of the UNISON branch.

Other moves to reconfigure hospital services in Wales have also run into opposition, including the plans to close Swansea's neurosurgery unit at Morriston Hospital and create a new specialist unit in Cardiff in 2011 to cover the whole of South Wales. Opponents have raised numerous objections, not least the vastly extended journey times for patients from further west needing urgent treatment, and an angry march on 29 April underlined the potential impact of this issue on the imminent Assembly elections (Evans CM 2007). After the subsequent change of government, with a new coalition of Labour and Plaid Cymru, Health Minister Edwina Hart instituted a review of the proposals, and opted to retain both units (Hart 2007).

This has been part of a wider rethink of policy, which began in June 2007. First Minister Rhodri Morgan, extending an olive branch to other parties in the protracted attempts to secure a new governing coalition, called a temporary halt to all hospital closures and reconfiguration. He further promised that changes already agreed in district general hospitals would not be implemented until promised community services were in place (BBC News 2007d).

Possibly in response to this change of government line, Andy Williams, the chief executive of the beleaguered Powys Local Health Board (which had been wrestling with a £3.5 million deficit) resigned. There had been vocal protests over plans to axe services in four small hospitals in Powys, and the Welsh Assembly Government had announced an inquiry into the way the LHB was being managed (BBC News 2007e, f).

The new political complexion of government in Wales appears to be well set out in the joint statement *One Wales* endorsed by Plaid Cymru's leader Ieuan Wyn Jones and Labour's Rhodri Morgan, with a section on health services which reaffirms a commitment to a distinctive model quite unlike the current version of the NHS the other side of the Severn Bridge:

> We firmly reject the privatisation of NHS services or the organisation of such services on market models. We will guarantee public ownership, public funding and public control of this vital public service.

Stressing that the ownership and financial basis of the NHS does matter, the *One Wales* statement goes on to promise:

> We will move purposefully to end the internal market.

> We will eliminate the use of private sector hospitals by the NHS in Wales by 2011.

> We will rule out the use of Private Finance Initiative in the Welsh health service during the third term.

> We will end competitive tendering for NHS cleaning contracts.

Privatisation of non-clinical services had always been much more limited in Welsh hospitals than in England, but there has for some time been a movement to roll back the privatisation that did take place. In a conspicuous turnaround, the Swansea NHS Trust in 2006 defied the last minute threat of an injunction and went ahead with a new in-house hospital cleaning contract to replace the poor services delivered by ISS Mediclean (Lister 2005b). Around 480 domestic and portering staff working in the Morriston and Singleton hospitals transferred from Mediclean to the Trust. The resultant improvement in standards has been dramatic, and in November 2007, working to revised specifications and with more cleaning staff, the standard of cleaning in Swansea hospitals was showcased by the Welsh Audit Office as an example of good infection control (Swansea Hospitals Trust 2007).

In another sharp contrast to the top-down relentless "reform" and reconfiguration process that had triggered such angry protests across parts of middle England, *One Wales* promised a more thoughtful and responsive attitude:

> We will revisit and revise proposals which reconfigure individual services through single site solutions.

We will reinstate democratic engagement at the heart of the Welsh health service by putting the voice of patients and the public at the centre of what we do. We will reform NHS trusts to improve accountability both to local communities and to the Assembly government.

However this has not stopped Health Minister Edwina Hart rubber-stamping the merger of two giant South Wales Trusts, Swansea and Bro Morgannwg in April 2008 to form a new super-Trust with four major hospitals, 16,000 staff and a budget of £770 million. She had earlier approved the merger of Pontypridd and Rhondda and North Glamorgan Trusts to form Cwm Taf Trust in April 2008. There remains an unresolved question over the accountability of such large and geographically spread Trusts, and the longer-term drive towards rationalisation once mergers are carried through.

However, with a promise in the *One Wales* agreement to base future consultation documents on sound evidence, there is a possibility that the frenetic jargon and jumbled back-covering lists of *Designed for Life* and the evasions and vagueness of *Gwent Clinical Futures* could be superseded in Wales by a more serious attempt to engage with local communities, and set out to win and hold the confidence of NHS staff and service users rather than bully them into submission. That would certainly ensure clear red water between the policies of Cardiff and Westminster for some time to come.

Scotland

A similar political shift has taken place in Scotland, with the 2007 Scottish elections returning an SNP-led government which has also shifted, at least in words, leftwards from New Labour's model of market-based health care.

While Wales has set the pace on prescription charges, Scotland has used its devolved powers to introduce free personal care for older people at home or in nursing homes since 2002. With the National Health Service Reform (Scotland) Bill (2003) the Scottish Parliament has also gone the furthest down the line of scrapping the elements of the "internal market", and breaking down the purchaser–provider split, dissolving Trusts into 15 new unified NHS boards (Jervis 2008).

Historically Scotland has had the highest health spending of the UK nations, and the highest allocations of beds per head. However, since 1996 NHS spending has risen much faster in England than Scotland (up 30% by 2002 in England, but up by only 20% in Scotland). If health spending had been allocated in proportion to health needs (measured by standardised mortality ratios), Scotland's additional spending should have been 20% higher per head than England in 2002: instead it was just 16% higher (Alvarez-Rosete et al. 2005). There will be further pressure from 2008, because NHS spending in Scotland, as in Northern Ireland, faces a squeeze from next year under the plans set out by the SNP government, with a real-terms increase of just 1.4% to £11.2 billion, and relatively small increases for two more years. Spending plans include £97 million to phase out prescription charges and £270 million to reduce waiting times (Trueland 2007).

The pressure on hospital services generated by poor levels of general health and high levels of morbidity are clearly one factor in Scotland's much more intractable problems reducing waiting lists. While England is on target to ensure that no patient waits more than 18 weeks for treatment by the end of 2008, Scottish ministers have only promised the same by 2011 (Plumridge 2007).

Scottish Labour ministers initially set the pace after devolution in creating the new model of integrated health service and breaking from health reforms hatched up south of the border. Even while Scottish Labour MPs in Westminster loyally voted with Tony Blair and Alan Milburn to force through Foundation Trusts in England, Scottish ministers were insisting that they would not be introduced in Scotland. However, the integrated model has come under severe pressure, not least from the review of health services carried out in 2005 by Oxford University cancer specialist Professor David Kerr, *Building a Health Service Fit for the Future*. The proposals in Kerr's report included introducing a form of tariff funding, although not as part of a competitive market. But Kerr's *Fit for the Future*, like its namesake reviews up and down England, has also called for a switch of care from hospital to community and primary care level, and urged a fresh round of hospital rationalisation (Plumridge 2007).

Unlike its English equivalents, Kerr's report enthusiastically uses the "I" word: integration. This is a complete contrast with the market-style fragmentation and competition at the centre of New Labour reforms south of the border:

> At risk of seeming overly sentimental, I believe that a more truly Scottish model of healthcare would be to take a collective approach in which we generate strength from integration and transformation through unity of purpose. Patient choice is important, but the people of Scotland sent us a strong message that certainty carries greater weight – if we make a commitment to see or treat a patient on a specific date, we must honour this, and ensure the quality of care delivered.
>
> In practical terms, this implies investment in patient pathways that span primary and secondary care, networks of rural hospitals linked to and supported by the major teaching hospitals, rational distribution of services between neighbouring hospitals and national planning of complex service frameworks like neurosurgery and specialised children's services. I believe that Scotland is better suited to health improvement through collaboration and internal cohesion, making us externally competitive.
>
> (Kerr 2005)

However, this poses a problem for the politicians because, like a Scottish forerunner of Professor/Lord Darzi's more recent work in London and England, the central focus of Kerr's report flies in the face of popular opinion, attempting to displace popular and accessible District General Hospitals, and trying to change the behaviour of people who for generations have turned at times of emergency to accident and emergency departments. When push comes to shove these policies will always be hard to implement in the teeth of a sceptical electorate, especially when, like Kerr's report, the policies hinge on such utopian visions of out-of-hours and emergency services being delivered by GPs:

> Our work described above tells us that the majority of 'traditional' A&E activity can and should be delivered in local hospitals. It also tells us that it can only be sustained in those local hospitals by redesign. We are recommending a reprofiling of the current 'one size fits all' system where we squeeze a whole range of people, many of whom can be dealt with elsewhere, into busy hospital emergency departments.
>
> In its place we want to see a whole system approach to urgent care on the basis of our general principle of delivering care as locally as possible. The new system has GPs and nurse practitioners working alongside each other to maintain services in local hospitals.
>
> (Kerr 2005: 32)

Kerr's plans were initially backed by the Scottish National Party in opposition, and by Labour and the Liberal Democrats in government. However, that was two years ago, and the power has since changed hands at Holyrood. The SNP's Nicola Sturgeon is now Health Secretary, with a firm commitment and a mandate to halt the unpopular closure of A&E units at Monklands in Lanarkshire and Ayr, the cause of big protests. She promptly ordered NHS Lanarkshire and NHS Ayrshire to come up with new proposals which would keep the A&Es open, and set up a scrutiny panel to assess them. This concluded in November 2007 that the arguments for the Monklands closure were "weak". Another SNP MSP pointed out that – in a technique grimly familiar in the English NHS – the arguments to justify downgrading the existing A&E units had been presented in a biased manner "in an effort to push through the closures without proper scrutiny" (Schofield 2007).

More recently there have been big protests over plans to close down emergency medical services, coronary care and a high dependency unit at Vale of Leven Hospital in Dunbartonshire: mental health and maternity services are also being scaled down. The closures would mean some 6,000 patients a year would need to travel to Paisley for urgent treatment. NHS Greater Glasgow and Clyde in response have simply insisted that the hospital itself would not actually close. The plans were due to go before a scrutiny panel in September 2007 (Puttick 2007a).

If the Kerr plan, and plans claiming to be inspired by Kerr's plan, are now to be subject to this type of additional scrutiny, what other elements of the former Labour administration can be found in Scotland? There had never been any great effort made to recreate an English-style market in health care, not least because the heavy concentration of Scottish population and health services in Greater Glasgow and Lothian has meant that these are really the only health boards able to attract patients and revenue from outside their own boundaries, making any 'competition' completely and brazenly one sided.

Private involvement

Three main strands of Westminster health policy have made an impact on Scotland: PFI, treatment centres and the privatisation of primary care. Of the three, PFI is the one which has most powerfully located itself in the Scottish NHS, and will have a profound impact for decades to come. The first deals to build new hospitals in Scotland were among the very first PFI deals to be signed after Tony Blair's government took office, and the three completed projects at Wishaw, Hairmyres and Edinburgh have subsequently furnished numerous case studies to underline the flaws in PFI (Lister 2003a). More recently Edinburgh Royal Infirmary has been named as the second dirtiest hospital in Scotland (*Edinburgh Evening News* 2006), and in the autumn of 2007 was compelled to publish previously secret documentation revealing the terms of the contract with the PFI consortium, Consort (Puttick 2007b). Meanwhile, the contractual commitments involved in the PFI hospitals at Hairmyres and Wishaw, both in Lanarkshire, appear to have been a major factor driving the proposal to keep them open, but close the A&E at Monklands, another Lanarkshire hospital without such a hefty price tag for closure (BBC News Online 2006b). As in South East London and other parts of England, it seems that PFI is a powerful factor in shaping the profile of local services, to the detriment of the rest of the NHS.

Additional PFI contracts have been signed for a £180 million project to build new Stobhill and Victoria hospitals in Glasgow, and by the end of 2006, 20 new Scottish hospital projects were being planned or negotiated (Hellowell 2006). Early in 2007, NHS Forth Valley gave the go-ahead to a £300 million new hospital in Larbert to replace Falkirk and Stirling Royal Infirmaries, while NHS Greater Glasgow and Clyde contemplated a £500 million scheme for a new adult and children's hospital in Govan. Later, Allyson Pollock and Mark Hellowell in an article in *Public Money & Management*, warned that Scotland was on course to run up a £500 million per year bill for PFI hospital projects. In 2005–6, when only a few projects were up and running, Scottish health boards paid out over £100 million in "unitary charge" payments – equivalent to almost a quarter of the capital value of the hospitals. With the average lease lasting for 30 years, the PFI consortium could, on this basis, enjoy 26 years of profit. When as yet uncompleted hospitals come on stream, the annual bill will rise to over £500 million by the beginning of the next decade (Hellowell and Pollock 2007a; eGov Monitor 2007).

The SNP has proposed an alternative device to raise money for public sector projects in place of PFI: a Scottish Futures Trust would be established that would issue bonds enabling the provision of capital at a substantially lower overhead cost than PFI. However, this has been contested by Scottish Labour – on the basis that the Scottish Government has no legal powers to borrow money (surely ignoring the fact that PFI deals represent borrowing on a colossal scale). In June 2007 the Scottish Executive announced an end to "partnerships" with the private sector, and Health Secretary Sturgeon told the NHS Confederation that she was opposed to using public sector money "to help private companies compete with the NHS" (BBC News Online 2007).

Even if future plans for PFI are scaled down in Scotland, the hospitals already built mean that PFI is set to run as an income stream from Scotland's NHS for many years to come. However the Labour-led Scottish Executive had less success in promoting another core New Labour policy – private sector treatment centres.

Waiting list initiatives, which have eventually succeeded in scaling down Scotland's queues for care, have made extensive use of private clinics, commissioning some 3,000 operations from the private sector according to the Scottish Labour Party's 2005 manifesto for the Westminster elections (Evans JR 2007). So far, however, only one treatment centre, based in a disused 24-bed unit at Stracathro Hospital, near Brechin, Angus, has been commissioned, run by Amicus, a subsidiary of the South African private sector corporation Netcare.

The contract, signed in November 2006, is worth £15 million over three years for 8,000 operations including hip replacements, and makes use of local Tayside NHS consultants. Another parallel with the English method of health care policy has been the refusal of local management and Scottish ministers to reveal the costs of the operations performed, to allow any evaluation of whether the deal represents value for money. Tayside's Chief Operating Officer Gerry Marr is on record as insisting that:

> Our decision is based on legal advice. We have a legal obligation of confidentiality to Amicus and I cannot imagine any circumstances in which that advice would alter.
>
> (Evans JR 2007)

Ministers have said in reply to the SNP's John Swinney, then in opposition, that the private sector was to be used "to provide the opportunity to test the market in terms of innovative solutions which may be available through the independent sector which are not available in the NHS," although no details of these "innovations" have been revealed (Evans JR 2007).

With a contract so hedged about by secrecy, it is clearly very difficult to carry out any evaluation of the work that is done and the relative cost compared with an expansion of NHS facilities. There may be very good reasons indeed why the company and the NHS managers who negotiated with them want to keep the figures out of the public eye.

The privatisation of primary care services appeared to have come to a swift halt at the beginning of 2007, when a contract to run a Harthill Health Centre in Lanarkshire was awarded to a local GP rather than private contractor, Serco. NHS Lanarkshire had invited private sector bids to take over as an "alternative health provider". Health Secretary Nicola Sturgeon has followed this by announcing a very different scenario for the development of primary care services as part of the SNP's strategy *Better Health, Better Care*.

Her proposals do involve the development of an "immediate nurse treatment service" to be based in chemist shops, and developing walk-in GP clinics at railway stations and shopping centres (Puttick 2007c). Unlike the English policy and the more recent proposals from Alan Johnson and Lord Darzi, there is no proposal for the private sector to do any more than provide the premises for these services.

Clearly there could be a danger of treatment being more angled towards the prescription of drugs if the consultation takes place in a chemist's shop; but in the absence of primary care services many patients would in any event resort to over-the-counter purchases of remedies which may not be appropriate.

Social care

One area where the separation of policy has been most visible and long standing has been Scotland's determination to maintain a system of free personal care for older people, while in the rest of the UK this is subject to means-tested charges. Free nursing care was introduced throughout the UK in 2002, when the New Labour government implemented that aspect of the Royal Commission report (Bell and Bowes 2006).

The Scottish system of free personal care does not represent as big a difference from the English system as many believe. Payments for nursing care in Scotland (£65 per week in 2006) are half the maximum payable in England (£129), and Scottish people in nursing or residential homes do not receive the Attendance Allowance of up to £61 per week that their English counterparts can.

The £145 weekly payment for personal care (or £210 for those in nursing homes) falls short of the average care home costs of £440 per week, and Scottish Executive figures show that 41 per cent of residents in private and voluntary care homes were funded wholly or mainly by private means in 2001. Payments are means tested, so that older people with savings and assets in excess of £12,500 are required to pay on a tariff scale towards their care home fees: if they have capital of more than £20,750 they are required to meet the whole cost of their fees until the money has been spent down to that level. As in the rest of the UK, care home residents are expected to hand over all of their income towards the costs of the home, but allowed to keep a personal allowance of £20.45 per week (Counsel and Care 2007).

The system was originally costed at £125 million a year, but has increased to more than double that (£259 million) and is set to continue rising, although this is not a significant financial problem from a Scottish government budget of £12 billion.

However, a shock court ruling in October 2007 did throw doubt over the policy of free personal care for over 9,000 people who had made their own arrangements as "self-funders" in private nursing homes. Lord Macphail ruled that it was wrong for councils to pay their care costs. He argued that the "unusually complex" and "ambiguous" legislation intended to guarantee free care to all regardless of income did not do so; instead it obliged councils to cover care costs of pensioners living in their own homes, and those receiving public sector support (McDonnell and Robertson 2007).

The ruling has questioned whether councils have any obligation to continue funding people already in care homes: but it could also have the effect of delaying decisions and payments to new applicants. Nicola Sturgeon swiftly agreed to amend the legislation if required, but by the end of the year the SNP announced plans to review and consult on social care for the elderly (Hemmings 2007).

In Scotland and Wales it appears to be the pressure of relatively radical nationalist parties which has kept the flame of NHS values and old Labour universalism alight when the Labour Party has drifted towards the Westminster marketeers. In Northern Ireland, even more curiously, it is the combination of Unionists and Sinn Fein that is driving towards free personal care and free prescriptions. In each of these distinctive National Health Services it appears that popular pressure can have more visible and dramatic impact on ministerial decisions than in England, where New Labour's Westminster majority is bolstered by Scottish and Welsh MPs.

CHAPTER NINE

New dimensions in privatisation

Overview

TEN YEARS AFTER TONY BLAIR TOOK OFFICE pledging to sweep away the "costly and wasteful" internal market system, ministers are committed to imposing a market system that is even more costly and wasteful. They have almost trebled health spending, but increased tenfold the NHS spend on private sector health care, and in the process have fostered the artificial creation of a brand new private sector which has no viable existence in its own right, and is entirely dependent on government sponsorship.

Worse, the obsessive focus on market-style reforms and expanding the private sector means that the real achievements that have been notched up since 1997 – the dramatic reductions in waiting times and improvement in cancer, cardiac and other key areas of care – have been wrongly attributed by ministers and less discerning elements in the media to the "reforms", and not to the simple, old-fashioned expansion of bed numbers, staff and budgets that really did the trick.

New Labour seems to have lost the plot. Their "third way" mantra of rejecting "dogmatism" against use of the private sector has become a dogmatic insistence that the private sector has a key role to play – regardless of the lack of any real evidence in Britain or elsewhere to support this view.

Of course, ministers hotly dispute the use of the word "privatisation". They argue that the NHS as a whole remains a public service funded through taxation, delivering services free of charge at point of use. But in reality they have added a new dimension to the term "privatisation", which in the context of the National Health Service used to mean the contracting-out of non-clinical support services to private companies – a policy driven forward in the mid-1980s by a Thatcher government that always insisted that clinical care would remain within the NHS.

Competitive tendering was introduced across the NHS ancillary services in the mid-1980s. A terrible price was paid, in terms of the loss of a skilled and dedicated NHS workforce and declining standards of hygiene, for the minimal, largely short-term "savings" that were achieved, mainly through cuts in the numbers, pay and working conditions of already low-paid staff (Newbigging and Lister 1988; Lister 2005b).

The onslaught was largely on support services. Even when Kenneth Clarke embraced the notion of the Private Finance Initiative (PFI) as a means to privatise the provision of capital for NHS projects in 1993, he and successive ministers were at pains to stress that this would not involve the privatisation of clinical care.

New Labour has swept away this distinction. Under Blair and Brown, a growing number of services in hospital, community and primary care are also being handed over to private providers. Multinational firms are bidding for contracts to run GP surgeries, out-of-hours primary care, and a host of other services. GPs in turn are making use of their powers under Practice-Based Commissioning to award contracts for treatment to private companies in which they are shareholders (Blake 2007). The expansion of private sector provision has been far larger and more rapid than many expected. Under John Major's government prior to 1997 the NHS was buying no more than an estimated £96 million of operations a year from private hospitals, mainly through the activity of fundholding GPs; the entire private market in NHS services was less than £200 million a year (Timmins 2005b). But in 2007, contracts for patient care with private hospitals, treatment centres, diagnostic services, psychiatric services and nursing homes amount to more than ten times that total. This is over and above the continuing contracts for hospital ancillary and other non-clinical services "outsourced" since the mid-1980s, and the soaraway sums involved in PFI hospitals and primary care services privately financed through LIFT schemes, all of which have taken place since 1997 (Timmins 2005b).

The Tory government never succeeded in signing a single hospital deal under PFI, because ministers would not make sufficient concessions to ensure the private sector carried no real risk. Now PFI payments for the hospitals already completed are estimated to be already costing an extra £500 million a year above the equivalent cost through public financing, with many of the very biggest schemes still in the pipeline and yet to levy their first charges. The cost of PFI in the NHS has been officially estimated at a staggering £53 billion repayments on investments totalling £8 billion – with upwards of £20 billion available as a guaranteed profit stream for shareholders, and even more to be made in windfall profits from refinancing deals (Nunns 2007).

In addition, the first contracts are being signed for a second wave of "Independent Sector Treatment Centres" (ISTCs) which are expected to cover up to 200,000 elective operations a year, despite growing doubts on whether this additional capacity is genuinely needed, or whether the first wave ISTCs are delivering value for money (Timmins 2007e). The second wave ISTCs are now expected to bring the private sector total to around 370,000 patients a year – a significant number, although well short of the 500,000 originally proposed, and even further short of the 15 per cent of elective operations, as suggested by John Reid when he was Health Secretary (which would equate to 900,000 a year) or the suggestion of even higher numbers by Patricia Hewitt (UNISON 2007). The total spent on private sector treatment and diagnostics may fall short of the target £1 billion per year.

So is all the concern over the impact of the private sector exaggerated?

The answer lies not so much in the scale as in the impact of the new private sector on NHS Trusts. The impact on patient care has clearly been hugely inflated to justify the government's policies. Ministers claimed that the NHS could not deliver its ambitious targets to reduce waiting times without using "extra capacity in the private sector" – but they never bothered to explain why expanding NHS capacity would not be better value and more sustainable. They have wildly exaggerated the impact of the policies implemented so far, claiming in 2006 that:

> 400,000 people have been taken off hospital waiting lists since 1997. 114,000 – 1 in 4 – have had their operation in an ISTC…
>
> (Parliamentary Labour Party 2006)

In fact, the NHS carries out around 6 million elective operations a year. The pinprick of the 1.3 per cent of elective operations carried out in ISTCs must be set against the loss of revenue from NHS Trusts, which has begun to destabilise local NHS orthopaedic, ophthalmic and other departments, as cash is pumped out to private providers.

Even within individual specialties, NHS consultants have always disputed the significance of the contribution made by private sector units. Consultant ophthalmic surgeon Mr Simon Kelly for example has argued that the key to reducing waiting times for cataract was not the relative handful of cases treated in the new private sector, but over 300,000 operations carried out by NHS teams (Kelly 2005). And of course there is a premium price to be paid for the private sector's limited contribution. Ministers now admit that the average surplus paid on ISTC contracts is 11.2 per cent above NHS tariff – which effectively means that for every nine patients treated in ISTCs, the NHS could have afforded to treat ten, if the cash had been kept in the public sector. But of course the caseload is not comparable; the ISTC and diagnostic contracts specify that the private sector will accept only the most straightforward and uncomplicated cases, which are cheaper to deliver – and leave all the more expensive and risky cases to the NHS.

The size of the private sector and its contribution to the NHS caseload are still small, but its impact on the shaky finances of NHS providers has been disproportionately large. New Labour's private sector contracts have brought with them a requirement to restructure the financing of NHS Trusts, to allow a chunk of the public sector budget to be spent elsewhere. This is why ministers have imposed the complex and expensive system of "Payment by Results" which pays NHS Trusts on a fixed tariff per item of treatment delivered – but ensures that each and every patient who chooses or is directed to go elsewhere for treatment takes the money with them, and leaves a hole in the budget. PCTs have faced increased administration costs estimated at £90–£190,000 a year each to implement PBR (*HSJ* 2006), which also has a number of other negative side-effects. Not the least of these is a double perverse incentive to acute hospitals – to admit patients from A&E rather than to treat and discharge, and having admitted and treated a patient, to discharge them as soon as possible regardless of their condition, because the fixed fee does not recompense a Trust for additional days of nursing care for those who require it.

Either way, patients stand to lose out, while the Trusts have lost any certainty on the resources they will have and the level of services they can afford to offer, since a fluctuation in demand can result in an unexpected drop in revenue, or even a sudden surge of patients for whom there are insufficient resources. The loss of the block contract and the focus on the random element of "patient choice" has pulled the rug from under any concept of planning services to meet local needs. In this type of market there is no safe way to invest in new and improved equipment or accommodation, because future fluctuations could simply remove the income stream necessary to repay the loans. However all of these problems fall only on the NHS hospital Trusts. The private sector is exempt from Payment by Results. Instead, ISTCs get long-term contracts – many of them on a guaranteed "play or pay" basis, which mean private for-profit providers are assured of an annual payment regardless of how few patients opt for (or can be cajoled into using) their services.

Ministers say they want "contestability" with a "sustainable independent sector" as a means to improve NHS services (DoH 2005): but the "contest" is purely a one-way process. NHS Trusts and Foundations are explicitly barred from bidding for ISTC contracts, while the private sector gets subsidies for start-up costs, preferential rates, and is exempt from "Payment by Results". So *all* of the risk, uncertainty – and prospect of cutbacks and closures – remain firmly in the public sector. Large Trusts with £200 million and larger turnover are left to guess how much they will receive for patient care, while the private sector is encouraged to expand. As a result, the expansion of the private sector since 1997 increasingly threatens to take place at the expense of – and in place of – NHS provision, rather than delivering "additionality" by supplementing NHS capacity.

But of course the private sector cannot fully replace the NHS. It will not offer the comprehensive range of services, the A&E services, the treatment for complex and chronic illness. The private sector operates its own Inverse Care Law, focusing most of its resources on the least demanding and least risky treatments – which also tend to involve treating younger and fitter, and often wealthier patients. The premium payment to commission elective operations from ISTCs effectively diverts resources away from more serious and long-term cases, often older and poorer people, for whom only the NHS offers any care at all. If these services are forced to close, no "market" pressure will generate a replacement. To model the whole NHS around the ISTC model is to break up its universal and comprehensive character as a service.

The case for private sector involvement has always been ideological rather than financial – since, like most of New Labour's restructuring reforms, it has resulted in higher costs and overheads, and been delivered despite the absence of any supporting evidence to show its effectiveness. This helps explain how ministers have combined the double whammy of increasing spending to record levels while at the same time annoying, confusing and demoralising such large sectors of the NHS workforce.

No relief or rethink seems to be in sight. Pensions Secretary John Hutton in a speech to the CBI business lobby on May 16, argued that the 'reforms' imposed on the NHS and other public services, including "marketisation" and "an open-minded approach to who provides" have now been "built into the DNA" of public services, and "Gordon Brown has been at the heart of this process".

Cabinet Secretary Gus O'Donnell, speaking to a PricewaterhouseCoopers forum has also praised the role of market-style policies, insisting that "we need market incentives to improve efficiency". Apparently unaware of the contradiction, O'Donnell also admitted that an essential element to usher in the level of "choice" that Blair and Brown have promised is that "you have to have some spare capacity". Of course the existence of unused spare capacity – especially if some of it is additional capacity provided by the private sector at increased cost above NHS rates – is by definition *less* efficient than making full use of the appropriate amount of capacity. But in fact the new system of "Payment by Results" ensures that the NHS cannot afford to maintain any spare, unused capacity. Trusts are paid only for work they do, and only the private sector gets paid to maintain empty beds.

NHS Trusts, by contrast, are forced into contemplating cutbacks and closures when patients are diverted to private treatment centres. This is the backdrop to the round of rationalisation and closures that has been looming in the wings across much of England in the last two years, and which has been held back only by the political impact of strong local protests. New Labour seems set on a course of cutting back popular public provision... to make room for private companies that no campaigners have demanded or endorsed.

One classic current case study underlines the contradictions of New Labour's privatisation and "reforms". Despite having apparently complied with virtually every aspect of the government's regime of targets and reforms, Hinchingbrooke Health Care Trust (HHCT) in Huntingdon has become one of the most obvious victims of the market-style reforms introduced by New Labour:

- As a historically low cost provider, but unable to claim additional cash under the new tariff, HHCT has lost out under Payment by Results

- Its treatment centre – funded through PFI at a total cost of £93 million for a £22 million unit – has been starved of referrals, as PCTs have reneged on agreements

- Its caseload has been squeezed by Foundation Trusts in Peterborough and Cambridge

- Its budget is to be cut to allow the PCT to send NHS patients to private hospitals 30 miles away

- And the merger of Cambridgeshire's PCTs has lumbered Huntingdonshire's health services with new deficits, squeezing HHCT's budget.
  (Lister 2007h)

Efficient, low-cost NHS Trusts like HHCT have been denied any opportunity to compete on level ground with private providers: and as a consequence the public sector provision is being run down to create space for a new private sector.

Ministers are pressing ahead regardless. One indication of the direction of travel was the appointment of R. Channing Wheeler, a senior executive from the American health insurance market, to one of the top positions in the NHS management structure, commissioning services from private and NHS providers. Wheeler had been chief executive of a subsidiary of UnitedHealth, the most profitable private health care provider in the USA, collecting a seven-figure salary plus perks, and making handsome donations to the Republican Party. It seems he has fitted in well with the New Labour team and their pro-market advisors (Timmins 2007f).

The rest of this chapter will look at the main elements in New Labour's new market and its increasingly close alignment with the private sector, despite the complete absence of evidence to show that this can deliver the promised improvements in health services and patient care. The overview will begin with the privatisation of clinical care through independent sector treatment centres, and private diagnostic centres, the crisis in NHS treatment centres, the franchising of management of "failing" Trusts, and the privatisation of increasing sections of the NHS regulatory and management structure with the involvement of highly profitable management consultants.

The final section of the chapter will chart the development of the Private Finance Initiative and its equivalent in primary and community care, LIFT.

From concordat to treatment centres

When is a private hospital not a private hospital? When it is an "Independent Sector Treatment Centre" – the coy official New Labour-speak for privately owned and run units previously known as Diagnostic and Treatment Centres (DTCs). But while 20 NHS-run DTCs have been quietly established and are on course to operate successfully, a key element in the NHS Plan was to allocate a substantial share of the routine elective (non-emergency) surgical and diagnostic work to the private sector.

The Plan focused on creating a new "partnership" with the private sector – the same private sector that in the UK has routinely poached NHS-trained nursing and medical staff, and which around the world cherry picks the patients and the procedures which offer the most profits, leaving all of the costly, long-term and intensive treatment to the public sector, if they are provided at all.

Milburn's "partnership" began with the "Concordat", signed in the autumn of 2000, which proposed a greater use of private sector hospitals to provide treatment for NHS-funded patients. It was later admitted that premium payments averaging over 40 per cent above going NHS costs were paid to private hospitals under these arrangements – siphoning cash from the budgets of the Trusts which were already struggling to cope with local demand (DoH Commercial Directorate 2004). The inflated costs for these elective operations also served to switch funding from emergency care to elective, regardless of the level of clinical need.

A whole BUPA hospital in Redhill in Surrey was effectively hired to deliver treatment for NHS patients – though the costs of this deal were never publicly revealed. BUPA's standard costs for routine operations are well above those in the NHS. More recently the NHS Trust has taken over the whole operation, bringing the service back in-house (*HSJ* reporters 2007).

The Concordat was grasped as a lifeline by a private sector which has never broken through to command the involvement of more than one in eight of the British population, and was carrying vast numbers of under-used beds: but ministers wanted to go further and, even though there was probably enough spare capacity in the existing private hospitals to handle the extra workload, opted to sponsor the creation of a new private sector to compete with the NHS for up to 15 per cent of its total elective caseload (DoH Commercial Directorate 2004).

The use of existing private hospitals continued under the guise of "general supplementary" contracts (Secretary of State for Health 2006).

First wave DTCs

According to ministers the DTCs were to be different; they were to be new units, set up and run from the outset by the private sector. Under the original specification, they were supposed to bring all of the necessary staff with them, making no demands on the local pool of qualified health workers. This meant that many of the corporations submitting bids have been overseas or multinational companies. They were supposed to ensure "additional clinical activity, additional workforce, productivity improvements, focusing specifically on additional capacity".

> It will be a contractual requirement for providers to define and operate a workforces plan that makes available additional staff over and above those available to the NHS. ...We recognise that additional costs may result from our requirement for the independent DTC to provide staff that genuinely add to the NHS workforce... We will recognise these factors in our evaluation of value for money.
>
> (DoH 2002b: 6)

Of the preferred bidders, five were from overseas – from Canada, South Africa and the USA, and two British (DoH Press release 2003).

They were to treat only non-urgent cases where waiting times had been a problem, including orthopaedics (hip and knee replacements), ophthalmology (mainly removal of cataracts) and minor general surgery such as hernia and gall bladder removal. The profit-seeking DTCs would scoop up a share of the projected caseload of 250,000 procedures a year which would be delivered in this way – 135,000 extra operations, and 115,000 treatments diverted from existing NHS units "to free up NHS capacity" (DoH Press Release 2003).

The private units would have no obligation in terms of after-care: and they would be able to fix their own terms and conditions: they would be offering consultants four or five times the amount currently paid to NHS consultants.[20] To make matters worse they were also told that they would after all be free to recruit staff from the NHS (the BMA claimed up to 70 per cent of ISTC staff could be seconded from the NHS) – potentially stripping local hospitals of the staff they needed, and burdening them with sky-high bills for agency staff to fill the gap (BBC News 2003a).

While ministers initially claimed DTCs would be paid the same cost per case as NHS hospitals, preferred providers knew they were always going to be allowed a premium price plus the guarantee of a "take or pay" contract, which ensured they would be paid the full amount regardless of how few patients presented for treatment (DoH 2002c, d). Ministers have subsequently revealed that the average premium on first-wave ISTCs was 11.2 per cent above the NHS reference cost (Secretary of State for Health 2006).

It was also clear that the private sector would concentrate on the most profitable and simple cases, excluding any which might present any complications (as measured against the American Society of Anaesthesiologists (ASA) score (DoH 2005)), and as a result leaving the NHS with an increasingly expensive caseload. Furthermore the DTCs' start-up costs would be subsidised – giving them a greater chance of generating a surplus.

Unlike NHS units such as the Oxford Eye Hospital, where the revenue from cataract operations helped underwrite the running costs of a department delivering a full range of services, any surplus created by DTCs would simply be pocketed as profit by shareholders. Oxford Eye Hospital had been working to a plan of expanding its capacity to treat cataract and reduce waiting lists to three months by December 2004. Consultants faced with the launch of an unwanted new ISTC pointed out that there was "no capacity gap in Oxfordshire – in fact we can demonstrate over-capacity". A DoH document on capacity gaps the previous December had made no reference to Oxfordshire.

Rather than providing extra capacity to treat additional patients, the new DTC would transfer up to 50 per cent of NHS cataract patients into the private sector, at higher cost.

According to top consultants at the Eye Hospital, the consequence was likely to be:

• Restricted ability to screen and treat patients with other eye problems, many potentially more sight threatening than cataract

• The Eye Hospital would be left with a more complex and expensive caseload

---

20 A DoH circular insisted that it was not true that the ophthalmic surgeons to work in DTCs would be paid £450–500,000 per year "as some clinicians have decided to assume when reading the pricing proformas and spreadsheets." "These staff costs include the add on costs such as pensions, admin, travel, etc." In other words, the package for these doctors would be very close to £450,000. "In reality the ophthalmic surgeons are probably paid more than those currently in the NHS but they work a lot harder for it" (*Health Emergency* 58, 2003).

- Withdrawal from outreach clinics in surrounding towns (Banbury, Wantage, Abingdon, Bicester and Witney)

- A loss of specialist corneal diseases services – meaning patients would have to travel to London for treatment

- Questions over the viability of on-call services, A&E services and specialist services

- Training and research – which requires a minimum caseload – would be restricted, with the danger of losing accreditation for training

- It would become impossible to recruit a Professor, undermining the academic department

- Restricted choice for patients, since the full DTC contract would have to be paid for, regardless of how many people were treated: the PCT would need to pressurise cataract patients to use the private unit.

(Health Emergency 58, 2003)

The Oxfordshire deal, awarding the work to South African for-profit company Netcare, was forced through the local Primary Care Trusts with the full weight of the NHS regional and national bureaucracy behind it. Eventually the contract was scaled down from 800 to just 450 cataract operations a year – but by November 2005 only 50 of 323 available pre-operative assessments had been booked, and only 43 operations had been done out of 249 theatre slots available. Since the NHS was committed to pay the full contract cost, each operation in the DTC effectively cost the equivalent of six times the NHS national tariff (Hanna 2006). After the stand-off with SW Oxfordshire PCT in particular, which led to the removal of its chair and the resignation of a non-executive director in a bitter row with the Strategic Health Authority, ministers were keen to rewrite the rules and reorganise the NHS to exclude the PCTs from any future involvement in the decisions on DTC projects (Secretary of State for Health 2006: 15).

Elsewhere, too, the opposition to DTC plans was widespread. Private hospital chiefs were upset that new units were being built instead of filling up their existing empty beds. Tory Shadow Health Minister Liam Fox argued that the contracts were too expensive. Almost all organisations representing health staff opposed the new private centres; UNISON warned that they would drain resources and staff from the NHS. Even the Royal College of Nursing expressed concern over staffing levels. The BMA said the DTCs could destabilise the NHS. The Association of Surgeons in Training warned that the centres could do lasting damage (*Health Emergency* 58, 2003). NHS units have responsibility for training doctors and nursing staff, and need to maintain a broad mix of routine and more complex cases to ensure that junior doctors gain the necessary experience. DTCs, by creaming off a large share of the routine work, would disrupt this balance while simply poaching the staff already trained.

To make matters worse, despite the talk of an NHS Plan, the proposals for DTCs have run alongside contradictory government targets, pressure on local

Primary Care and Hospital Trusts to reduce waiting times to a maximum of six months by 2005, and even an injection of new funds into the NHS to enable it to expand its own capacity. However just as some of those investments were starting to deliver, a small group of bureaucrats at national level announced where the new private sector DTCs were to be. Local health commissioners were given no say. Where, as in the case of Oxford ophthalmic services, PCTs objected, they were slapped down.

One of Patricia Hewitt's very first pronouncements, just hours after taking office in May 2005, claiming to be a "listening Health Secretary", was a new allocation of £3 billion for the purchase of additional treatment from the private sector. This second major round of tendering for private contracts opened in the autumn of 2005. The tendering documents made no bones about the long-term plan:

> A key factor in this Plan is the Independent Sector (IS) Procurement Programme, the purpose of which is to provide additional capacity, expand new ways of working and develop a sustainable IS market. The Plan anticipates that by 2008 the IS will provide an increasing volume and range of both elective procedures and diagnostics tests for NHS patients.
>
> (DoH 2005)

To make it quite clear that the driving force is privatisation and marketisation rather than expanding capacity, the reduction of waiting lists came third in the Department of Health's "primary objectives", which are itemised as:

- To help to create a sustainable, VfM [Value for Money], IS market in the provision of elective care to NHS patients

- To provide more choice for patients and real contestability in elective services

- To support implementation of the 18-week waiting time target, which comes into effect from December 2008.

The document went on to assert that the creation of this new competition would somehow "improve productivity and VfM in NHS-run services" (DoH 2005).

There was no evidence to support this assumption: indeed the first round of treatment centre contracts had not been completed, with some services yet to come on stream, and there had been no systematic evaluation of their effectiveness or value for money.

Expanding the private sector

The government plan to funnel new money preferentially into the private sector rather than adopt the cheaper and easier policy of expanding NHS provision, was leading to a dramatic expansion of commercial medicine. From a relatively small and marginal operation running with only around half of the beds occupied in its (generally very small) hospitals, feeding off historic NHS waiting lists, the private health care sector in Britain was seeing a big injection of cash and a massive increase in the numbers of NHS patients being treated in private beds. The Healthcare Commission had predicted that traditional paying patients would represent just over half of the caseload in private beds, with as many as 45 per cent of private sector operations paid for by the NHS, figures close to the forecast of Tony Blair that the NHS would soon be purchasing 40 per cent of the operations carried out by private hospitals (Mulholland 2006; *Health Emergency* 62, 2006). This was effectively a huge cash subsidy to force the expansion of a private sector which would inevitably draw on the same pool of human and financial resources as the NHS.

As the Department's own document explained, the new schemes had gone well beyond the notion of expanding NHS capacity, and were now seeking to transfer existing NHS work to private treatment centres. This was the pretext under which the staffing restrictions could be eased:

> Providers will be able to use NHS staff when providing the services for schemes where there is transferred activity.

> Where there is transferred activity it is expected that the amount of NHS staff time available to the Provider (as a proportion of the Provider's total staffing requirement) will be approximately equal to the amount of transferred activity as a proportion of total activity to be delivered by the Provider.

> (DoH 2005)

However the new proposals also made it easier to employ NHS-trained professional staff even where there was no transfer of activity:

> Providers will only be prohibited from recruiting NHS staff in specialties facing workforce shortages. Work is ongoing to identify any further shortage professions;

> All doctors, nurses and other healthcare professionals (whether or not in shortage professions) will be permitted to use their non-contracted hours to work for Providers, subject to first fulfilling their NHS commitments.

It was not just NHS staff who were to be handed over to fuel the private sector expansion. NHS buildings, some of them brand new, were also to be offered up to sweeten local deals. According to the same tendering document:

- A brand new state of the art NHS treatment centre in Birmingham, not even yet open, was to be handed over to private operators

- Also facing privatisation was a specialist unit in the new PFI-financed New Forest hospital in Lymington

- In South Yorkshire NHS catheter laboratories in Rotherham and Barnsley could be handed over as part of a cardiology contract

- "Spare surgical capacity" in NHS hospitals in the South West Peninsula could also be made available for private companies carrying out NHS-funded operations

- And a huge renal dialysis contract covering much of the north of England could see dozens of NHS units handed over for private operators to refurbish and run for profit.

> (DoH 2005)

Primary Care Trusts had been under instruction to send at least 10 per cent of their NHS elective (waiting list) operations to private hospitals by the end of 2005, but soon after taking office Patricia Hewitt set course to increase this still further, towards a longer-term target of 15 per cent, and insisted that there would be "no arbitrary limits" on the share of the market that private providers could capture (UNISON 2007).

The target figure of diverting 15 per cent of NHS elective caseload to private sector providers may have seemed arbitrary, but it reflected a secret survey of the scope for a new market in health care that had been drawn up the previous July by the Department of Health's Commercial Directorate, headed up by American import Ken Anderson. The survey began from the basis that ministers wanted to build up sufficient capacity in the private sector to generate "contestability" – a real fear that NHS Trusts that failed in the new market could be allowed close down, with the private sector picking up the services they could not provide (DoH Commercial Directorate 2004). The Commercial Directorate concluded that a market involving 15 per cent of NHS elective operations would be sufficient to secure the long-term involvement of four rival private companies. What this survey and the bid for "contestability" did not even attempt to address was the knock-on impact on the wide range of emergency and other services which have only ever been available from NHS hospitals, and which the private sector has shown no interest in providing.

Critics of the plans warned that if large numbers of patients were encouraged as individuals to opt for a private sector provider, they could unwittingly trigger the financial collapse and possibly closure of local health services or whole NHS hospitals – even those which are doing well under the current system. Hospitals which lost a slice of their elective care would see their unit costs go up, as existing capacity would be used by fewer patients, and as the NHS would be left to deal with the cases which the private sector does not wish to treat. The BMA warned that even hospitals which lost as few as 10 per cent of their elective patients to the private sector or to other NHS Trusts could be forced to close departments, or close altogether. Hewitt warned that any 'failing' NHS hospitals – those that lost out in this new, unfair competition with the private sector – would be closed down (*Health Emergency* 61, 2005).

Seeing through the scanner contracts

The privatisation of diagnostic services had also begun: private sector MRI scans had also been purchased for NHS patients – again on a long-term, generous contract which allowed Alliance Medical Limited, the contractor, to cherry pick only the most straightforward and uncomplicated scans, leaving the remainder to the NHS, while collecting full payment despite falling well short of targets for completed scans. Towards the end of 2007 an internal Department of Health report strongly criticising the quality of diagnostic services delivered by Atos Healthcare to eight PCTs in the North West was released under Freedom of Information legislation. The company delivered poor quality ultrasound images

– with 43 per cent not good enough to allow staff to draw correct conclusions – lacked proper supervision and failed to deliver a radiologist's report before returning images (Evans O 2007). The *Health Service Journal* also reported growing speculation that several of the diagnostics contracts proposed back in 2005 might finally be killed off (Mooney 2007c).

NHS treatment centres squeezed out

Even where public capital had already been invested in state of the art NHS-run treatment centres there was no long-term guarantee that these would remain viable or operational. Some were already in trouble. While the privately run treatment centres received long-term guaranteed income on a "take or pay" basis, and had been allowed to charge higher than NHS reference costs, none of these conditions applied to the 20 pioneering NHS treatment centres that had been established with few fanfares, but proved themselves highly effective and popular with patients – while remaining firmly integrated with the wider NHS.

While NHS consultants had been instructed by managers to pass over a share of their waiting list workload for treatment in private sector units, there was no such pressure to maintain the flow of patients to NHS units.

The blatant bias that was shown in favour of private providers was exposed by the problems faced by pioneering NHS-run treatment centres. These included the Ambulatory Care and Diagnostic (ACAD) unit at Central Middlesex Hospital; Kidderminster, where a new £14 million NHS treatment centre was seriously under used while a new ISTC was set up on the same site; the brand new, publicly funded £16 million South West London Elective Orthopaedic Centre (SWLEOC), based at Epsom General Hospital; and Ravenscourt Park Hospital, another orthopaedic centre in NW London, which had been leased from the private sector in 2002. By mid-November 2004 the ACAD had spare capacity to treat 3,000 more patients, Hammersmith Hospitals had 4,000 spare slots, and the new unit at Kidderminster Hospital had scope to treat 2,000, because the promised referrals from the NHS had not arrived. Payment by Results meant that every promised patient not referred left a gaping hole in the accounts. SWLEOC was £4 million in the red by 2005, and Ravenscourt Park a massive £12.5 million. Even the powerful University College London Hospital (UCLH) was warning that it may have to scale down its treatment centres if the odds remained stacked against them; but Foundation Trusts like UCLH remained banned from bidding for the provision of the next round of treatment centres (*Health Emergency* 61, 2005).

Early in 2005, the Epsom and St Helier hospitals NHS Trust told staff that an advert had been placed in the official EU Journal inviting private companies to bid to take over the management of SWLEOC. The decision appeared to flow from national level, and there was speculation that a similar fate might also befall Ravenscourt Park. In the event, Ravenscourt Park closed in 2006 and has since been sold to developers, closing a chapter in the NHS provision of treatment centre services in north London. By contrast, the campaigners who intervened at a Trust board meeting proved successful in stalling the efforts to hive off SWLEOC, which is still operating and delivering high-quality NHS care as this book is completed.

Cutting back the plans

2007 saw some pruning on the original plans for ISTCs: Hertfordshire scrapped a planned "surgicentre" for Hemel Hempstead as too expensive compared with NHS treatment, and NHS London axed a controversial £35 million scheme for a south London ISTC, to the profound annoyance of Clinicenta, who had been in the frame for the contract. The deal would have struck a heavy financial blow at most London Trusts and Foundation Trusts south of the Thames (Moore 2007a; Carlisle 2007c). Only six of the promised 24 second wave ISTC schemes had been signed, and six had been cancelled, with slow progress on some of the remainder. However, this has proved not so much the ministerial change of heart that the private sector had feared and union leaders longed for, as a pragmatic recognition of the financial problems facing already troubled local health economies.

By the autumn of 2006 it had become obvious that many treatment centres were delivering far short of the contracted numbers of treatments, and an in-depth investigation by the *Health Service Journal* suggested they were delivering as few as 60 per cent of their target (Moore 2006a). More recent figures have shown little improvement, with the *HSJ* finding 50,000 operations paid for and not delivered (Moore 2007b). The Department of Health eventually published its own figures in November 2007 showing that five of the 27 phase one schemes were performing at 60 per cent or less of contracted levels, with the Will Adams unit in Medway managing just 48 per cent. In the West Midlands a new diagnostic service run by Care UK was axed just after opening, after just 5 per cent of the expected patients opted to use it.

On the plus side for the private sector, in the north west the same NHS regime had just instituted a monitoring process to check that PCTs were sending sufficient patients to the privately run integrated clinical assessment and treatment service (ICATS) negotiated by the Department of Health, which is to cost a staggering £104 million a year – despite the fact that acute hospital Trusts in the north west argue it is not needed to meet the 18-week waiting time target (Mooney 2007d). Lord Darzi was also on the case, adding his support to the ISTCs and linking up with Alan Johnson in proposing new link-ups with the private sector to deliver primary care, 100 new GP practices and 150 new "polyclinics" (Timmins 2007g).

Franchising out NHS Trust management

The NHS Plan in 2000 began to lay the basis for separating out Trusts into a two-tier system by promising to reward the best-performing 'green light' hospitals with additional resources and "earned autonomy", while threatening those which were struggling to meet targets and scoring yellow or red lights on external inspection visits with varying degrees of escalating intervention, culminating in the imposition of a new management. In the NHS Plan there was just a hint that this intervention might not be from NHS managers, but from outside the NHS, when it suggested:

> Clinicians and managers from 'green' organisations could be deployed for this purpose. Alternatively expressions of interest could be invited from elsewhere, and subject to a tender from an approved list.
>
> (DoH 2000b: 66)

Eventually these proposals developed into a star ratings system, under which the most successful three-star Trusts were to be allowed to become Foundation Hospitals – with a variety of new freedoms, including the right to set up "non-profit" private companies or establish partnerships with private sector providers, while those failing to cope with pressures and meet targets would be subjected to an escalating process of intervention, potentially culminating in the "franchising" of their management to external organisations.

Ministers probably thought this all sounded dynamic and determined: however the experience of "franchising" out the management of failing NHS Trusts to managers from elsewhere, whether NHS or private sector was far from positive.

The most notorious failure was at the Good Hope Hospital Trust, the first to have its management franchised to a private company. The three-year contract between the GHH Trust and Secta to manage the financially challenged 550-bed hospital began amid a welter of optimistic publicity in September 2003, but was terminated eight months early at the end of 2005 after Anne Heast, the Secta employee appointed to the chief executive role, left for another position within Secta's parent company Tribal Group. The running of the hospital was handed to the management of Birmingham Heartlands Hospital Trust.

During the contract the company had successfully increased its own fees by 48 per cent in the first year, but this was clearly not performance-related pay. Instead, by the time the Trust's acting chief executive, Secta's Anne Heast, finally cleared her desk the Trust was in dire financial straits, losing money at £1 million per month, heading for a £47 million deficit, and threatening the entire local health economy.

An Audit Commission report on the franchise agreement revealed a managerial shambles, with no financial strategy in place, and branded the franchise agreement as a costly failure:

> During the period of the franchise, the cost of the chief executive to the Trust was £225,000 per annum. This is approximately £60,000 to £80,000 more than would be paid for a direct appointment. In addition, in excess of £1 million has been spent on interventions during the contract period.
>
> The franchise arrangement, despite significant effort on behalf of the Trust and private sector company, was only partially successful and introduced significant additional costs to the Trust.
>
> (Audit Commission 2006)

Inadequate provision within the contract meant the Trust itself could not terminate the contract early or enforce penalty clauses.

Shortly after the deal ended, managers at the hospital agreed on radical cost-cutting measures including a loss of beds, wards and buildings, to make potential savings of £21 million a year. The hospital said the measures were needed to prevent a worst-case scenario deficit of £47.5 million the following year: quite a legacy from a pioneering privatisation of NHS management.

PCT gives commission to big business

2007 was the year in which – after almost two years of hesitation – the Department of Health began to apply open pressure on PCTs to bring in private companies to advise them on commissioning, and warned SHAs that they would be measured on the number of PCTs that were implementing the Framework for Procuring External Support for Commissioners (FESC) (Mooney 2007e). Even in advance of the publication of a DoH list of approved companies it was clear that PCTs were expected to comply. The final list of 14 trusted firms – three of which were US insurers whose trustworthiness was strongly questioned in Michael Moore's film *Sicko* – was unveiled by Health Secretary Alan Johnson in October.

In September the financially challenged Hillingdon Primary Care Trust, which at one point had been recommended to privatise 90 per cent of its staff, confirmed that it was to bring in management consultants from BUPA to help it commission services (Mooney 2007f).

Hampshire PCT appointed Roger Hymas, a strategy advisor from US health giant Humana as its director of commissioning. Hymas had not even gone through the motions of leaving the company, but moved over on a two-year secondment to help carve up the £200 million a year Hampshire health budget. Humana and the PCT chief executive both insisted that there was no conflict of interest involved in allowing such a senior private sector fox into the NHS henhouse (Mooney 2007g).

Regulator privatised

Meanwhile concerns over the future direction of Foundation Trusts were heightened by reports in the *Health Service Journal* revealing that Monitor, the 'independent regulator' charged with overseeing Foundation Trusts, had itself been largely privatised. Two-thirds of Monitor's £15.5 million first year budget had been spent on hiring private management consultants from the USA, flying in American whizz-kids from McKinsey consulting – including Chelsea Clinton. The following year's annual report showed a similar reliance on external consultants, consuming 68 per cent of Monitor's budget (*Health Emergency* 61, 2005; Monitor 2006).

The USA has the most expensive, least inclusive, most privatised and most bureaucratic health care system in the world, spending $1 out of every $3 of health spending on administration – $400 billion a year. It is not clear what useful lessons McKinsey might have been able to teach the NHS, or the organisation supposed to keep a watch on the activities of Foundation Trusts.

It turns out that McKinsey and fellow management consultants from Accenture, Deloitte, and AT Kearney were also picking up over 40 per cent (£67 million) of the £160 million budget of the Department of Health's own commercial directorate, charging fees as high as £2,000 per day (Carlisle 2007a). By 2006 the NHS was spending more on consultancy than the whole of UK manufacturing industry (Reed 2006).

Throughout 2007 there were steadily increasing indications of the rising pace of privatisation in primary care. On Easter Sunday four areas were named as seeking expressions of interest to run GP services, and PCTs were telling *Public Finance* magazine that the pressure to privatise was coming from the centre, with PCTs using any opportunity to go around local existing providers and bring in the private sector (Gainsbury 2007a). By November, as the primary care market continued to grow, Heart of Birmingham PCT was breaking new ground and seeking to out-Darzi Darzi in its proposals to press gang 76 GP practices into 24 franchises, to be run from polyclinics which could be offered up to "trusted" High Street store companies such as Asda, Tesco or Virgin. The PCT document argued that:

> There is a growing interest in primary care as a future market from a number of non-health organisations such as Virgin, Tesco and ASDA.
>
> It is hoped that in the heart of Birmingham, some GPs, particularly younger ones, new entrants and portfolio professionals, will see a franchise model as an attractive option.
>
> (Nowottny 2007)

For more on primary care see Chapter ten.

In primary care, as in elective surgery and diagnostics, the expansion of the private sector at the expense of the NHS did not flow from any external market pressures, and was not based on any normal organic process of growth: it was purely and simply the product of New Labour government sponsorship. If they had not invented the need for the private sector, and diverted resources to help build it, it would never have existed. The same was definitely true of the Private Finance Initiative.

The rise and fall of the Private Finance Initiative

The sixth decade of the NHS was the one which saw the implementation by Tony Blair's New Labour government of the Private Finance Initiative (PFI), the policy devised by Conservative ministers. The then Chancellor Kenneth Clarke told the CBI Conference in December 1993 was seen as a means to "privatise the process of capital investment" in public services.

For the first seven years of its life as a policy, PFI in the NHS was the subject of furious but entirely abstract debates. Outline business cases had been constructed and laborious and expensive discussions had been had with would-be private sector partners – but nobody had yet built a PFI hospital. Indeed, the Conservative government had failed even to secure a single signed financial close contract to build a hospital under this scheme. Even when New Labour took office in 1997 pledged to rescue the policy and make it work, there were another three years of speculation before the issues became more concrete and immediate.

However, the main discussion over PFI was very far from being abstract or purely ideological. The best-argued criticisms of the policy have always gone well beyond generalisations to point to the inevitability of increased costs, the consequences of squeezing down bed numbers and scaling down the size of buildings to make them less unaffordable, the unrealistic and ludicrously optimistic projections of increased efficiency and throughput from the new hospitals, and the likely impact of these expensive experiments on other local health services (Price 1997; Pollock et al. 1997; Gaffney and Pollock 1997; Gaffney et al. 1999a; Lister 1998b).

The need for any kind of speculation and guesswork is now long behind us: in the seven years since the first PFI-funded hospitals opened their doors to patients an increasing body of information has accumulated to demonstrate the high costs and doubtful value of financing new hospitals through PFI, and new primary care and community facilities through the equivalent system known as LIFT (Local Improvement Finance Trusts).

One spectacular failure sums up the dangers and problems of the entire policy of PFI. The £93 million PFI-funded Queen Elizabeth Hospital in Woolwich opened in 2002: by 2005 it had been officially declared "technically bankrupt" as a result of the sheer size of its ballooning PFI debt (Audit Commission 2005). The 'unitary charge' (effectively the lease payment by the NHS Trust for use of the PFI-funded hospital and the supply of non-clinical support services) amounted to 14.6 per cent of the Trust's income – and the payments for the building alone, index linked each year, amount over 35 years to more than five times the initial cost of the project (Picture of Health 2007: 3).

Two years later, as this book is completed, the knock-on effects of the inflated costs of Queen Elizabeth and two other PFI hospitals in South East London have generated a combined "unpayable" accumulated deficit of £180 million, with Bromley Hospitals Trust alone notching up a staggering £99 million in debts (Palmer 2007; Iggulden 2007). Lewisham, the third PFI hospital in the area, also faced deficits, and has been running a brand new PFI-funded building with a whole top floor – "a large part of the new capacity" – left empty to reduce costs, while the new building, on a fixed 30-year contract had increased the Trust's occupation costs by around 50 per cent (Picture of Health 2007: 6).

PFI contracts are notoriously inflexible, with heavy penalty payments to deter any early cancellation, regardless of the changing needs of the NHS. In the case of South East London the combined effect of the PFI-induced deficits in three Trusts has been to force proposals for the closure of services in a fourth hospital – Bexley's Queen Mary's Hospital, Sidcup, a Trust which had achieved a dramatic financial turnaround, and was not facing large deficits, but did not have the dubious 'protection' of a PFI contract that would incur huge penalty charges for closure (Gainsbury 2007b; Lister 2007d).

This meltdown in South East London is just one of the most recent and dramatic expressions of the rumbling crisis unleashed by PFI. Another example is the chaos in University Hospitals of Coventry and Warwickshire Trust following the opening of the new £410 million Walsgrave Hospital on the outskirts of Coventry in July 2006, boasting 1,250 beds, state-of-the-art equipment and 27 operating theatres. This monster PFI project – the biggest so far operational after London's UCLH – emerged after years of negotiations which began with plans for a £30 million refurbishment of Coventry's two crumbling hospitals (Monbiot 2007). The new "superhospital" carries with it a £52 million annual unitary charge (index linked, to £56 million this year) – equivalent to 13 per cent of the Trust's £400 million turnover. The Trust's most recent Annual Report confessed to an underlying cash shortfall of £74 million – in addition to the need to generate savings of £30 million a year (University Hospitals Coventry and Warwickshire 2007). This has already brought ward closures, the threat to 200 jobs, with a letter going to all staff asking if they would volunteer for redundancy, early retirement, a cut in hours or up to two weeks unpaid holiday a year. In addition, sky-high car parking charges increased to £10 per day, with no exemptions for disabled badge holders. However, the 2008–9 financial year will see the savings target cranked up again to £40 million, with the threat of even more job cuts (Scott 2007); yet even now the hospital is in the bottom ten in the country for waiting times (Monbiot 2007).

Underlying these pressures in Coventry, London and elsewhere is the fact that PFI has forced up the overhead costs of dozens of Trusts across the country... at the very time that the government's controversial new system of "Payment by Results" has imposed a fixed tariff of payment. The PBR tariff assumes a far lower (5.8 per cent) level of spending on buildings and facilities than many PFIs are obliged to pay (Gainsbury 2007c, g). As a result the soaring costs of these projects – for which payments are index linked and take the form of a legally binding top-slice from the budgets of Trusts and primary care providers for 30 or more years ahead – have begun to undermine services and force cutbacks elsewhere in the local health economy.

By far the largest commitment has been to hospital building, where the private sector has continued to stack up a combination of contractual and additional windfall profits from their relatively limited direct investment. Official figures have revealed projected repayments totalling a staggering £53 billion on capital projects costed at just £8.5 billion[21] (Mulholland 2007). Since most PFI schemes

---

21 The problems are especially sharp for district general hospitals, 41 of which have signed PFI deals for hospital buildings with a headline value of £4.8 billion, while the Trusts face payments under PFI totalling £28.5 billion (Gainsbury 2007b).

show a split of roughly 2:1 in the unitary charge between the availability charge and the facilities management contract, this suggests that over and above the costs of building and maintaining the hospitals and delivery of non-clinical services, the private consortia are set to cream off a surplus of at least £23 billion for the 80 or so hospital schemes already operational or under construction.

Labour ministers have repeatedly defended their policy of seeking to build hospitals using PFI by claiming that it has enabled them to embark upon the "biggest ever programme of hospital building in the NHS". Their NHS Plan (2000) called for a total of 100 new hospitals by 2010. The sums of money involved in such an investment programme are obviously larger than the previous major programme of hospital modernisation, the 1962 Hospital Plan for England and Wales, almost 40 years ago, when the value of money was rather dramatically different. However, the 1962 scheme, eventually approved by the then Conservative government on the urgings of Minister of Health Enoch Powell, was hugely ambitious for its time. It spelled out proposals for 90 new hospitals and another 134 major redevelopment programmes. The 280-page Plan also listed a further 356 smaller schemes and acknowledged the need for many more smaller schemes "which represent a large volume of modernisation and upgrading" (Ministry of Health 1962).

The Hospital Plan was initially costed at £707 million – the equivalent of £2.85 billion in 2002. It was almost three-quarters of the entire NHS budget of that year (£971 million); a similar proportional share of NHS spending today would amount to a £67 billion investment in new buildings. Between 1962 and 1971, £500 million was to be to be spent – an average of £50 million a year, more than double the going rate at the time. Indeed the Conservative election manifesto had included a commitment to double the NHS capital programme, while Labour in opposition had called for spending of £50 million a year (Webster 1996: 99).

The Hospital Plan recognised that such a massive leap in public investment would represent a major change of policy, after years in which NHS capital to modernise the aged building stock nationalised in 1948 had been in desperately short supply. In 1962 the government was spending a much smaller share of national wealth on the NHS, just 3.4 per cent of GDP – compared with 7.8 per cent today (Commons Health Committee 2006). Within this limited pot of cash, NHS capital budgets in turn consistently accounted for less than 3 per cent each year (though allocations had increased slightly, peaking at £24 million in 1960–1). This was well below the level of around 5 per cent that had been recommended back in 1956 by the Tory government's own Guillebaud Committee. As a result, there was not enough capital to enable any substantial modernisation or even systematic repairs to buildings which were often unsuitable for modern medicine; 70 per cent of hospitals taken over by the NHS in 1948 had fewer than 100 beds, and 20 per cent of the building stock was found to be over 100 years old in 1962.

The situation called for a major change of policy but perhaps surprisingly, given Enoch Powell's right-wing leanings and the dominance of a Conservative government, the entire 1962 investment programme was to be funded by the government from general taxation – and the completed hospitals would as a result be assets wholly owned by the NHS. (It is an irony that many of the latter-day PFI deals have only been possible for Trusts on the basis of trading in some of the property assets inherited from a more prudent and long-sighted policy in previous decades.) The entire debate in 1962 was framed by the prevailing consensus around the NHS as a key component of welfarism. There was no serious discussion of seeking the finance from elsewhere: the only debate within the Tory cabinet was over how much or how little should be invested in the modernisation of the NHS.

The Hospital Plan also looked forward to the likely patterns of population and health needs in 1975, and pioneered the concept of the District General Hospital of 600–800 beds covering a catchment population of around 150,000 as the key building block for acute (short stay) hospital services. This is the very pattern of provision that is now being called into question on such sketchy evidence by Lord Darzi, other academics and NHS managers, and – more significantly – by the growing financial pressures on the NHS.

The 1962 Hospital Plan involved a six per cent reduction in numbers of acute hospital beds, but (reflecting the medical model of the time) a 35 per cent *increase* in numbers of maternity beds. The process would close 1,250 hospitals, most of them small or very small. But in mental health the Hospital Plan also commenced the shift from institutional to community-based care, proposing a drastic cut in hospital bed numbers. It also took an important step towards setting up a nationwide plan and a coherent policy. It laid down norms for minimum levels of bed provision per head of population for each specialist service, and addressed the issue of staffing levels, both within the NHS as it then was, and within the Local Authority Health and Welfare Services (many of which are now council social services). This was an important step along the road to more equal allocation of resources according to population, breaking from the previous pattern of huge inequalities. This planning system is of course today being sacrificed to the New Labour notion of a market.

The Hospital Plan recognised that the schemes would take time to get up and running, and assumed spending of £200 million in the first five years rising to £300 million in the following five years. It accepted that "the sums which will eventually become available may be somewhat more or less, dependent on the state of the economy" (Ministry of Health 1962). In fact the costs were much higher than expected – but a change had been made.

Only six new hospitals had been built between 1955 and 1965: but between 1966 and 1975 another 71 were started – and some completed, changing the shape of health care for a generation. By 1968 large schemes (carrying out building work costing over £1 million a year) accounted for more than half of the NHS capital programme. There were 66 of these schemes – six of which were projects planned to cost over £10 million. Capital expenditure that year was almost 10 per cent of current NHS spending, and it continued to rise to a peak of

12.8 per cent in 1973–4, before being cut back again to 9.9 per cent in 1974–5. Cost estimates were distorted by high levels of inflation in the increasingly turbulent economic situation. The new Royal Free Hospital with its tower block was completed in 1973 at what today seems an incredibly modest cost of £20 million!

The 1970s saw a change in the economic climate, and a retreat by successive governments from investment, not only in the NHS, but throughout the public sector. Government net capital spending plunged from a peak of £28.8 billion in 1974–5 to just £12.5 billion in 1979–80, and fell again to a nadir of just £1.9 billion in 1988–9. Only in one year during the 1980s (1983–4) did public sector capital investment reach £10 billion. Though it rose again briefly to double figures (with a peak of £14.2 billion in 1992–3), it fell back again sharply in the second half of the 1990s. (Figures are all at 1999–2000 prices.) (HM Treasury 2001)

This cut in government spending was accelerated in the 1990s by the introduction of the Private Finance Initiative from 1992, which was accompanied in the case of the NHS by a steady reduction in government capital allocations. The 1995 budget projected successive cuts in NHS capital spending – by 17 per cent in 1996–7, another 5 per cent in 1997–8, and 6.5 per cent the following year. PFI investment was supposed to increase year by year, from £47 million in 1995–6 to £300 million in 1998–9 (DoH 1995b). But PFI – and NHS land sales, which had become a regular feature of the Tory government's asset-stripping approach to the NHS – weren't the only ways in which governments found ways to masquerade as investing generously in the NHS, while injecting comparatively little new capital.

During the mid-1990s the establishment of NHS Trusts within the Tory "internal market" reforms brought the introduction of *capital charges*, which were to be levied on each Trust's land and property assets. This meant that a growing percentage of the NHS budget each year was generated *internally* from these capital refunds. Beginning at 1.2 per cent of NHS total spending in 1993–4, these capital refunds steadily increased in scale as new Trusts were formed and more began paying charges on a greater share of their assets. By 1998–9 capital refunds amounted to a hefty 8 per cent of the NHS budget (DoH 1998b).

So despite the appearance of allocating large sums for investment in new hospitals and other NHS facilities, and despite the apparent upturn in allocations since Labour took office in 1997 (Denham 2000), in practice the government began by injecting even less public capital for major hospital projects in real terms than the miserly amounts available in 1961. Indeed in the two years 1997–8 and 1998–9, the injection of Treasury capital for Hospital and Community Health Services (HCHS) was more than outweighed by the cash generated from land sales and the refund to the government of capital charges paid by NHS Trusts on their assets. Far from pumping in desperately needed capital, the New Labour government effectively pocketed a *surplus* from existing NHS assets in these two years – of £139 million in 1997–8 and £348 million in 1998–9 (Gaffney et al. 1999b).

Since PFI got going the real figures have also been disguised by the inclusion of PFI money under the general heading of "health capital investment" – which soon made up around a quarter of the claimed total (DoH 2002b). However, the extent to which PFI can be seen as NHS investment at all is not clear, given that the assets to be constructed do not belong to the NHS. Instead the (inflated) cost of paying for the hospital projects financed through PFI would be met from NHS revenue budgets over the next 25–30 years. The investment was not a public sector capital asset, but a long-term public sector revenue liability.

Despite the claims by the DoH that PFI is simply "one of the weapons in our armoury of procurement tools", the pool of NHS capital was inadequate to offer Trusts a real choice of whether or not to seek private finance. This squeeze, tighter than ever since 1992, meant that PFI was seen by NHS managers as the only game in town. Only six major NHS-funded schemes, totalling less than £300 million, were given the go-ahead in the five years from 1997. This followed a long lean spell for NHS investment under the Tories. From 1980 to 1997, only seven publicly funded schemes costing more than £25 million were completed (Gaffney et al. 1999b).

Since PFI came on the scene, New Labour ministers have made no secret of their preference for PFI as a means to finance NHS projects; a massive 85 per cent of all new capital investment in the NHS has been coming from the private sector. Critics have argued that any short-term benefits of PFI are outweighed by the long-term costs. In 2001 the *annual* cost to the NHS of PFI payments involved in leasing these privately owned, profit-making hospitals, and buying ancillary services from private contractors, was projected to reach £2.1 billion by 2007 (Pollock 2001). However, many schemes have been much slower to completion, and the figure has not yet reached that level. Nevertheless, researchers from Manchester Business School have calculated the extra cost of financing the new hospitals through PFI at £480 million a year, from which companies can expect to pocket a rate of return well above the 15 per cent level which the Treasury described as "too high" in 2005. They also questioned the longer term affordability of PFI schemes which commonly consume upwards of 10 per cent of a Trust's income (Gainsbury 2007d).

Unlike capital charges, the payments to PFI consortia represent a net flow of cash and capital *out of* the NHS and into the coffers of banks, building firms and their shareholders. In the longer run it is possible to see the process of renewal of NHS buildings through PFI, coupled with the disposal of NHS "surplus" assets, leading towards a situation like that in social care, where the estimated value of assets involved was £13.3 billion in 2000, £10 billion of which were owned by the independent sector.

In 2000 the estimated net book value of Health Authorities and Trusts was around £23 billion, with primary care assets valued at £2.2 billion. The estimated cost of replacement was over £75 billion. But with NHS PFI projects likely to total £7 billion by 2007, inroads were being made. Existing NHS assets are still being sold off, (estate worth an estimated £1.58 billion was identified as surplus in preparation for the NHS Plan) while little new public investment has been injected into health care facilities and buildings. The NHS Plan in 2000 looked forward to a situation where by 2010 "40% of the value of the NHS estate will be less than fifteen years old" (DoH 2000b: 44). Since virtually all new buildings were to be PFI financed, this suggests a dramatic penetration of public assets by the private sector.

The Department of Health's Investment Strategy pointed out that:

> One of the legacies of the under investment throughout the nineties is the sharp increases in backlog maintenance levels over the latter half of the 1990s. Between 1995–6 and 1998–9 backlog maintenance increased by around 40%. In 1998–9 it was £3.4 billion.
>
> (DoH 2000c)

But this scale of backlog maintenance and the lack of NHS capital funding have proved handy additional levers to force Trusts down the road favoured by ministers, supplying some of the most potent arguments by Trusts seeking to justify embarking on costly and controversial new-build PFI schemes rather than refurbishing and redeveloping existing NHS assets. How have the PFI schemes delivered for Trusts that have tried to make them work?

Increased headline costs of schemes

PFI hospital projects have become notorious for the massive level of increase in costs from the point at which they are first proposed to the eventual deal being signed.

In part this is because PFI consortia are keen to make each scheme as big as possible, and also because private firms prefer to buy and then build on greenfield sites and lease buildings back to the NHS rather than refurbish existing NHS hospitals.

Among the more dramatic increases in prices from original plan to PFI deal are:

- Greenwich: up from £35 million in 1995 to £93 million in 1997
- UCLH, London: up from £115 million to £404 million
- Leicester: up from £150 million in 1999 to £286 million in 2001
- South Tees: up from £65 million to £122 million
- Swindon: a £45 million refurbishment of Princess Margaret Hospital in Swindon turned into a £96 million new hospital on a greenfield site out by the M4
- The Worcester Royal Infirmary, a project which was originally estimated at £45 million when it was first advertised for PFI tenders in 1995, was eventually given the go-ahead at a total cost of £110 million.

The first 14 PFI deals escalated in cost by an average of 72 per cent, from a total of £766 million to £1,314 million by the time they were approved (Price 1997).

This inflation has obviously had an impact on the final bill to be paid. The new Dartford Hospital was originally projected to be "at worst cost neutral", but it soon emerged that purchasers were going to have to foot the bill for an extra £4 million a year if the Trust were to be enabled to pay the PFI costs (National Audit Office 1999).

The costs of PFI also impact on other local services. In South Manchester, a deal through which mental health beds in the PFI-funded Wythenshawe Hospital have been sub-let to Manchester Community and Mental Health Trust resulted in a hefty £5 million annual rent which soaked up almost ten per cent of the Trust's revenue in 2004, effectively "crippling the mental health economy" (MCMHT 2004).

Rate of return for private investors

PFI consortia don't build hospitals for the sake of our health. They want profit for their investment – and lots of it. A *BMJ* article in 1999 pointed out that shareholders in PFI schemes "can expect real returns of 15–25 per cent a year", and went on to explain how little actual risk was involved for the companies in PFI consortia (Gaffney et al. 1999a). In Barnet, the second phase of the new general hospital, originally tendered at £29 million, went ahead at a cost of £54 million, with capital borrowed at 13 per cent over 25 years.

Margins for PFI consortium partners

But the profits flow to the private sector at every level in PFI. Building firms, banks, business consultants and other PFI hangers-on are eagerly anticipating a generous flow of profits as the first hospital schemes take shape. An investigation in the *Health Service Journal* showed building contractors "expecting returns of up to 20 percent a year on the equity stakes they hold in the project companies" as soon as the building is complete and Trusts start paying up for the use of the new buildings. Consultancy firms, too – architects, engineers and surveyors – are pocketing above average fees for work on PFI schemes. As the *HSJ* article pointed out: "there is little chance of the construction industry losing interest in PFI hospitals" (*HSJ* 1999).

And once the building is finished, maintaining and providing services in the buildings will deliver comfortable, guaranteed profits of up to seven per cent for firms holding service contracts. The first two waves of PFI hospital schemes all involved the privatisation of any non-clinical support services that were not already in the hands of the contractors.

Fewer beds

The first wave of PFI hospitals were by no means as expensive as the later schemes were to become; but they became notorious for the scale of the cuts in bed numbers they represented, with reductions in frontline acute beds ranging from 20 per cent to 40 per cent. PFI planners wanted to axe almost 40 per cent of beds in Hereford (from 414 to 250) (Smith 1999) and North Durham (from 750 to 450). The newly opened North Durham Hospital was plunged into an immediate beds crisis, while Hereford was forced to hang on to its crumbling war-time hutted wards for years after the brand new, smaller hospital opened up next to them. Two other PFI hospitals embodying large-scale bed reductions in Dartford and in Carlisle, have also struggled from the outset to cope with pressures on the depleted numbers of beds remaining.

These bed numbers were based not on the actual experience of frontline Trusts dealing with current levels of caseload, or on any actual examples of hospital practice in this country, but on the wildly over-optimistic projections of private sector management consultants working for PFI consortia. In Worcestershire the health authority forced through plans for a PFI-funded Worcester Royal Infirmary which would cut 260 acute beds – over 200 of them in Kidderminster – as well as beds in Redditch – a county-wide cutback of 33 per cent (Lister 1998c). This caused a desperate shortage of beds, while the PFI hospital forced the Trust deep into the red.

Lesser, but significant bed reductions were also involved in most of the PFI schemes that have been completed. Bromley's new £121 million hospital – which has since developed the country's largest-ever Trust financial deficit, was to have 13 per cent fewer beds than the hospitals it replaced.

After the findings of the NHS Beds Inquiry – commissioned by the Labour government to report on the adequacy of bed numbers – concluded the NHS was well short of the necessary number of acute beds, Alan Milburn become more sensitive to the charge that PFI was further reducing frontline capacity. After intervening to force the University College London Hospital scheme in central London to be expanded to include additional beds (at dramatically increased cost), Milburn insisted that new PFI schemes must at least match the existing numbers of acute beds (Commons statement, 15 February 2001). This in turn led to a further escalation in the costs of the next generation of PFI schemes.

Consultancy fees/negotiation costs

The first 15 PFI schemes for new hospitals spent a combined total of £45 million on advisors, with costs varying between 2.8 per cent and 8.7 per cent of the capital cost of the project. These costs are heavily inflated by the need to strike legally binding deals with private sector firms in what are often very complicated deals (UNISON 2000). The contract for Coventry's Walsgrave Hospital – long before financial close – added up to a colossal 17,000 pages in 1996, at which point the two consortia vying for the deal reportedly asked for government cash to pay lawyers to read it all! (Health Select Committee 2002)

Delays in major projects – and in smaller ones, too

The complexity of the procedures and process of PFI and the negotiations that it involves has brought a new level of delay to schemes which might otherwise have proceeded with public funding. In East Kent NHS Regional bosses warned that the plans for a new PFI hospital to replace four existing hospitals – the projected cost of which had already almost doubled to £102 million – could take four to seven years to complete the complex PFI process: the project has still not been signed.

Even more serious were delays in projects which are smaller, and which do not involve high-profile general hospitals. In London the Brent, Kensington, Chelsea and Westminster Mental Health Trust wanted to improve its community services, at a cost of around £24 million: but the project had been log-jammed since 1998. In June 2001 the local health authority was told that:

> The Regional Office has said that the Trust must establish whether there is private sector interest in funding and managing the proposed new facilities. …What seems clear is that the development at Woodfield Road could be more attractive to the market because this is a new development. Schemes that involve refurbishing facilities are less attractive. However the scheme is a small one in cost terms and may be below the level at which most companies would be interested.

If the Trust had to advertise the scheme for PFI bidders, the HA was warned that:

> Clearly this could add several months to the timetable. If any part of the scheme is then funded privately the Trust estimates this will add a delay of another 12 months.
>
> (KCWHA 2001)

Staffing levels reduced

In Bromley, the Full Business Case projects savings in staff costs of £2.9 million a year, which arise, among other things, from "the reduction in the number of beds and theatres. 136 jobs are expected to be axed, including 34 nurses and 8.5 doctors, while the reduction in qualified nursing is to be compensated by a higher ratio of health care assistants". (Bromley Hospitals Trust 1998)

Privatisation of support services and staff

In the first few PFI hospital schemes, staff working in non-clinical support services have been routinely "sold on" to private contractors providing "facilities management" for the PFI consortium. Their pay and conditions were safeguarded only by the fragile TUPE (Transfer of Undertakings) rules, which protect only existing staff – leading to a two-tier system in which new employees are on different term and conditions – and which can easily be circumvented by unscrupulous employers.

After the 2001 election, Alan Milburn – in the aftermath of nearly a year of strike action by support staff at Dudley Hospitals Trust fighting their compulsory transfer to a private contractor as part of a PFI deal – announced three pilot schemes, in which support services would be separated from the financing of the new building. There followed negotiations with the unions on a Retention of Employment agreement, by which NHS staff would be seconded to the management of the private sector.

Loss of additional income (car parking, shops, catering, etc.)

Car parking charges and rent from shops, cafes and restaurants on the hospital site, which might previously have gone to the Trust, become another income stream for the consortium under PFI. These are just some of the changes that will be ushered in when private firms own the hospital and its surrounding facilities.

Squeeze on clinical staff

The inclusion of all non-clinical support services in rigid, legally binding "unitary payments" effectively top-sliced from Trust budgets under PFI creates a new pressure on staff in clinical services. Clinical services become the only area of Trust spending where Trust managers can seek the "cost improvements" and "efficiency savings" which they are required to make each year by government and by NHS purchasing bodies. As the Wellhouse Trust was told in the negotiations over the new Barnet General Hospital (where even medical records have been incorporated into a PFI contract in a new computerised system):

> Part of the price... has been to agree to an indexation regime which has no in-built cost improvement and is linked to the published RPI index... The Trust will not therefore be in a position to impose Cost Improvement Programme targets across most of its support and operational services. ...The scope for future mandatory CIP targets will be limited to clinical services and to the few support services remaining under the management of the Trust.
>
> (Green B 1997)

Squeeze on community and other services

If more has to be spent in paying inflated costs of building new acute hospitals through PFI, less cash is left in the pot to finance other aspects of health care in each area. As we have seen, many of the first wave of PFI hospitals have had to be heavily subsidised by local health authorities in order to make them affordable. The Worcestershire scheme meant that an extra £7 million was allocated to acute services to enable the Trust pay for the new hospital: this had to be found by squeezing cash allocations for mental health, community services and primary care.

Poor quality buildings

Unveiling the latest round of PFI schemes receiving the rubber stamp, Alan Milburn argued that:

> For too long investment in NHS infrastructure has been a low priority when it should have been a high priority. Capital investment in the NHS was lower at the end of the last Parliament than it was at the beginning. The consequences are plain for all to see. Buildings that are shoddy, equipment that is unreliable, hospitals that are out of date. In too many places the environment that staff work in and patients receive care is simply unacceptable.
>
> (DoH Press Release, 15 February 2001)

But the experience has been NEW buildings which are shoddy and NEW equipment that is unreliable – at a higher price than before. After just a few months of the first PFI hospitals coming on stream there were problems in Carlisle, in Dartford, in North Durham, and less-publicised problems with the fabric and design of the building in many other PFI hospitals. Many of these are itemised by staff interviewed in PFI hospitals by this author in 2002 (Lister 2003a, b).

Smaller schemes can prove pro rata even more disastrous than larger ones, and the combination of PFI with mental health services has proved to be just as hazardous as the more routine deals in the acute sector. In the autumn of 2003 a devastating report by private consultants for East London and City Mental Health Trust laid bare a whole raft of major problems that had hit a new £12.5 million mental health unit in Newham built using PFI. The report, a copy of which was later leaked to London Health Emergency, made it clear that the new building was too small, in the wrong place, poorly designed, poorly built, and suffered from poor quality support services from the private consortium.

- Almost every paragraph of the 36-page report from consultancy firm Hornagold and Hills pointed to another basic flaw in the process that had led to the Newham unit's completion

- The bidding and negotiating process was delayed, but even after two years the contract did not adequately specify the obligations of the PFI consortium

- No details were specified of acceptable room temperatures or lighting levels

- The architects' full fees were not paid, and so the architects did not inspect works, certify completion or identify defects

- No drawings existed of the finished building

- The original design provided no office space at all – and the resultant reorganisation to squeeze in offices left some admin staff having to pass through wards to go in and out

- The ward arrangement made gender segregation impossible

- Cold water tanks on the ground floor meant that all water had to be pumped into the building, and at opening there was a 'total failure of water supply'

- The wrong specification baths were used, but the proper replacements were too big to go through the doors

- The wrong specification windows were used: standard windows are unsuitable for a mental health establishment, and have suffered damage and broken handles

- A number of toilets were not connected to drains, "leading to obvious problems"

- The site was polluted and released methane, raising serious hazards for smokers

- Floor coverings were defective, alarm and call systems unreliable, emergency systems non-functional, staff were ill informed and alienated, and the contractor has been 'uncooperative and adversarial'.

(Hornagold and Hills 2003)

Worryingly, managers clearly wanted to keep these real problems quiet, which would potentially prevent other PFI schemes from learning any lessons from the Newham fiasco.

Land assets stripped: NHS as tenant

Many PFI deals are part-funded by handing over to the consortium "spare" NHS land and building assets released as part of the new scheme. Although this defrays some of the initial costs – and therefore reduces the monthly "unitary charge" which it must pay, the Trust then becomes a tenant, renting its key acute facilities from the private sector.

This has important consequences for the future:

1. Once the NHS assets – paid for over the generations by the taxpayer – have been passed over in this way, the Trust no longer has any scope to use them in future service developments. At the end of the contract period, the NHS Trust is likely to be in a weak position to negotiate over a further extension of the lease agreement.

2. The PFI deal effectively locks the Trust into a long-term commitment to maintain services around the new hospital or PFI-funded facilities – no matter what changes may take place in local health needs, medical techniques or population over the next 25–60 years. The flexibility of owning land and buildings and being able to take decisions over how they should be used is seriously reduced.

3. A third major problem comes when the package of land and property is traded in as part of a PFI deal at much less than its eventual market value. Edinburgh's Royal Infirmary PFI involved handing over property assets that turned out to be worth as much as the new hospital, but only a fraction of this value came back to the Trust. (Lister 2003a)

Refinancing: another private sector rip-off

Huge bonus profits can be made by PFI companies which refinance the deal as soon as the most risky phase – of constructing the hospital – is complete. Octagon, the consortium that financed and built the £220 million Norfolk and Norwich Hospital refinanced the deal and scooped a bonus £115 million – almost half the initial cost – in windfall gains. Just £34 million of this was shared with the Trust, and that to be paid in the form of a £1.7 million cut in the annual fees for use of the building and support services. The remaining £81 million has no doubt been wisely invested by Octagon's gleeful shareholders. The deal, later branded by the Tory head of the Commons Public Accounts Committee as the "unacceptable face of capitalism" was even more amazing when we realise that the five firms behind the Octagon Healthcare consortium invested just £30 million of their own money in the project (Hawkes 2006c; Smith 2001).

Another NHS hospital which has generated a healthy hand out for shareholders is Dartford, where a third of the refinancing gain was shared with the Trust, but the Trust found its 28-year contract extend to 35 years as part of the deal. As more PFI hospitals come on stream, we can expect more refinancing deals to surface, within which the NHS Trusts will receive at best only a portion while shouldering much of the real risk, underlining once more how unequal is the "partnership" and "risk sharing" between public and private sectors.

"Hidden", non-financial costs

• Planning distorted

Under PFI, NHS managers and professionals play no role in planning hospitals: this is delegated to the private sector. Instead the Trust draws up an invitation to negotiate and an "output specification", which does not state how many beds should be provided but the anticipated level of clinical activity. It is left up to any consortia which respond to the invitation to propose the numbers of beds and scale of the services to be provided.

But any publicly funded option must show itself to be comparable to PFI in "efficiency" and value for money: the inevitable consequence in the first round of PFI deals was a Dutch auction on bed reductions, led by the most gung-ho private sector management consultants.

In Worcestershire, for example, the management consultants drawing up the scheme pointed out – without any evidence to support their assertion, other than other PFI schemes – that "many acute service reviews and proposed hospital business cases have assumed that future targets of between 8–10 beds per 1,000 inpatient episodes are feasible". These assumptions amounted to a 40 per cent increase in throughput for each bed in the new Worcester Royal Infirmary. It was on this same fragile basis that health chiefs decided they could close down 229 acute beds at Kidderminster Hospital, even though their own advisors warned that achieving these bed capacity targets across the county "would be a major challenge" (Lister 1998b).

Throughout the NHS, bed throughput had largely levelled off at around 56–7 patients per bed per year. The PFI plans for Edinburgh Royal Infirmary aimed to increase this to a massive 88; but the Worcestershire plans aimed at almost doubling the national average, to over 100 patients per bed per year. The driving force in this was PFI (Price 1997).

Such a big increase in throughput per acute bed in Worcestershire or elsewhere could only be achieved by discharging more patients to less intensive, intermediate or step-down beds. But this calls for additional investment in community health services and an expansion of these beds. Unfortunately this investment was less likely to be forthcoming because of the increased costs of renting and running the PFI hospital.

• **Accountability weakened**

Secrecy is a key ingredient in the whole process of PFI. Once a decision to negotiate has been taken, all of the detailed discussions about the shape, size, cost and service profile of the hospital take place behind firmly locked doors. In 1998 Health Secretary Alan Milburn announced with a flourish that Trusts would be required to publish "all the key PFI project documents. This includes documents covering existing PFI deals. This gives local people and local staff a new right to know about the future of their local health service" (DoH Press Release, 8 April 1998).

The reality has been very different. Deals are being done with no publicity until after the details have been agreed and binding agreements made. Often the details are still withheld from the public even after a deal has been closed. Even MPs have found it hard to get at the facts. When the Commons Health Committee asked for details on the Norfolk and Norwich PFI scheme in 1999, they were given copies of the "full business case" with large sections withheld as "commercial in confidence". And when BBC documentary producer John Mair tried to find out 18 months later what the unitary charge was going to be for the N&N, he found a discrepancy of over £13 million a year between the lowest estimate (£22.8 million) and the highest (£36 million), and even over how many years the charge would be payable. Chief executive Malcolm Stamp was unable to answer the question, or put a price on the whole deal (*Public Finance*, 1–7 December 2000).

As the National Audit office found in the case of the Dartford PFI hospital, there is ample scope for purchasers and NHS Trusts to make very large and expensive mistakes with little detailed scrutiny until it is far too late to affect decisions that then last for 25–60 years (National Audit Office 1999). Eight years later little has changed: even as this book is completed details of a £300 million PFI scheme signed by Mid Yorkshire Hospitals Trust five months ago (July 2007) are being withheld as "commercial in confidence" after months of fruitless trade union requests under freedom of information legislation.

Worcestershire Health Authority, unable to give convincing answers to awkward questions from local campaigners on how a much smaller PFI-funded Worcester Royal Infirmary could cope with county-wide demand, refused in its response to the consultation even to mention that the questions had been asked by local statutory organisations. It preferred to fight campaigners all the way to a judicial review – and then hide behind the cavalier ruling of a reactionary judge rather than answer or give details.

How does PFI show "value for money"?

• **Untested assumptions**

As we have shown above, the inability of the first PFI hospitals to meet pressures for emergency and elective work with substantially fewer beds has already been exposed. In North Durham, within 12 weeks of the new hospital opening there were calls for an additional 42 beds to be provided to prevent patients enduring 12-hour waits in A&E (Lawrence 2001). But their expected ability to deliver dramatic increases in efficiency has always been seen as key to the affordability of PFI hospitals, and the principal way in which they can defray the additional money they cost the Trust.

As the full financial cost of operating the new system – including the use of increased numbers of community beds and services – is counted, the underlying false assumptions will be fully revealed as well as the heavy price of PFI.

The next generation of PFI hospitals, embodying Alan Milburn's call for schemes to be at least "bed neutral", or embody an increase in bed numbers, will find it even harder to show that they offer value for money.

- **NHS innovation excluded**

Any Trust seeking PFI investment has to depend upon the private sector to suggest the best way of meeting estimated clinical activity, leaving scope for 'innovative' developments. By contrast, any public sector comparative scheme is required by the Treasury to be "based on the recent and actual method of providing that defined output (including any reasonable and foreseen efficiencies the public sector could make)" (Public Accounts Committee 2000).

- **Cooking the books: "Public Sector Comparator"**

Every PFI scheme is supposed to prove that it represents value for money by being contrasted with a "Public Sector Comparator" (PSC). But it is clear from the outset of such an exercise that the comparison is not between like and like. The investment of energy and commitment into selling the PFI scheme to secure the only likely source of funding will not be matched by the ritualistic development of a hypothetical and unloved alternative, whose main virtue is to appear less attractive.

Government guidance spells out that the public sector scheme is not a real plan for a real hospital but just a fig leaf to hide the blushes of the PFI plan: "The purpose of the PSC is to provide a benchmark against which to form a judgement on the value for money of PFI bids" (Public Accounts Committee 2000).

- **Discounting the future**

One of the manipulative techniques that works consistently to the advantage of a PFI deal in comparison with the PSC has been the calculation of the "net present costs". This assumes that money spent now is worth more than money spent in five, ten or 20 years time – and that the full costs of a hospital development will be paid in the first few years of the scheme (when the value is highest) while the costs of a PFI deal can be defrayed over the whole life of the contract.

The exercise was for several years made surreal by selecting an arbitrary, and high, level of six per cent per year – well above current and projected levels of inflation – as the basis for discounting the value of future payments (which in any event are index linked, and do not diminish but increase each year to keep pace with inflation).

- **"Risk transfer"**

To further stack the odds in favour of the PFI option, the costs of the Public Sector Comparator (PSC) are commonly loaded to compensate for "risks" allegedly transferred to the private sector consortium under the PFI deal. It is often only after this and other statistical sleight of hand that the PFI option can be shown as even marginally better value than a publicly funded scheme.

The central risk in this phase is that of cost over-runs. But while the average over-run of eventual building costs in NHS projects has been between 6 per cent and 8.5 per cent for the last 10 years, PFI business cases assume much higher levels of 12.5 per cent – or up to 34 per cent in the Norfolk and Norwich Hospital (Pollock 2004). Other "risks" which are given a notional cash value and added to the cost of the public sector comparator are either similarly inflated or fictional – such as the £5 million added to the Carlisle PSC to compensate for the "risk" that clinical cost savings would not be made, despite the fact that the consortium was under no obligation to compensate the Trust if this occurred (Pollock 2004).

- **Subsidies – open and covert**

To further stir the pot of obfuscation on the genuine comparative costs between a privately funded hospital and a publicly funded project, a variety of subsidies can be openly or covertly slipped in.

As with the examples of Worcestershire and North Durham, the subsidies may be implicit, in the requirement for a large increase in spending on community hospitals and community health services to create a new system of care that may or may not allow the new hospital to deliver its target of much more rapid throughput.

Or subsidies may take the form of smoothing payments from a special fund held by the NHS Executive, effectively providing a direct subsidy for the introduction of the PFI scheme where it is clear that there is insufficient cash in the local kitty to pay the increased costs.

However, as PFI hospital Trusts such as Dartford, Queen Elizabeth and Bromley now know to their cost, these smoothing payments can be ended by government as easily as they are put in place, leaving the Trusts to pick up the remaining bill.

The rising tide of PFI costs

The combined unitary payments on the six PFI hospitals which were already operational in 2001 added up to £83 million a year, giving a total payable of £2.4 billion – *six times* their capital value of £423 million. The annual fees on the next 14 schemes in the queue for which details were available added up to £250 million a year, giving a total cost of £7.9 billion – over *five times* the capital value of £1,507 million.

The argument that support services are included in this overall cost falls flat when we contrast this cost of financing a project through PFI, in which every £1 million of capital eventually costs £5–6 million, with a standard six per cent mortgage. Every £1 million could be financed this way over 25 years for just £1.94 million, less than double the amount borrowed, and with no obligation to buy any other services, and freehold tenure of the assets at the end of the deal.

To make matters worse, some small-scale deals which ought to have been affordable from one-off capital funds were also signed as PFI deals, to be paid off over 25 or 30 years, with a resultant cost as high as 24 times the value of the scheme.

- Queens Medical Centre catering: value £1 million, total cost £23.8 million
- North Birmingham Mental Health: value £12.4 million, total cost £163.5 million
- Royal Wolverhampton Radiology: value £10.9 million, total cost £70 million
- Rotherham Priority Elderly MH: value £2.1 million, total cost £16.9 million
- North Bristol Brain Rehab unit: value £4.9 million, total cost £42 million.

(Lister 2001)

The more money that is squeezed out of the NHS in PFI payments to bankers and private providers, the less that remains to treat patients, pay clinical staff and develop modern, appropriate services.

Growing awareness

As the facts have emerged to show the real costs and pitfalls of PFI, and the costs of new PFI projects have rapidly increased, more mainstream critics have joined the trade unionists, campaigners and radical academics in pointing out that this emperor has no clothes.

Early in June 2002, the NAO's deputy controller and auditor general, Jeremy Colman, questioned the way in which PPPs, and PFIs before them, have been shown to represent better value for money than more traditional sources of public infrastructure procurement. Speaking to the *Financial Times*, he argued that much of the financial analysis weighing PPP projects against so-called "public-sector comparators" ranges from the "spurious" through "pseudo-scientific mumbo-jumbo" to "utter rubbish".

"People have to prove value for money to get a PFI (or PPP) deal", he told the *FT*.

> If the answer comes out wrong, you don't get your project. So the answer doesn't come out wrong very often.

(Timmins 2002)

That same month, Audit Scotland published a study of six of the twelve current PFI schools projects – covering schools in Falkirk, Glasgow, Stirling, Highlands, Edinburgh and West Lothian – and found that in all six cases operating costs were higher than a publicly funded comparison, while borrowing costs were also higher than if the councils had simply borrowed to finance the schemes themselves (Audit Scotland 2002).

In July 2003, the Commons Public Accounts published a highly critical report on the first 400 PFI schemes so far signed, effectively arguing that the public sector – and the taxpayer – was being conned. The Committee's chairman Edward Leigh MP – a right-wing Tory, sympathetic to the private sector – warned that:

> In too many cases value for money declines after contract letting, and the approach of many authorities to managing their contracts is seriously deficient.
> (Moore W 2002)

A September 2002 survey of nearly 200 Association of Chartered Accountants members working in the UK public sector, including the NHS, local government, central government, education, charities, the police and prison services, found that a majority of its members think PFI is such poor value it should not be used. Only 2 per cent felt strongly PFI was having a beneficial effect on public services, whereas 57 per cent did not believe that PFI generally provides value for money. The same percentage agreed that, as PFI is often the only available source of investment in public services, public-sector organisations are prevented from achieving value for money. And 58 per cent did not believe that PFI schemes are objectively tested on whether they provide value for money.

In early 2004 a growing number of PFI-funded hospitals had opened... and a 'snap shot' survey of ten first-wave PFI hospital Trusts in England and Scotland by *Health Emergency* newspaper found many hospitals struggling to cope with the pressures of demand for emergency and waiting list treatment. Most faced soaring debts and chronic bed shortages: combined deficits added up to almost £50 million (*Health Emergency* 59, 2004).

- At the £93 million Queen Elizabeth Hospital in Greenwich, management had already resorted to the desperate measure of closing a ward in the two-year-old hospital to save money towards its £6 million deficit – despite the fact that this would add 600 more patients to its waiting lists.

- The more recently opened West Middlesex Hospital in Isleworth, West London had also announced that a ward would close at the end of March, with staff redeployed to save money towards the Trust's £2.5 million deficit, even while patients waited hours on trolleys for admission due to lack of beds.

- And at least one Trust, County Durham and Darlington Acute Hospital NHS Trust, had publicly admitted its new £97 million University Hospital of North Durham had been built with too few beds.

Health Emergency which carried out the survey warned that while PFI hospitals had already been struggling, and often failing to meet government targets on waiting times, their position was likely to worsen when new arrangements for "Payment by Results" within the NHS were introduced.

Because the PFI contract involves the Trust paying a monthly index-linked fee to the consortium to cover the lease of the new building and the provision of all non-clinical (ancillary) services and maintenance, if the Trust runs into financial difficulties the only parts of the budget the Trust itself still controls are clinical services: doctors, nurses and patient care.

The underlying problem has always been that PFI hospitals are inherently very expensive buildings, in which the apparent price was artificially reduced by making them smaller than they needed to be, and by temporary government handouts.

But while the first wave hit problems, the scale of difficulty facing the second wave of PFI hospitals seems likely to be even greater. These hospitals are much bigger, often with as many or even sometimes more beds than the buildings they replace – but are massively more expensive, and therefore even less affordable by NHS Trusts.

By early 2004, according to reports collated by *Health Emergency* from national and local press coverage:

- Hundreds of patients waiting for treatment at Worcester's new £97 million PFI-funded hospital were having their operations cancelled because of a rise in emergency admissions, and inadequate numbers of beds, chief executive John Rostill had publicly admitted. The knock-on effect was contributing to the Trust's financial deficit, projected to reach £15 million by April 2004.

- An estimated 11 per cent of Hereford's hospital's beds were "blocked" by patients who should have been discharged to care elsewhere, while community hospitals were reported by the Primary Care Trust to be "stuffed to the gunnels".

- England's biggest operational PFI hospital, the £229 million Norfolk and Norwich Hospital was facing an underlying deficit of £6.5 million and an overspend of £1.5 million on its planned budget. Penny-pinching economy measures included scrapping the supply of biscuits and bottled water to the boardroom, and a drastic 120 per cent increase in staff car-parking charges.

- Scotland's flagship PFI hospital, the £184 million Edinburgh Royal Infirmary, was also leaking funds below the waterline with an £8.5 million deficit by April 2004 – an improvement on earlier forecasts that the gap could be as wide as £13 million. A report by the Auditor General warned at the end of 2003 that the Lothian University Hospitals Trust's debts could spiral to reach a staggering £180 million by 2008. The hospital had also been dogged by a series of problems flowing from the poor design and quality of the building, including power cuts, leaks in the roof, ventilation failures, and abandoned attempts to computerise patient records.

- Swindon's £180 million PFI-financed Great Western Hospital had been forced to add a 36-bed orthopaedic ward and 26-bed ward, and opened a discharge lounge to ease pressure on beds.

By 2005 the underlying problems of affordability in the mega-PFI deals burst to the surface. The ill-conceived Paddington Health Campus was finally put out of its misery by an increasingly irritated Strategic Health Authority and the health minister in June 2005. It had an unbridgeable affordability gap which had at one point exceeded £40 million a year, and the overall cost peaked at close to £1 billion. The project had been under intensive negotiation and development work for seven years, but was bedevilled by policy changes at national level, including ministerial instructions requiring increased space between beds and a higher proportion of single rooms. It never even achieved planning permission (National Audit Office 2006). This fruitless project soaked up management time and cost a staggering £14 million before it was axed. *Public Finance* magazine summed up the lesson:

> In the end, history may view the scrapping of the Paddington scheme as the first PFI casualty of the new health care market.
>
> (Ward 2005)

With Blair's third election victory secured, a new Health Secretary, Patricia Hewitt, triggered rumours that ministers were about to call time on a number of other large-scale hospital projects to be funded through the Private Finance Initiative. Hewitt called for a review of the soaraway costs of the £1.2 billion Bart's and The London PFI Hospital project and top DoH officials warned of the danger of investing in costly "monuments" which would quickly outgrow their usefulness (White 2005). Bart's and Paddington were far from the only problems to be tackled. The rocketing cost of PFI schemes raised questions of whether Trusts could implement the latest schemes and stay viable under Payment by Results.

When the first wave of PFI hospitals had been signed off under Frank Dobson in the late 1990s the average capital cost of a new hospital was £75 million. This had since spiralled into the stratosphere, with a number of schemes running above, or close to, £1 billion, and several more in excess of £400 million. The costs were staggering. Annual payments on a £420 million scheme in Central Manchester came out at £51 million per year, index linked, over 38 years, £30 million of which was the 'availability charge' for the building itself (Lister 2003d).

The soaraway Bart's and London project had grown to a total capital cost of at least £1.89 billion – almost £500 million of which comprised interest and fees. The annual payment started off at £115 million a year, index linked – with £67 million of this being the rent ('availability charge'). This meant that the taxpayer would have forked out well over £5 billion for the two hospitals over the following 40 years, while the Skanska Innisfree consortium would pick up guaranteed profits from legally binding payments equal to 23 per cent of the Trust's annual turnover (Lister 2005a).

This type of increased overhead costs – and restricted capacity – had already helped to force most of the operational PFI hospital Trusts deep into deficit. Where new PFI hospitals were rubber stamped, they were likely to drain vital resources from community health care and mental health budgets, leaving a lop-sided pattern of care for a generation to come.

These economic facts of life had forced the decision to axe the Paddington Health Campus project – and subsequently brought the demise of several more lumbering giants. University Hospitals of Leicestershire Trust has finally seen its ballooning PFI scheme, which started out at a projected £150 million, scrapped after the costs rose more than sixfold – to a staggering £761 million, and then to £920 million, even after the numbers of beds in the scheme had been whittled back down (Hawkes 2007). In February 2001, Leicester Trust managers had drawn gasps of astonishment when the projected cost of their plan rose to £286 million. By recent standards that was a bargain that should have been snapped up.

In 2006 ministers did eventually decide to rubber stamp schemes for three more mammoth hospital projects costing a total of well over £2 billion, to be financed under the Private Finance Initiative (PFI). The first big announcement came in March when, after prolonged delays and a top-level review, Patricia Hewitt finally ended the constipated silence over the future of the £1.9 billion plan to rebuild Bart's and the London hospitals – and gave the nod to a plan that nobody wanted. Two hundred and fifty beds – 20 per cent of the planned capacity – were to be axed, with three floors of the new buildings to be "shelled" (left empty) to wrestle down the capital cost of the scheme by £160 million.

So these new mega-hospitals will have fewer beds than they do now, explicitly breaching the assurance of previous Health Secretary Alan Milburn that any second-wave PFI hospital would have to have at least as many if not more beds than the services it replaced.

The "unitary charge" to be paid to the PFI consortium, Skanska Innisfree, will be reduced by £20 million a year – but remains a staggering £96 million a year, index linked over 35 years – equivalent to a massive 20 per cent of the Trust's turnover last year. Even if we assume the rent element will also be reduced by the same proportion, this means payments of at least £55 million a year – 11.4 per cent of the Trust's total income. This leaves the Trust no leeway to deal with future financial pressures.

These payments will have to be taken from other parts of the East London health economy, plundering budgets for primary care, mental health and community services. The new University Hospital for Birmingham had rocketed again in cost from a Final Business Case projection of £543 million in 2005 (UHBFT 2005) to a staggering £697 million when finally signed off by health minister Rosie Winterton in April 2006 – more than double the projected £291 million cost of the scheme when it was put out to tender in the Official Journal of the EU four years earlier (DoH 2006b; Lister 2001). Press statements avoided the thorny question of how much the hospital will cost the Trust over the 35 years of the PFI contract (estimated at £50 million index linked over 35 years in 2005).

Meanwhile things lurched from bad to worse in Worcestershire, where the £100 million PFI hospital that famously triggered the closure of A&E and inpatient acute beds at Kidderminster Hospital – and cost the local Labour MP his seat when he supported the closure –remained mired in crisis. Lacking beds, space and cash the Worcestershire Acute Hospitals Trust was staring down the barrel of a £31 million deficit on a £250 million turnover. Chief executive John Rostill was quite open in pointing the finger at the added costs of PFI as the root of the historic debt, but the cash pressures had been compounded by the lack of beds, which had forced the Trust to pass waiting list patients over to costly private hospitals. Seven hundred jobs were to be axed, along with beds and services as the Trust tried to balance the books. It was a similar tale of woe in the North East, where the merged County Durham and Darlington Trust, spanning two PFI Hospitals in Durham and Bishop Auckland, was shedding 700 jobs and axing services in a bid to cut spending by £40 million.

In the midst of the 2006 summer holidays, blithely optimistic New Labour ministers rubber stamped another clutch of six PFI hospital schemes worth almost £1.5 billion, although several of them had already been drastically hacked back to make them appear more affordable.

- The cash-strapped University Hospital of North Staffordshire Trust, whose near £400 million PFI scheme originally called for index linked payments of £53 million a year, was given the go-ahead for a scaled-down £272 million scheme.

- Walsall Hospital Trust had downsized its plans to try to make the PFI project affordable. The £140 million scheme given the nod by health minister Andy Burnham in August will increase costs by £13 million a year for the next 30 years, at a time when PCTs and ISTCs are scaling down the use of NHS hospital care.

But while some Trusts are counting the costs of successful bids, others are surveying the wreckage as cherished schemes crashed to earth with nothing achieved.

- In the summer, Colchester's Essex Rivers Trust scrapped a £167 million scheme, after warnings from finance chiefs that it could lose up to 20 per cent of its elective budget to a new ISTC planned for Essex, and lose more from its income under the controversial Payment by Results system. The Trust faced an immediate claim for up to £10 million in compensation to the jilted PFI partners (Moore 2006b).

- Also in the Home Counties, East and North Hertfordshire slashed back plans for an ambitious £550 million hospital in Hatfield, and attempted to hatch up a cheaper £400 million alternative – which has now also been discarded as unaffordable under government guidelines for PFI (Moore 2006c).

The new PFI-funded Queen's Hospital in Romford, which opened in late 2006 to replace Oldchurch and Harold Wood hospitals, has just 939 beds, with an option for another 60 – compared with the previous provision of 935 beds. The top floor remains unused for lack of the cash to staff it and run it. Harold Wood Hospital – once touted as the proposed site for a single-site hospital for Barking, Dagenham and Havering – closed at the end of 2006, with its site earmarked for a major housing development. This has resulted in much greater problems of access to care for residents in the outer areas of Havering and the London end of Brentwood.

But even as local MPs belatedly question whether the new hospital will be large enough to cope with the health needs of an ageing local population, plans are being laid to divert even more patients to Romford as part of the Trust's "Fit for the Future" proposals for a population of 700,000 in three London boroughs. The plans have been driven by the massive financial crisis confronted by the Barking, Havering and Redbridge Trust (which now picks up the bill for the £238 million hospital in the form of annual index linked payments of £36 million for 30 years, on top of an underlying cumulative deficit of £43 million), and by the adjacent Whipps Cross Hospital Trust.

All of the crazy alternatives that have been put before the "consultation" process would mean the run-down of existing hospital services to centralise care at the new PFI hospital, regardless of the problems of access and its lack of spare capacity to cope. One scenario would reduce Whipps Cross to an "ambulatory only" hospital, but it seems that the favoured option is to downgrade King George's Hospital in Ilford, which was only completed in 1993, to an "ambulatory care" centre, with a privately run treatment centre on site siphoning out vital revenue from the NHS Trust.

The treatment centre, due to open up in February, is scheduled to take over 11,000 elective cases a year, every one of which will result in a loss of revenue to the BHR Trust and further destabilise NHS care in NE London.

By June 2007 it was clear that the PFI hospital building programme had been slashed back drastically, to the tune of £4 billion from an original £12 billion, in the previous 16 months:

- Projects in Plymouth, Aintree, South Devon and north east London (Whipps Cross) – adding up to more than £1 billion – had been scrapped

- Others had been brutally cut back: Maidstone (£200 million cut); Hillingdon (£200 million cut); Hertfordshire (the £550 million project for East and North Herts had been replaced by a £250 million refurbishment plan); PFI projects in Liverpool had been almost halved from £700 million to £390 million (Timmins 2007h)

- Seven other schemes, in Kent, Bristol, Gloucester, Teesside, Mid Yorkshire, Middlesex and Essex (Chelmsford) have since been scaled down by about 15 per cent in an effort to make them more affordable (Gainsbury 2007e)

- Another PFI project that was later to be axed as unaffordable under the current drive for cash savings and centralisation was the £350 million "critical care" hospital planned as a replacement for services at Epsom and St Helier hospitals in SW London (*Sutton Guardian*, 11 September 2007).

In the same month, a published National Audit Office survey found that four out of nine PFI schemes failed to deliver good value to taxpayers – three of the four being NHS projects (Gainsbury 2007f). Another, unpublished NAO survey was uncovered that showed serious problems in a large majority of 19 NHS Trusts whose PFI schemes were scrutinised from 2005. Out of 19 Trusts, 13 were operating at bed occupancy levels above the NHS target of 85 per cent because bed numbers had been based on unrealistic assumptions of changes in patient care; and 15 felt restricted on getting value for money on small scale works such as shelves and notice boards (Moore 2007c).

The following month the collapse of Metronet, the PFI provider with contracts to upgrade six London Underground lines, threw more than the maintenance and improvement of the network into crisis. The stark reminder that the public sector is never fully absolved of risk under PFI raised more questions over the supposed value for money of high cost schemes (Gosling 2007; O'Grady 2007). In September came a fresh warning of soaring costs as more NHS PFI hospitals come on stream, with a report researched by Edinburgh University academics warning that this could push unitary charge payments across the NHS from £480 million a year to £2.3 billion over the next eight years (Hellowell and Pollock 2007b).

In November it became clear that a number of the new PFI hospitals under construction would follow the inglorious examples of Lewisham Hospital and Queens Hospital in Romford, by "shelling" some of the new space – i.e. keeping it closed, to reduce running costs. Bart's and the London had reduced its unitary charge in this way – to £98 million a year. Birmingham's new £697 million hospital, too was to have almost 10 per cent of its beds "shelled" (Moore 2007d).

PFI has been the fig leaf behind which the government has hidden its refusal to invest in the long term future of the NHS, with just 4 per cent of the capital for new hospital projects coming from the Treasury. And throughout the 14-year process, PFI has been costing millions for management consultants, accountants, lawyers and endless NHS management time. One of the reasons for ministers getting cold feet over signing off recent rounds of PFI hospitals is not so much the fear over the future affordability of such massive projects, but fear of one of the consequences of the accelerating pace of privatisation of health care under New Labour.

Ministers have become ever more obsessed with the notion of the NHS acting not as a provider of services but as a continental-style insurance fund, purchasing ("commissioning") health services from a range of (increasingly private or privatised) providers. On this model, it makes no sense to keep forking out large sums to rent buildings for the NHS to deliver care, when PCTs could simply turn to the private sector to deliver these services, with companies building and maintaining their own "Treatment Centres".

Their plans to float off all major NHS Trusts as free-standing "Foundation Trusts" accountable only to Monitor (the largely privatised independent regulator) will mean that fewer hospitals will be able to negotiate PFI deals. These deals all rely upon the underlying guarantee that the Secretary of State for Health will be obliged to step in and compensate the PFI consortium if a Trust goes seriously bust. If the Secretary of State is no longer responsible for the hospital, there is no basis for this guarantee, and the PFI consortium could be exposed to risk.

Admittedly this would leave huge gaps in care, since the private sector has shown no interest in delivering much of the bread and butter work of the NHS – emergencies, chronic conditions, and complex cases. However, ministers appear to have abandoned all but the most rhetorical commitment to planning or equitable access to care as they plunge eagerly into creating a barely regulated market system that seems destined to bankrupt a substantial number of NHS hospitals and even more local specialist units.

They have shown no regard for logic, evidence or even internal consistency as on the one hand they have urged Trusts down the path of hugely expensive PFI projects to fund new hospital buildings, and then on the other moved the goalposts on the financing of NHS treatment by introducing the Payment by Results system. This is already beginning to destabilise NHS hospitals, and will have the most serious impact on PFI-funded hospitals with inadequate bed numbers and sky-high overhead costs.

The answer to the need for investment and development to facilitate twenty-first century medicine with improved access for all was never PFI, which threatens decades of financial dislocation to health care. We still have to demand that the government scraps the PFI policy as a failure, brings the existing projects into public ownership, and steps in to loan the cash to build the new NHS hospitals that we all agree are needed for the future.

CHAPTER TEN

The evolution of primary care

PRIMARY CARE IS MOST SIMPLY SEEN as the first level of care which most patients can access, a "gateway" through which they must pass if they are to be referred for any elective or more specialist treatment, other than attending a hospital accident and emergency department. The definition of primary care services has been summed up by Julian Tudor Hart as:

> Medical and nursing care provided in the community from family doctors' surgeries or health centres, and other sources of health professional advice to which people have direct access, such as chemists, dentists and opticians.
>
> (Hart 1994: 118)

Gordon (1999) argues that primary care:

> can be described as a network of community-based health services that covers the prevention of ill-health, the treatment of acute and chronic illness, the promotion of health, rehabilitation, support at home for frail people, the management of long-term ill-health, and terminal care.
>
> (Gordon 1999: 3)

At the centre of the ethos of quality primary care is the notion of a continuity of personal care. This involves having a defined list of patients for a particular doctor, or group of doctors, and a practice-based team, including nurses and therapists, with whom the patient can become familiar.

These characteristics of primary care indicate that it is as unsuitable as any other aspect of health care for delivery in a free and competitive market. To work effectively, primary care services need to be planned jointly with community-based services and key social services, and with hospital care available as and when required, with planned and coordinated discharge of patients once their hospital care is completed.

The possibility of this type of relationship with the patient was opened up in the NHS in 1948 by the elimination of consultation fees and other devices which had excluded many people with the greatest health need. The NHS enabled those with long-term conditions to return as necessary for monitoring and treatment.

In other words, GPs have developed in a profoundly contradictory way: they have jealously guarded their status as "independent contractors – private sector businessmen" (Meads 1999: 38); yet the progressive development of primary care that has taken place since 1948 flows above all from their role in delivering a public service, through their involvement with the NHS. As Julian Tudor Hart puts it, they act as "private purveyors of *public* service" (Hart 1994: 98). Klein points out that the great initial achievement of the NHS was in liberating GPs and other doctors from the mechanism of the market, cutting the links between the practice of medicine and the income of the doctors – "thus removing any perverse incentives for either the selection or treatment of patients" (Klein 2006: 155).

However, the past 60 years have seen primary care evolve in different ways. On the one hand, there have been glimpses of the potential for the holistic, personal and integrated service that the best NHS professionals have aspired to develop; but especially in recent years, there have also been stark warnings of the danger that a reversion to a health market run on commercial and pecuniary lines could roll back and negate the gains that have been made. No section of the NHS workforce has been more cynically manipulated and used than the primary care team, headed, inevitably by general practitioners. Since 1948, GPs have by turns been appeased, marginalised, exploited, feted, courted, abused and even attacked by a succession of governments pursuing different agendas.

Where it has suited ministers, GPs have been well rewarded, and treated as vital, altruistic and public-spirited components of a great NHS team; but where ministers have wanted to distance themselves from GPs they have stressed their role as independent contractors. This version presents GPs as "private sector" providers on relatively lavish pay scales, functioning largely outside the control and governance systems that apply to their salaried hospital colleagues.

Bevan's compromise

The initial treatment of GPs by ministers in the mid-1940s revolved around their influential position in the BMA at the time Bevan was negotiating with the profession on the establishment of the new NHS. While junior doctors recognised the establishment of a National Health Service as opening up a new, nationwide career structure and opportunity to progress, and consultants were bought off with similar prospects plus the promise of pay-beds and part-time contracts, the GPs were the last group of medical professionals to keep on fighting and rejecting Bevan's proposals (Timmins 1995; Rivett 1998).

Progressive models for the development of primary care could be found as early as the Dawson Report of 1920. This bravely flew in the face of contemporary professional prejudice against local authorities, to suggest the establishment of council-funded primary health centres employing between six and twelve salaried GPs, and offering an additional range of related services – dental care, ophthalmology and pharmacy services combining curative and preventive medicine. These ideas were taken up by the Socialist Medical Association, later the Socialist Health Association, an affiliate of the Labour Party (Allsop 1984; Pollock 2004; Hart 1994).

These proposals were put forward, in slightly modified form, in the initial proposals for the establishment of the NHS: even the idea of a salaried service enjoyed massive support among GPs in the armed forces in 1944 and among medical students in 1948 (Pollock 2004). However, it was the backward-looking and narrow-minded GPs who then set the pace for BMA policy, and they rejected even the notion of a basic salary.

Egged on by the right-wing press and by Winston Churchill's Conservative Party, which opposed the NHS Bill in Parliament, the BMA's GPs dug in to wage an opposition which ran right up to the launch of the NHS in July 1948 (Timmins 1995). In his efforts to bring them on side, recognising that the system could not operate without the local provision of primary care services, Bevan conceded the principle that GPs would remain independent contractors and the basic salary was made optional. Indeed, the only principle which Bevan insisted upon was an end to the sale and purchase of the "goodwill" of GP practices – effectively selling on their patients as a commercial going concern. Even this progressive reform was lavishly compensated with the payment of £66 million to be shared between the 18,000 GPs who signed the NHS contract (Klein 2006; Pollock 2004).

Even though they had been finally enticed and pressurised into signing up for the NHS, GPs and primary care services remained at first very much the poor relations, a separate section with little public profile or political influence (Gordon 1999). More than 40 per cent of the GPs were then working in single-handed practices, and many of those in inner-city areas were in extremely poor premises, lacking any funding to facilitate improvements: but capital funding was one of the weaknesses of the early NHS, which did little to improve the stock of hospitals and other facilities until the 1960s. However, the 1952 pay settlement did give GPs an increase designed to move their incomes closer to those of hospital consultants, and also made loans available for new and refurbished premises, and this encouraged the development of group practices (Pollock 2004). During the 1950s and 1960s new, exciting work was also done on developing a theoretical basis for expanded general practice and a vision of GPs working in a more integrated way with the wider NHS – with the launch of the Royal College of General Practitioners in 1952 and the development of "a professional culture of audit and vocational training far ahead of the hospital sector" (Gordon 1999: 7).

Perhaps the biggest step forward in the development of primary care as an integral component of the NHS came in the 1966 Doctors' Charter, drawn up by a prominent member of the Socialist Health Association, Hugh Faulkner. This offered GPs a weighted capitation fee that gave greater rewards for caring for older people and for practices in less desirable areas, but also opened up subsidised loans for new premises and reimbursed 70 per cent of the costs of employing additional support staff – although Hart argues that this still left almost a third of the costs of support staff with the GPs, raising the danger that they would run their practices with too few (Hart 1994; Pollock 2004). Local government money also became more freely available to fund the building of health centres, and 731 of them were operational by 1977, accounting for 17 per cent of GPs (Lister 1988). There was a "renaissance" in general practice, with medical schools opening departments of general practice and new models of care that were "recognised as probably the best in the world" (Gordon 1999: 8). But the process was inevitably uneven, with many backward-looking GPs, especially those in deprived under-resourced inner-city areas, acting as individuals, clinging on to old and discredited ways of working. Gordon argues that the gap between the best and the worst primary care probably widened in this period of advance (Gordon 1999). As late as 1979, 15 per cent of GP practices were still run single-handed.

Throughout the first four decades of the NHS, GPs remained bound by a contract which obliged them to provide 24/7 cover to the patients on their list: however, GP services, run through separate Family Practitioner Committees, were outside of any collective planning process by the district health authorities. One compensating advantage of this semi-detached relationship was that primary care budgets, then largely centred on the costs of prescriptions, were not subject to the regime of cash limits which were applied with increasing rigour to the hospital sector from 1976 onwards.

Reorganisations in the 1970s eventually worked to integrate other services which are properly part of primary care, but which had been assigned to local authority control when the NHS was first established. District nursing, health visiting, midwifery, maternity and child welfare, vaccination and immunisation programmes – all were belatedly brought in to the NHS in 1974, and with them large numbers of nurses and other health professionals who have since been seen as integral to primary and community-based care (Gordon 1999; Timmins 1995).

The Conservative market reforms

It seems beyond a coincidence that the political argument preceding the implementation of the Tory internal market in 1989–90 coincided with a major trial of strength between the government and the GPs, which culminated in the imposition of a new contract that GP delegates had voted to reject. Certainly many of the GPs who joined the popular local campaigns against the *Working for Patients* White Paper, and subsequently against local hospitals "opting out" to become NHS Trusts, saw a connection between the two. They linked the new, competitive, cash-oriented mechanism of the internal market – with its separation of purchasers (health authorities and fundholding GPs) from providers (NHS Trusts) – and the imposition on GPs of a contract which tried to use cash incentives to persuade them to offer services such as minor surgery and chronic disease management, and required many of them to change the way they worked, without offering any significant additional resources – effectively demanding "more work for the same money" (Rivett 1998: 411).

The contract was unpopular, and became the focal point for wider subsequent demoralisation and dissatisfaction: it had undermined GPs' "sense of being in control of progress":

They saw themselves as moving from being the champions of primary care to being servants of the new Family Health Services Authorities (FHSAs). They saw few additional rewards for good practice, but much additional bureaucracy.

(Gordon 1999: 9)

Changes in the contract that had the implication of reducing consultation times, and thus undermining the qualitative element of primary care, were followed by market-style reforms. These proposals seemed to create new perverse incentives for fundholders to withhold treatment from the more needy patients and seek out a list of fitter, younger patients more likely to result in an unspent surplus at the end of the financial year. This created a new uncertainty in the patient–doctor relationship. No longer could a patient be certain that decisions were being taken solely in his/her interest: now the financial situation of the practice, even the personal financial gain of the GP, could be seen as a possible factor underlying a decision. Worse, each item of treatment was being transformed by these changes back into a financial transaction, a commercial issue, even though the patient was not being required to pay up front for their treatment.

There was also an underlying assumption in the fundholding proposal that GPs had time and energy to spare for the extra managerial and administrative work involved, such as ringing round a range of hospitals seeking the best (and cheapest) deal for patients. This was especially unlikely for inner-city GPs, many of whom were still in small or single-handed practices, swamped by a tide of ill health and human misery flowing from unemployment, poverty and poor housing. With hospitals themselves also under pressure and short of funds and resources, for these GPs it was often a struggle to find even one hospital bed for a patient needing emergency admission, let alone a choice.

A primary care-led NHS?

In 1992 the Tomlinson Report on London's NHS, borrowing arguments put forward earlier in 1992 by the King's Fund argued – without a shred of evidence – that improvements in primary care services would reduce the demand for acute hospital beds. This pious hope of a large-scale switch of services from hospitals to GPs, coupled with a change of behaviour by patients, was soon to be embraced by Health Secretary Virginia Bottomley and projected as a policy for the whole NHS – although unfortunately the additional resources for primary care were to be derived by first scaling down the hospitals, a formula that has brought conflict and public disquiet (DoH 1993b). By 1994, the NHS Executive was trumpeting the new buzz-words "primary care-led NHS" (NHS Executive 1994b; Bloor et al. 1999).

Henceforth, confused managers in health authorities throughout the country would tell even more confused staff and sceptical local people that the NHS was to be "primary care led". This was later interpreted by Ham and others as a new 'consensus' (Ham 1996; Meads 1999). Nobody troubled to define this new jargon term, or to address the problem that GPs and other primary care professionals were not directing the new system, or making the policies: resources were to be diverted from hospital care into various primary care schemes – whether GPs liked it or not. As Meads points out:

> The NHS was seen as being defined in relation to the power of one of its constituents (over the rest). For those who were direct employees of the NHS, the effect in many places, particularly those where the quality of primary care was inadequate, was to engender downright alienation and hostility. That GPs with their independent contractor status could be legitimately regarded as partially detached from the NHS, or, even worse, as the vanguard of the independent sector paving the way for ultimate privatisation clearly for many spelt disaster.
>
> (Meads 1999: 28)

The real push for privatisation which Meads raises as an issue was to come later, under New Labour. But it was clear that, far from "leading" the changes that were being forced through in the NHS, GPs were in fact being left to pick up the pieces left behind as health authorities and Trusts wrestled with cash limits, taking decisions in secret sessions without the slightest reference to the wishes or needs of GPs.

Indeed, inner-London GPs were among the foremost opponents of the Tomlinson Report and the government policy which flowed from it. A BMA meeting of inner-London GPs in December voted to reject "The flawed premise that an improvement in primary care and community services can substitute for secondary care," and called for "a moratorium on hospital mergers, closures and bed cuts" (Stanton 1992). Other advocates of primary care also distanced themselves from the logic of Tomlinson (Royal College of General Practitioners 1993; Holland 1992). As is usual with opponents of government policy, their voices were ignored.

Problems with primary care

Despite the new rhetoric of a primary-care-led NHS, all was not well among the GPs. By the summer of 1994 it became clear that fewer doctors were entering general practice, and health academics warned ministers that there was "a problem of morale" (*Guardian*, 24 June 1994). The new NHS chief executive, Alan Langlands, admitted that GPs faced a "paper overload" in the new, market-style NHS. Dr Ian Bogle, chair of the BMA's GP committee warned that doctors were being turned into a "demoralised and demotivated workforce".

A consolation for GPs was that there were promising pickings if they decided to become fundholders. The figures were starting to become available. It emerged that the government had been handing out £16,500 a time in lump sums as a down payment to any GP who expressed an interest in fundholding – money that was theirs to keep. Several practices had reportedly picked up this largesse more than once, and no less than £2.3 million had been handed over in this way in 1991–2. It would be followed by another cheque for £30,000 as a start-up gift for any that joined the scheme (*Sunday Express*, 23 January 1994).

There was an added incentive in that practices could retain any unspent surplus from their annual budget. Figures obtained by Alan Milburn MP showed that 585 fundholding practices had retained a total of £28 million in 1993–4. Health authorities had no power to retrieve unspent allocations, which averaged £48,000 per fundholder in the second year of the scheme. In North East Thames region, fundholding GPs held onto more than £1 for every £6 allocated, equivalent to £77,000 per doctor (*Guardian*, 23 December 1993, 28 February 1994).

There was growing anger, too, at revelations of the predicted two-tier service emerging within the NHS. A BMA survey of 173 hospitals in 1994 found 73 of them were offering preferential services to fundholders' patients, 41 of them promising "fast-track", more rapid admission (BMA Press statement, 8 December 1993; *Guardian*, 10 December 1993). The administration of the contracts between a growing number of fundholding practices and the NHS Trusts from whom they purchased services also became increasingly complex and expensive.

Meanwhile, those GPs who had valued the degree of organisational independence that primary care enjoyed from the local health authority saw the Family Health Services Authorities merged in 1996 with the District Health Authorities – and with it the submergence of virtually all of the leading FHSA managers. One study cited by Gordon showed that in just seven cases out of 87 mergers was the new chief executive a former general manager of an FHSA (Gordon 1999: 16).

Despite these obvious problems, the involvement of an ever-growing proportion of GPs in the fundholding project served to soften up the political opposition. In 1997, in the run-up to the general election that was to bring Tony Blair to office, a Primary Care Bill which opened up the possibility of a new kind of GP contract, Personal Medical Services, was rushed through Parliament with all-party support. This allowed local-level negotiation on terms and conditions for individual GPs or whole practices, conditional on them delivering quality standards and meeting local needs: PMS also allowed GPs to opt for salaried status, the first substantial development along these lines since 1948.

The policy was aimed at filling gaps in provision in deprived and under-doctored areas – but one unwelcome innovation was that it rolled back the principle of funding GPs for the overhead costs they would encounter in providing care: instead, each PMS contract offered a cash-limited global practice budget, from which all costs and salaries had to be met. This, like fundholding, transferred risk to the GP (Pollock 2004: 146; Meads 1999). This legislation was inherited by New Labour ministers Frank Dobson and Alan Milburn when they took office from May 1997. It was one of the features they opted to retain as they set about reviewing and dismantling some of the Tory government's market-style policies (Meads 1999).

Primary Care Groups explored

The attitude to PMS set the tone for the new government's approach. The Dobson reforms which followed New Labour's landslide victory in the 1997 election set out to tackle the fundholding system that they had criticised so effectively in opposition, but in such a way as to retain the purchaser–provider split which was always the kernel of the Tory "internal market". At the same time, Labour ministers have been unremittingly eager to maintain the references to "primary care" in the many and frequent changes that have taken place in the last ten years.

The interim solution was a change of rhetoric from "purchasing" to "commissioning", and from "competition" to "cooperation" (DoH 1997a). For primary care there was to be a transition from fundholding to Primary Care Groups, which seemed to have some potential as an inclusive way of drawing GPs into decision-making on services alongside local health authorities. However these proved to be limited in scope, and short-lived: the consultation on their replacement by Primary Care Trusts generally began within a year of the launch of the PCGs.

The initial plan proposed that there would be around 500 PCGs in England, each covering a catchment population of around 100,000, and covering all of the GP practices within its area. They were to replace the old complex system in which 3,500 GP practices (about half) had become "fundholding" practices with their own budget to buy non-emergency hospital care for their patients. Each PCG board would have a cash-limited budget to buy all of the treatment required by all of the local population. Each Primary Care Group would have a "governing board" of between 9 and 13 members – about the same size as a health authority, including:

- 4–7 GPs
- 1–2 nurses
- 1 social services officer
- 1 "lay member"
- 1 non-executive health authority member
- 1 PCG chief executive.

(NHS Executive 1998)

Ministers claimed that this would put doctors and nurses "in the driving seat" of decision-making: but there was never any doubt that PCG boards would be dominated by GPs – and more specifically by the GPs from the larger and better-resourced practices, many of them former fundholders, who had the time and inclination to engage in PCG business. Indeed, the newly appointed National Director for Primary Care in England was a high-profile former fundholder, Dr David Colin-Thome (Pollock 2004).

The experience of putting GPs in charge of health budgets had previously been far from positive. Fundholding had brought the bizarre spectacle of many GPs from already prosperous practices piling up surpluses of cash left over from their more generous budgets, while their less-well-resourced inner-city colleagues struggled to deliver services and local hospitals and community services faced cutbacks. In many areas a two-tier NHS developed, in which the patients of some fundholders were able to jump the queue of local waiting lists, while their neighbours on the lists of non-fundholders had to wait for months or years because their health authority had exhausted its budget.

Many GPs also had an appalling track record as employers of support staff in their own practices. And ever since 1948 this group of professionals had refused to be employed by the NHS, insisting on their status as "independent contractors", making GPs the least accountable of any NHS professional group. What was new was the idea that GPs, through PCGs, be given the leading voice on the allocation of NHS resources – with potentially huge implications for thousands of staff working for local NHS Trusts.

The White Paper and subsequent guidance set out four distinct levels at which Primary Care Groups might decide to operate, culminating in a Primary Care Trust, which would span the purchaser–provider split, commissioning care from hospitals while also providing primary and community services. These Trusts would be able, among other things, to "run community hospitals and other community services". All health authorities were required to establish PCGs operating at least at Level One from April 1999 (NHS Executive 1998).

Although there were signs that some "empire-building" GPs already aspired to the top level, the legislation had not yet been put before Parliament, suggesting that this stage might take some time: it eventually became clear that Primary Care Trusts, despite the name and the apparent promise to GPs, would *not* be primary-care-led bodies at all, but a reincarnation of the District Health Authorities with only a relatively marginal input or control by local GPs.

GPs: in the driving seat?

The variable number of GPs to sit on PCGs ran alongside the government decision that GPs should be allowed a guaranteed majority on PCGs if they chose: seven GPs would be sufficient to outvote all of the other participants. Government guidelines insisted that as an overriding principle nothing should be done that might "negate" the majority of GPs.

However, the new system consolidated the regime that had prevailed under fundholding and PMS – now incorporating the whole of primary care within the global cash limits that had applied to the hospital sector for over 20 years.

> In the future there will be one stream of cash-limited funds flowing through Health Authorities to Primary Care Groups. …It will align clinical and financial responsibility so that those who prescribe, treat and refer have control over the financial decisions they take.
>
> (DoH 1997a: 70)

There would be a downward pressure on prescribing costs and limited options to match services to local needs, with very little extra cash in the national pot.

The most influential member of each PCG board was the chief executive, who became the officer responsible for the budget of around £300,000 a year for the PCG management, and up to £60 million a year for commissioning services. PCG chief executives were to be the only board members working full time on PCG issues and able to follow every aspect of the work.

Time and again, references to doctors were coupled with a ritual reference to nurses. The stock phrase promised nursing staff a place "in the driving seat": but there were to be at most two nursing representatives on any PCG board, while the dominant role of GPs was written into the new structure from the outset (NHS Executive 1998). It was always clear that the relationship between GPs and nursing staff is not a relationship of equals. Any community nursing staff wishing to argue at board level for policies which ran counter to the GP reps – who may currently, or in the medium-term future, be their employers – would have to take their courage in both hands.

While nurses were given a token involvement, the many other professionals who provide key components of primary and community services in each area – dentists, pharmacists, optometrists, occupational therapists, podiatrists, physiotherapists and speech therapists – were among those excluded from any but the most marginal involvement in the new structure.

But the PCGs were under no obligation to meet in public or to invite in the local press, and faced little or no public accountability. The DoH guidance note claimed that "wider public involvement in the PCG board" would occur "through three routes":

• One of the non-executive directors of the health authority would be appointed by the HA as a director of each PCG

• The Local Authority would nominate a social services officer to sit on the board [significantly this would be a manager, not an elected councillor or a representative of social workers]

• A "free standing lay member" would be appointed by the health authority "following an open and fair process which might involve local public advertisement" (NHS Executive 1998).

In other words the "wider public involvement" consisted in adding another meeting to the diary of somebody already on a quango (the HA non-exec member), and appointing another individual who was seen as acceptable to the health authority.

The HAs themselves were to become "leaner" bodies, and fewer in number.

> Health authorities... over time will relinquish direct commissioning functions to Primary Care Groups. ...Fewer authorities covering larger areas will emerge as a product of these changes.
>
> (DoH 1997a: 22)

Do GPs make good planners?

Most GPs come into primary care in order to work closely with the relatively limited numbers of patients on their practice list. Few GPs will have any wide experience or training in management, and even the largest and most effective fundholding practices only had experience of purchasing elective hospital services for up to 12,000 patients: none had any experience or expertise in planning the full gamut of services required for the much larger population, averaging 100,000, of a PCG (Pollock 2004).

The White Paper stirred up the division of interest between the primary and secondary care sectors when it claimed, without offering any evidence, that hospitals had been deliberately admitting patients to boost their contract income when the patients would be better looked after elsewhere. Ministers appeared unaware of the fact that in the five years after Virginia Bottomley adopted the primary-care-led model, an ever-increasing number of patients – many of them reportedly with minor ailments suited to primary care services – had been attending A&E departments and minor injuries units, while hospitals with fewer beds had struggled to cope with soaring numbers of emergency admissions; or if they were aware, the failing was put down to the hospitals rather than a chronic weakness and failure to develop adequate primary and community services to support people at home. Even ardent proponents of fundholding and the "primary-care-led NHS" have been forced to recognise a failure to deliver any reduction in emergency referrals, which has remained as a problem ever since (Meads 1999: 41).

Many of these admissions turn out to be emergency *medical* cases – frail elderly patients who, despite the rhetoric from ministers, were clearly not being supported by primary care or community-based services. It was becoming increasingly difficult to recruit GPs, especially to inner-city areas, while numbers seeking GP training had fallen by 21 per cent in the decade to 1996 (DoH Press Release, 22 May 1997). But the heyday of GP control was already passing.

Primary Care Trusts

From 2002, Primary Care Groups were replaced by Primary Care Trusts, local commissioning bodies which within a few years were expected to control upwards of 80 per cent of the total NHS budget for primary, community and hospital services.

From the outset it was clear that these organisations would be very different in structure and control from the PCGs. GP involvement was pushed right back to the periphery. According to the Department of Health guidance a PCT board should typically consist of 11 members:

- Chair
- Five lay members (which could include local authority elected members)
- Chief executive
- Finance director
- Three professional members drawn from the Executive (typically clinical governance director, one GP and one nurse).

Separate from the board would be the Primary Care Trust Executive (later renamed the Professional Executive Committee (PEC)) which was to have "a professional majority" as well as including the chief executive (the accountable officer) of the Trust, and the finance director.

The interim Level 3 Primary Care Trusts were to have an Executive consisting of:

- Up to seven GPs
- Two nurses
- A professional with public health and health promotion expertise
- A social services officer.

The more developed Level 4 PCT – the system that would take over the purchasing function from health authorities – would have a PEC with up to 10 clinicians, with "significant representation from general practice balanced with local nurses and other community professionals, public health expertise and Social Services" (NHS Executive 1998).

It is immediately obvious that the separation of the PEC from the PCT main board opened up a substantial gap between the professionals and the actual decision-making body: in practice PCTs would take all of their key decisions through the main board. GP control and involvement passed swiftly with the demise of the PCGs, and normal NHS business resumed rapidly with the consolidation of PCTs as health authority-like bodies, which then proceeded to merge into larger and less accountable bodies: as Pollock points out:

> GPs, having helped in paving the way for market-oriented reforms, would now be relegated to the back seat again.
>
> (Pollock 2004: 145)

The early promise that PCTs would exercise substantial local autonomy was thrown into question by the Department of Health's insistence that Oxfordshire PCTs had no choice but to agree to the establishment of a controversial private sector treatment centre delivering cataract treatment, despite PCT concerns that it would undermine the financial viability of Oxford's existing NHS Eye Hospital (Carvel 2004).

> The widely-held view that PCTs have failed adequately to establish themselves as effective purchasing bodies forcing maximum value from hospital Trusts led to fears that these organisations would in turn be reorganised and merged into new, larger and less accountable bodies after the 2005 election – as in fact proved to be the case.

However, the PCTs were not the only way in which GPs were to be marginalised and primary care services ripened up for the privatisation which many had begun to fear. The 2002 GP contract broke the principle of primary care services that had been a badge of honour since 1948: GPs were allowed to buy themselves out of any obligation to provide 24/7 services to the patients on their list. This commitment had already been diluted by the development during the 1990s of GP cooperatives and "deputising services": but all of these had been organised by the GPs themselves. Now the 2002 contract allowed them to renounce a share of their income in exchange for handing over the responsibility for out of hours cover to the local Primary Care Trust – and very large numbers of GPs were swift to do so.

As Pollock points out, this revision to the contract effectively ended the GPs' monopoly on the provision of primary care services: from here on in, the PCTs were in overall charge, and they would be encouraged to look to a variety of providers – including for-profit private companies and multinational corporations – to deliver these services (Pollock 2004). This line of approach was further facilitated by the Alternative Provider Medical Services contracts, which PCTs were encouraged to draw up with a range of external providers from 2006. PCTs were given discretion to "unbundle" aspects of the GP contract to offer a more attractive package for private-sector bids: up to a third of PCTs expressed an early interest in putting at least some GP services out to tender (*Pulse* 2006a). Nor did the Department of Health guidelines and model contract stipulate that services should be delivered at any fixed or comparable rate, opening up the possibility of private and voluntary sector providers charging well above the going rate for NHS contracts (DoH 2006c).

However keen they may have been to bring in private providers, the potential generosity of this scheme towards private companies has been limited by the cash-limited funding available to PCTs: attempts to bring in private companies to deliver primary care in 30 "under-doctored areas" hit problems in December 2006 because the PCTs involved could not afford to meet the price demanded by the providers (*Pulse* 2006b). But there was a further lure to attract private-sector involvement in primary care, which at the level of an individual or group practice might seem to offer relatively limited potential for profitable involvement. The Primary Care Trusts had been established with a perspective of taking control of up to 80 per cent of the NHS budget, which was continuing to rise dramatically year by year to 2008: but the Department of Health was looking to devolve the "commissioning" function even further, prodding GPs and PCTs towards the implementation of practice-based commissioning, in which a proportional share of the PCT commissioning budget would be controlled by each participating GP practice.

Health Minister John Hutton announced the plans in 2004 and hoped to have every practice implementing PBC by 2008: but he also made clear that there were strings attached – the practices involved would be even more tightly scrutinised:

> Clearly in return for the significant new freedoms that PBC will bring I do believe that it is fair and reasonable for PCTs to expect that primary care services will operate to the appropriate level of customer service and convenience. …

> There will also be effective safeguards to ensure value for money and the proper use of public funds. Practices will have the responsibility of balancing their budget over three years and PCTs will have the right to intervene if public money is being used inappropriately.

> (Hutton 2004)

Hutton's ambitious plans appear to have proved far less than realistic: by the end of 2007 an Audit Commission report suggested that only modest and uneven progress was being made in implementing PBC, and that the limited progress that had been achieved had come at a cost of £98 million in payments to induce GPs to participate. The report also identified a number of issues in which there had been especially slow progress, notably securing genuine engagement of GPs, PCTs being unwilling to relinquish their control over commissioning, and a lack of sufficient information (Lewis et al. 2007). Once again, a reform based on assumptions and a questionable evidence-base is being expensively introduced to deliver as yet unproven results.

PBC also opened up the tempting prospect that a private company, by establishing itself as a provider of primary care, could not only pick up a guaranteed surplus for undertaking the contract, but also begin to influence the allocation of funding both at practice level and through the PCT, where budgets totalled hundreds of millions.

Choice for patients – but not for PCTs

By the end of 2005 Primary Care Trusts were firmly established as part of the centralised government control over the NHS: as such they were obliged to offer almost all patients a "choice" of providers – including at least one private hospital – from the time they are first referred, while from 2008 onwards any patient was to be allowed to choose any hospital which could deliver treatment at the NHS reference cost (Stevens 2004). Irrespective of what patients (or their GPs) may choose, ministers made clear that they wanted at least 10 per cent of NHS elective operations to be carried out by the private sector in 2006, rising to 15 per cent by 2008 (Ward 2005). The Commons Public Accounts Committee warned that the policy could give GPs perverse incentives to refer patients to hospitals which did not have adequate facilities or medical support.

All change for PCTs: another reorganisation hits the NHS

In July 2005, just weeks after Tony Blair secured his historic third term with a substantially reduced majority, NHS chief executive Sir Nigel Crisp issued a circular to all NHS managers entitled 'Commissioning a Patient Led NHS'. This pressed for mergers of SHAs and PCTs, and for the separation of PCTs' commissioning role from their direct provision of services, and in doing so marked a real acceleration of the national drive towards the fragmentation, privatisation and marketisation of the NHS (Crisp 2005). Clearly the NHS needs some form of mechanism to make local services accountable to local people: and while the 2005-style PCTs were far from perfect in this regard, the new, larger, and more remote PCTs proposed by Crisp threatened to make matters even worse, while offering no compensating improvements. Unions and campaigners were concerned that fewer, larger, and less accountable PCTs would be more vulnerable to future pressures from above to privatise, hive off or close down services (Lister 2006b, c).

As if to bang home the point, London's new Strategic Health Authority got into action… by seeking to ration referrals to hospital by London's GPs. News of the cash-led scheme, which would process each GP referral through a team of bureaucrats in a "referral management centre" broke in a leaked document, in which managers discussed plans to restrict Londoners to the lowest 10 per cent of hospital referral rates anywhere in England (Revill 2006). The London-wide clampdown on GP referrals and consultant-to-consultant referrals was imposed by top civil servant John Bacon. NHS bosses offered no evidence to show why the lowest levels of hospital treatment in England would be appropriate for the population of London, which is far and away Europe's biggest city, with a chronically poor infrastructure of primary care, community services and social services, and a huge pool of poverty, ill health and deprivation. Emergency attendances and emergency admissions have been rising year by year in London, much faster than the national average, despite empty promises of a new "primary care-led NHS" (*Health Emergency* 62, 2006).

With GPs under pressure not to refer patients to consultants, the principle of a consultant second-opinion, part of the fabric of the NHS, was also slung out of the window along with "choice". An article in the *British Medical Journal* exposed the lack of any evidence that the new system, which had "appeared overnight in an evidence-free zone" could deliver any positive benefit for patients (Davies and Elwyn 2006).

Privatisation was also a current and pressing issue in the NHS across England. Even during the consultation process on the Crisp proposals steps were taken towards the privatisation of GP services in Derby and in North Derbyshire to UnitedHealth Europe[22], a subsidiary of one of the biggest and the most profitable of the health care corporations in the USA. Well-informed rumours began to circulate that more GP practices could be hived off in similar fashion to private corporations, or for-profit groups of GPs (Nunns 2006).

A popular local campaign was waged in the former mining village of Langwith, supported by the Keep Our NHS Public campaign: this showed clearly that there was little or no local support for the plan to wheel in a major US corporation to deliver primary care. Local views had been arrogantly ignored by the PCT, which refused to engage in discussion or debate, but proceeded on the most perverse basis to exclude existing and established local GPs from the shortlist in Langwith, and then to pronounce UnitedHealth Europe, which at that point had no staff, no functioning services, no local links or experience and no track record of delivering primary care in the UK, as having topped the list as preferred provider. In the event this local privatisation was halted by the tenacious and courageous legal challenge mounted by a local pensioner Pam Smith, after an initial setback in the High Court was reversed on appeal. However, a few miles away in Derby, where no such resistance was organised, the privatisation was rubber stamped, and United secured its first foot in the door of primary care in England (Barrett 2006; Nunns 2006).

---

22 UnitedHealth Europe was then chaired by one of Tony Blair's former health advisors, Simon Stevens, who has since taken a post with the parent company in the USA (Revill 2007).

Darzi and primary care: the Jekyll and Hyde question

Another substantial debate on primary care services opened up when Professor Ara Darzi's 124-page report *Healthcare for London: A Framework for Action* was launched on 11 July 2007. It addressed some long-standing and important weaknesses in health and health care in the capital, and offered a few fresh ideas, although one which appeared more radical, the proposal for a new network of "polyclinics," turns out to be a rebranded rehash of ideas for "community hospitals" or primary health care centres going back through the 1960s to the Dawson report of 1920 (Darzi 2007a; Pollock 2004).

At first sight, Darzi's report appeared to some to present a detailed strategy to address chronic inequalities in health care provision. However it has left many important questions unanswered as a laborious and costly (£15 million) process of "consultation and implementation" grinds into action across the capital, to conclude by March 2008. And subsequent statements and publications from Lord Darzi, elevated to junior minister by Gordon Brown's summer government reshuffle, gave rise to more serious concern that even the positive and progressive proposals in the London document may simply be a decoy to distract attention from an agenda of increased privatisation in primary and secondary care. There are too many inconsistencies and missing factors in the Darzi report for it to be the finished article: there is no road-map towards implementation, the costings do not appear to be realistic, one key group of staff (GPs) have yet to be convinced of the merits of the central proposals, and too many real and pressing problems are wished away or simply ignored.

Darzi's London plan is certainly far more than a recipe for privatisation. Insofar as it contains concrete proposals and examples, his report only singles out examples of good practice in NHS treatment centres and units, and the main focus of the report is on the development of the NHS as a public service. However, Darzi has raised the possibility that some polyclinics, for example, might be owned and run privately by GPs – and his interim report on the NHS in England looks quite unambiguously towards private-sector solutions to shortages of GPs, the improvement of GP premises, and new elective treatment centres (Darzi 2007b).

In London, Darzi needs a lot of GPs on board to make his plans work. He proposes to replace many traditional A&E services with a combination of improved out-of-hours GP services, and a number of "urgent care centres," some of which may be downsized A&E units, others based in new "polyclinics". 150 polyclinics are proposed across the capital, at an estimated annual cost of £3.1 billion: this would bring a root and branch reorganisation of most primary care services in the capital. But of course it would also cause havoc in the hospitals.

Darzi accepts without question the market-style reorganisation that has taken place since the NHS Plan in 2000, despite the fact that these measures have already substantially restricted the ability to plan the type of modernisation and reform he is proposing. His London report, for example, proposes that 41 per cent of hospital outpatient appointments should be transferred to polyclinics (and primary care): but under Payment by Results this would slice a massive £330 million from hospital budgets, while a fresh approach to axing "unnecessary" outpatient visits could remove another 20 per cent of existing caseload, and cut hospitals' income by another £160 million.

Darzi also argues in his report (page 90) for a far greater extension of outreach working by NHS staff from polyclinics, with clear implications for the primary care workload in London: "NHS staff will be going into people's homes to keep people out of hospital".

This is extending into the area of social care. But on the ground the reality is alarming. Throughout England two-thirds of councils have now restricted eligibility to social care to virtually exclude all but the bed-bound: and London's boroughs have been among the meanest in raising charges and imposing ever more draconian eligibility criteria.

- Brent and Lewisham have trebled charges for some services

- Harrow has slapped a £20 charge on its day centres

- London boroughs implementing tighter interpretations of the means test for charges include Harrow, Camden, Islington, Merton and Richmond

- Wandsworth has slashed its subsidy on each hour of home care from £3.21 to just 1p, while tightening its eligibility criterion from "moderate" to "substantial"

- Redbridge too has increased criteria from "substantial" to "upper substantial", yet DoH definitions stipulate that "substantial" means "abuse or neglect has occurred or will occur and/or there is, or will be, an inability to carry out the majority of personal care or domestic routines" (*Public Finance*, 16 March 2007)

- Lambeth has pushed through cuts which restricted services to those with "critical" needs – withdrawing support from 750 frail older people, while more than doubling hourly charges for home care, increasing meals on wheels costs by 54 per cent and slapping a massive £35 fee on previously free day centre services.

This collapse of social service support for all but the most frail older people across much of the capital represents a major challenge to the NHS, and to primary care services as well as the hospitals. Any attempt to revamp the system without addressing these key questions is likely to run into problems.

Darzi predicts that "Community Care" services in London will handle a vast and expanding caseload, and that use of primary care will increase exponentially over the next ten years – by 75 per cent to more than 48 million consultations a year. This is linked with the assumed transfer of a growing volume of work from hospitals to primary care, but it does also assume a relatively rapid and complete culture-shift by London's population to accept the new system.

So getting London's GPs on board will be vital if they are to be recruited to work in a completely new way in the planned polyclinics, which cannot run without them. A serious discussion with the BMA and with local medical committees would have been a sensible way to work towards a common view, but the Darzi approach is to impose the new plan from top down. The intervention of a high-profile specialist hospital doctor seeking in this way to force GPs into line has already angered some of the more conservative elements.

Polyclinics: the case examined

One new concept stands out from the report: the suggestion of a network of 150 "polyclinics" to serve the capital's 7.5 million population: on closer examination a polyclinic appears to be a combination of a super-sized health centre, a minor injuries unit, a small-scale outpatients department and a base for community health services.

In early debates with NHS London it has been one of the first ideas to be diluted and rephrased, and it has become obvious that the concept as spelled out in the Darzi report and technical paper is controversial even with the managers charged with carrying it through. However, since the idea seems likely to remain a talking point for some period to come, it is useful to analyse its implications for primary care.

According to the GP magazine *Pulse*, the proposal amounts to "herding GPs into polyclinics":

> The Healthcare for London report, written by Professor Sir Ara Darzi, the newly appointed health minister, proposes merging hundreds of GP practices in the capital into a network of so-called 'polyclinics'. SHAs elsewhere in the country are now closely studying the controversial new model, which could lead to the relocation of thousands more GPs.
>
> The new sites would offer extended opening hours and provide up to 50% of outpatient treatment currently carried out in hospitals.
>
> The BMA warned that polyclinics would 'destabilise and fragment' existing GP and hospital services, and GPC acting chair Dr Laurence Buckman said they were reminiscent of something from communist Soviet Union. 'This review does not bode well.'
>
> Dr Tony Stanton, joint chief executive of London-wide LMCs, said it would 'destroy the very bedrock of British general practice' if most surgeries were relocated to polyclinics.
>
> Dr Michael Dixon, chair of the NHS Alliance, also attacked the proposals, adding: 'I don't think it's what patients or GPs want. We need an increased focus on continuity and personal care.'
>
> (*Pulse*, 13 July 2007)

One factor driving the hostile response from GPs could be the studied vagueness over how the proposal would be implemented: it is not clear from Darzi's report whether the polyclinics would be run by PCTs, or free-standing units of the NHS, each run with an overall management employing a staff, including dozens of salaried GPs, or whether the polyclinics would effectively operate as gigantic health centres, drawing together a large number of local GP practices under a common roof, with shared support services. The first two of these options would effectively spell the end of the treasured "independent contractor" status they have jealously guarded ever since 1948: the second option would be a less traumatic change for GPs but would offer different problems in organisation and management.

Polyclinics versus A&E?

Much of the Darzi plan amounts to yet another attempt (after many others have failed) to switch patient care away from hospitals (and especially from A&E) to a variety of alternative venues. In the mid-1990s the fashion was for "Minor Injury Units" – often as a transitional step towards closing a full-scale A&E, and frequently coupled with proposals for more out of hours services to be provided by GPs: Darzi's version is "urgent care centres" attached to polyclinics as well as hospitals. However, as with so many of his proposals, we are not told how many such units are required or where they would be: nor would all of them be open 24 hours.

Nor are by any means all A&E attenders "inappropriate": Darzi's own figures in the technical paper (page 15) show that of 3.5 million A&E attendances in London's hospitals in 2005–6, over 40 per cent were "major" episodes – classified as "emergency admissions, trauma"; if 581,000 fractures are added, it means almost 60 per cent of the total had good reason to come to a hospital for treatment rather than a minor injury unit. This undermines Darzi's prediction that as many as 50 per cent of A&E attenders could appropriately be diverted to polyclinics.

Key numbers that don't add up

Darzi's report appears to propose that each polyclinic should offer supporting services including:

• Minor procedures
• Urgent care
• Diagnostics (pathology and radiology).

However, the report and the "Technical Paper" (Darzi 2007c) offer very few hard facts to show that the cost and space implications of this have been taken on board. It suggests each polyclinic would employ an average of around 90 medical and nursing staff, including 35 GPs and 3–4 consultants, be located in rented accommodation, and run on a budget of around £21 million a year – a total investment of £3.1 billion annually when all are open. The scale of the new polyclinics and their substantial projected caseload for primary care services would mean that they would need to enlist a total of over 5,200 GPs to full-time work – slightly more than the 2007 complement of GPs in London.

However, the culture of work in polyclinics would be vastly different from most current general practice: Darzi specifies a polyclinic would need a minimum of 43 consulting rooms, while at present almost 500 London GPs are currently working in single-handed practices, and fewer than 300 London GPs are part of large practices with 10 or more doctors. While there are always a few exceptions to the rule, and one or two GPs have been involved in drawing up the Darzi plan, there is no sign so far that GPs in general will respond positively to proposals which would in many cases lead to a reduced status, a requirement to work in a big team, and a loss of identity and control over standards for smaller but committed practices which have worked for many years to develop and improve their services.

The qualitative element of continuity of patient care seems to be almost completely obliterated by the polyclinic plan. The projected caseload of each polyclinic is enormous even at the primary care level – with an estimated 226,000 consultations averaging a staggering 620 per day, every day throughout the year. Even with no gaps between patients, and working on Darzi's estimate of 15 minutes consultation time, this stacks up to 93 hours of GP time and 57 hours of Allied Health Professional time EACH DAY – requiring 13 GPs and 7.5 AHPs to be available even if they did nothing else but process patients. And all of these figures assume that a third of primary care would remain in GP practices outside of the polyclinics.

In fact, polyclinics would handle even more than this: an average polyclinic is also expected to deal with 25,000 outpatient appointments a year (480 every week of the year); plus 21,000 "A&E" ("urgent care centre") cases – 57 every day of the year; and 41,000 community care episodes – almost 800 per week, over and above home visits.

Activity on this scale, managing and arranging payroll, training and other support for 100 or more staff, and ensuring reliable and punctual operation of a wide range of treatments, consultations and tests, represents a major management challenge. Inadequate resources for management, and insufficient experienced and qualified secretarial and clerical staff would be a short-sighted economy that would rapidly threaten chaos. It seems obvious from the figures that Professor Darzi has seriously underestimated the numbers of non-clinical staff needed to ensure that the new polyclinics would work as they should. His projected total "administrative overhead" is just £1.26 million per polyclinic: but it seems that at least £900,000 of this would be rent, leaving just £326,000 for IT services, admin and clerical staff and management to run a £20-million-a-year operation. That would equate to just 13 clerical staff on £25,000 a year – nowhere near the level of managerial and support staff that will be needed.

Darzi's financial projections exclude any capital costs for building and equipping new polyclinics: instead his figures for "administrative overhead" include an assumed annual lease payment – but this in turn hinges on the availability of 150 sufficient suitable premises for indefinite rent. However, the sheer scale and complexity of the buildings required must raise genuine doubts over the possibility of securing anything like the number of ready-made premises that Darzi proposes. Polyclinics require 43 consulting rooms, space for at least 100 to wait, another 1,000 square metres for office and other admin space, circulation space, etc. – plus the fact that any integrated X-ray facility, for example, would need to be housed in a lead-lined room. Cue the private sector and combinations of LIFT, PFI and multinational health corporations to fill the gap – at significant further expense.

While the daunting workload of primary care and community care services questions the quality of services that the polyclinics would be able to deliver, the extremely small and fragmented caseload for some other services also raises serious doubts over quality. The average polyclinic is projected to carry out just 336 "minor elective surgical procedures" a year – that's just 6.5 per week, and especially if the work is shared out, it is nowhere near enough to enable medical staff to develop specialist skills. Worse, the average polyclinic is expected to carry out just 19 "emergency surgery procedures" a year (Darzi 2007c: 25).

Projections for emergency medicine also make it clear that only a handful of patients each week would be receiving treatment at polyclinics, raising the question of whether it would not be safer and better all round to leave these procedures in hospitals where more experienced and specialist staff are on hand, seeing many more cases day by day. Ironically the Darzi report itself repeatedly stresses the problems of staff seeing too few patients to develop skills:

> There is evidence that specialist units performing larger numbers of cases achieve better results, particularly in more complex work.
>
> (page 22: 42)

> Hospitals in London are not able to take advantage of the latest advances in medical care, as specialist staff and facilities are spread across too many sites.
>
> (page 24: 44)

> A recent meta-analysis in the *British Journal of Surgery* has found that there is a positive relationship between volumes of specialist surgery and three key outcome indicators (mortality rates, reduced lengths of stay and complication rates).
>
> (page 70: 178)

It is on the basis of this that Darzi goes on to insist controversially that "The days of the district general hospital seeking to provide all services to a high enough standard are over" (page 71). So why should GPs in polyclinics now be expected to deliver adequate standards of treatments which until now have always been provided by specialist surgical staff in hospital?

Dreams of preventive utopia

Nobody can object to efforts to prevent unnecessary hospital admission: but health promotion campaigns have shown time and again that they require a long-term and consistent input, and that achieving long-term change is difficult or impossible where the patient concerned has not accepted the need for change. So it is quite unrealistic to expect rapid and measurable results from the well-intentioned proposals set out in the Darzi Report, which states that:

> Community healthcare staff… should work with public health colleagues to seek out people at high risk of smoking and obesity (e.g. through deprivation indices). They should then provide tailored advice and support to help people to improve their diet, take more exercise and stop smoking. This is likely to require effort to reach out, recall and follow people up who may be reluctant to access services or keep up with the programmes.
>
> (page 72)

Nobody would oppose a campaign to reduce smoking or obesity: but Darzi offers no evidence that such tactics have been successful in changing the long-standing, often socially rooted behaviour of people unwilling to change or engage with services. This seems to be a sure-fire formula for failure and demoralisation, which may perhaps be garnished with some self-deception in the form of carefully juggled statistics and "targets" to conceal the actual situation.

A growing market in primary care

According to a major survey by Allyson Pollock and colleagues, about 30 companies had already secured commercial contracts to deliver primary care services in England by March 2007: they ranged from GP-owned companies to international health care corporations (Pollock et al. 2007).

The pace of private-sector intervention continued to increase, and at the end of 2007 Heart of Birmingham PCT announced its plans to force 76 GP practices into 24 polyclinic-style franchises which would be offered up to Tesco, Asda or Virgin as commercial ventures. The PCT plan was eagerly welcomed by the West Midlands Strategic Health Authority, and seen as a model for other cities (Nowottny 2007).

In another worrying development, 73 local GPs in Merseyside were revealed by Channel 4 News to have used their powers under practice-based commissioning to award a dermatology contract to a private company in which they had shares. The switch of services to the private provider, charging £25 per case below the local specialist NHS unit, was forcing it to cut back in services, raising the danger that specialist care for more complex and serious cases may no longer be available locally. The PCT stridently denied the obvious conflict of interest (Blake 2007).

Conclusion: not what the doctors ordered

Six decades on, the NHS has still not established a coherent and workable framework for primary care that allows GPs and other professionals to develop the qualitative and consistent relationship with patients, or organises and resources a network of services to enable primary care to deliver its potential.

Instead this vital sector, which deals with over 90 per cent of the day-to-day contacts between patients and the NHS, but which in many areas must also work to address deep-seated social inequalities, has been subjected to a succession of half-baked market-style "reforms" and a patchwork process of privatisation that has served to demoralise some of the more progressive and committed professionals while opening the door for some of the most individualistic and self-seeking GPs to pile up personal profits and wealth.

The underlying contradiction in government policy is that a fragmented, competitive and partly privatised primary care system will undermine any of the government's continuing attempts to reduce hospitalisation and speed the discharge of patients after treatment. Once again the left hand appears oblivious to what the right hand is doing – while Lord Darzi mounts a sideshow, trotting out a succession of interesting ideas with little or no actual purchase on reality.

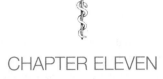

CHAPTER ELEVEN

The NHS in an international context

MANY ENTHUSIASTS FOR THE NATIONAL HEALTH SERVICE see it as a distinctively British phenomenon, flowing from British culture and institutions and the politics of British rather than European social democracy; but this is something of an illusion. Of course, some of the political factors which made the establishment of the British NHS possible in 1948 were national in origin, and therefore specific to time and place. But Britain was by no means the only country looking for solutions to the same social problems in the post-war period. Governments were looking to placate and incorporate potentially militant working class organisations, and to gather some authority and acceptance of the post-war settlement. It is perhaps more accurate to see the NHS as one part of a much wider international awakening of political leaders to the need for some form of collective provision of health care, one which brought almost simultaneous developments towards health services and health care systems in many other countries, both in Europe and around the world.

In the pre-history of scientific medicine and modern-day health services, religious orders had for centuries provided primitive forms of care. They developed "hospitals" as shelters for the needy which, from the sixteenth century, increasingly became seen as places to care for sick people. Cities on the continent of Europe tended to have larger public hospitals than Britain. The sixteenth century onwards saw many countries (including England) develop various forms of "poor law" provision to give some form of support to the destitute. By the eighteenth century, Sweden had already established a system of salaried district physicians (Freeman 2000).

During the second half of the nineteenth century a number of countries could be seen to make more advanced moves towards collective health-care provision than Britain. In Sweden, county councils were responsible for hospital care from 1864, while in Italy communes were obliged to provide medical care for the poor from 1865 (Freeman 2000).

Britain was by no means the first European country to move towards social insurance for health care, nor was the pace set initially by left-leaning political parties. It was Russia's Czar Alexander II who led the process, when in 1864 he established public medical care for the poor, to be administered by local district assemblies (zemstvo). Twenty-five years later, one in six Russian doctors were employed in the zemstvo system, and in 1913 there were over 4,300 rural medical stations, providing 49,000 hospital beds, delivering free health care by salaried health professionals[23] (Tragakes and Lessof 2003). Bulgaria established state-funded free hospital care for the poor after the fall of the Ottoman Empire in 1879, and later carried a law on public health care in 1903 (Hinkov et al. 2005).

The next system offering health benefits to a section of the workforce came in Germany in 1883, as Chancellor Bismarck's authoritarian regime attempted to bind sections of the most skilled workers to the newly unified state, and blunt the appeal of the rapidly strengthening trade unions and the social democratic party. Italy and Austria also followed soon afterwards (1886, 1888), followed then by Sweden (1891), Denmark (1892), Belgium (1894) and France (1898). The UK, Ireland and Switzerland adopted similar proposals only in 1911 (Pierson 1998).

The period between the wars is summed up by Pierson (1998) as one of "consolidation and development" of welfare states including health care, and Freeman (2000) notes extensions in insurance coverage in France, Italy and Sweden in this period. In 1938, New Zealand became the first to introduce comprehensive welfare-state provision, including medical and hospital care and health promotion. One exception to the rule was the USA, which in the 1930s also saw a substantial growth in social insurance; but the welfare provision that developed there was above all dominated by the issues of unemployment and pensions rather than health care.

While the US trade unions and both major US political parties took a strongly anti-communist line, and tended to regard any proposals for "socialized medicine" or even "single-payer insurance" as "Bolshevism", the USSR from 1918 had rapidly built and consolidated its own "Semashko" system of health care. This was centrally funded and controlled, provided free medical services for everyone, and was able to implement drastic epidemic control measures to tackle what had been rampant outbreaks of tuberculosis, typhoid fever, typhus, malaria and cholera. It also made huge inroads into controlling and preventing these infectious diseases by adopting community prevention approaches, routine check-ups, improvements in urban sanitation and hygiene, and quarantine of those infected. Nikolai Semashko's system centred on the principles of: government responsibility for health; universal access to free services; a preventive approach to "social diseases"; quality professional care; a close relation between science and medical practice; and continuity of care between health promotion, treatment and rehabilitation. From 1928 onwards, the Ministry of Health established a network of polyclinics to provide health services for industrial workers and farmers. However, only in 1937 were the Bismarck-style social insurance funds established in 1912 finally abolished, with hospitals, pharmacies and other health facilities nationalized and brought under district

---

23 However, it should be noted that this offered just one doctor per 6,900 people, and 1.3 hospital beds per 1,000 population – with few of these available in the rural areas (Tragakes and Lessof 2003).

health management (Tragakes and Lessof 2003: 23).

As a result, these were a relatively recent memory by the time Bevan proposed his nationalisation eleven years later: but by then there were also political developments in Eastern Europe which might have appeared to underline the notion of a 'socialist' model. The period following the Second World War is frequently depicted as "The Golden Age of the Welfare State" (Pierson 1998), drawing together a variety of developments in broadly the same time frame, some of which developed under very different political dynamics. Pierson argues that views of the post-war development of welfare states are substantially moulded by readings of the British experience which appear to exaggerate the pace, scale and novelty of the measures introduced:

> Great emphasis is placed upon the consequences of the Second World War... the 'messianic' quality of Beveridge and his proposed reforms... and the subsequent development of a broad cross-party consensus "Butskellism" in favour of compromise of the interests of capital and labour, within which the welfare state was a crucial component.
>
> (Pierson 1998: 122)

Pierson goes on to question each of these suppositions, pointing out that far from all of the experiences of government intervention had been positive during the war; that Beveridge could more accurately be seen as a codifier and consolidator of existing systems than an innovative architect of a new social order; and that the "consensus" – such as it was – centred on a very limited commitment to welfare state provision which left British social spending lagging well behind most other developed economies for the next 40 years. This was certainly true of health spending, which has only moved substantially upwards towards the European average in the period since 2000 (OECD figures). However, it is clear that the moves to establish the NHS in Britain came at a point of growing interest and commitment to such policies around the world. This moment also coincided with a historic defeat for the parties and politics of the far right, and a growth in prestige and influence for both the Soviet Union – that had carried the brunt of the military effort in defeating the Nazi war machine – and the Communist and social democratic parties across Europe.

In many cases countries were responding to the end of occupation or the fall of a fascist dictatorship. In 1943, as Mussolini fell from power, Italy consolidated a number of company insurance funds into a single health insurance fund (Donatini et al. 2001). Belgium adopted a new Social Security Act in December 1944 which advocated universal access to social security and made all social insurance funds, including unemployment, health and disability insurance, compulsory for all salaried employees, and created a central institution to collect the contributions and the National Fund for Sickness and Disability to manage health insurance (Corens 2007).

France, freshly liberated from German occupation, saw a reform and generalisation of national health insurance in 1945. The authors of this reform had been "inspired by the Beveridge Report" (Sandier et al. 2004: 8) but were unable to extend the scheme to cover farmers and the self-employed until the 1960s, with additional sections of the population included in various further measures. In 1947, the government of the Netherlands legislated to extend health insurance cover to pensioners who had previously had none (den Exter et al. 2004), and Austria consolidated and extended its social insurance for health care which already covered two-thirds of the population (Hofmarcher and Rack 2006).

Also in 1945, Australia introduced social insurance for health care (Pierson 1998). Sweden's National Health Insurance Act was passed in 1946, the same year as Britain's National Health Service Act (Freeman 2000). The late 1940s and early 1950s saw moves towards publicly funded health coverage in Canada, led by a number of provinces: this led to a 35-year process of development towards the landmark 1984 legislation (the Canada Health Act) that established the principles of today's universal, tax-funded Medicare system.

Buying time: the right wing and health insurance

However, the establishment and maintenance of health insurance appears to span normal political divides. In Spain, where General Franco's fascist dictatorship remained in place at the end of the Second World War after the defeat of Hitler and Mussolini, the regime had also retained the previous system of social health insurance established under the republic, and run through the social security system. This left the public sector in control of upwards of 70 per cent of hospital beds and facilities, employing 70 to 80 per cent of doctors and commanding 75 per cent or more of the available health budget (Duran et al. 2006).

In Portugal, the Salazar dictatorship carried legislation in 1946 to establish a Bismarck-style health insurance scheme for workers and their dependents, delivering services free at point of use. Subsequent changes in the law brought in wider groups in addition to the industrial workers (Barros and Simões 2007). Japan, which sided with the Axis powers in the Second World War, has had a Bismarck-style system of health insurance since the 1920s. This currently retains no fewer than 5,000 separate insurance funds, most of which buy services from private non-profit providers which account for 80 per cent of hospital provision – although investor-owned hospitals are prohibited, and private health insurance is marginal (Imai 2002).

Stalinist regimes and health care

Much of Central and Eastern Europe after 1945 had fallen under the military and political control of the Soviet Union or the Socialist Federal Republic of Yugoslavia, headed by Marshal Tito. Most of these countries had operated some form of the Bismarck-style system that had been widespread in the Austro-Hungarian Empire (though often covering only a small minority of the population), and these in turn were then shaped by the new regime.

In Hungary, for example, the post-war "communist" regime nationalised the insurance funds and the hospitals in 1948, as part of a wider nationalisation of the economy at large. Private health enterprises, such as insurance companies and private general practices, were dismantled. Instead, centralized state services were set up in their place to deliver a free and universal health care service. Public health measures and action against infectious diseases, including immunization, did produce positive results, as they had in the Soviet Union. The 1949 Constitution declared health to be a fundamental right, and as a result the Ministry of Health funded and delivered health services including hospitals, polyclinics and district doctor services (Gaál 2004). Similar changes were also imposed on Czechoslovakia in 1948 and 1952 (Rokosová and Háva 2005). In Bulgaria, 1948 was also the year in which the country was switched to a Semashko-style health care system, which nationalised hospitals and pharmacies and replaced the family doctor system with polyclinics (Hinkov 2005).

In Poland, the equivalent changes came earlier (1945). They were distinctive in the Eastern bloc in that not all private practice was abolished, and that there were subsequent moves to decentralise control (Kuszewski and Gericke 2005).

In Romania, a Bismarck-style system that had covered just five per cent of the population between the wars was replaced in 1949 with a Semashko system, giving universal coverage and free access to services. The system centred on:

> government financing, central planning, rigid management and a state monopoly over health services. Also notable were the absence of a private sector (as the private system was abolished) and the fact that all professionals in the health system had the status of salaried civil servants.
>
> (Vladescu et al. 2000: 5)

In 1949 came the Chinese Revolution, and with it, in the early days of the new regime, a turn towards Soviet-style health care provision. There was a fivefold expansion of urban hospitals, a dramatic expansion of numbers of doctors and pharmacists trained by medical schools, and an extension of health care facilities into major industries and government departments, again mostly located in the cities[24] (Bloom and Tang 2004).

The Stalinist regimes of Eastern Europe could be seen to have carried through the nationalisation of health care partly as a means to achieve a degree of legitimacy and public support from an otherwise sceptical and still politically repressed working class; and also partly as a way to eliminate another focus of power and wealth for private capital, and thus strengthen their initially unstable position as bureaucratic rulers over a newly nationalised economy, buttressed by Soviet military power.

---

24 Although these policies delivered remarkable improvements in the health of urban populations and the working class, they did little to remedy the health problems faced by the rural peasant population. In 1965, Chairman Mao explicitly criticised the unequal allocation of services and triggered the programme that led to the training of "barefoot doctors" and the combination of public health measures and medical intervention that had positive impact in the countryside, but which serviced to undermine some of the systems that had worked well in the cities (Bloom and Tang 2004).

Exceptions and late developers

There was a seemingly worldwide confluence of ideas in the post-war period towards a common conception of increasingly universal health services in such widely divergent political settings. This suggests that it reflects a generalised response to a commonly perceived problem or pressure. Indeed, it would appear that no political regime which has the means to do so, and which wishes to remain in control for any length of time, can avoid maintaining or establishing some form of social provision to fill in crucial gaps left by the unfettered capitalist "market" in health care.

Perhaps here it is the rare exceptions that prove the rule. The USA, for example, is today unique among the wealthier countries in still having failed to establish any form of social insurance system that could support the 45–50 million low-income Americans with no health cover. It has been argued that this is down to the relative weakness of the trade unions or "labour movement" in the US, and to the resulting lack of any significant social democratic party in recent years (Navarro 1983, 1992). Yet this ignores the political orientation of the leadership of the trade unions: for considerable periods since the First World War, they have been in a very strong position to secure concessions and reforms, but have explicitly taken sides *against* the establishment of any form of "single-payer" or universal system of health insurance.

It also ignores the very significant economic concessions that were made to the trade unions to head off what appeared to be a rising tide of militancy in the immediate post-war period, including a massive strike wave in 1946. The big corporations had been able to maintain undisrupted and highly profitable production throughout the war, and thus had a position of global dominance in the post-war years. They were consequently in a strong position to buy off the unions with generous pay increases – including a remarkable 'escalator clause' in some agreements which provided long-term protection against inflation (the first of these signed by General Motors with the United Auto Workers in 1948). There were even packages including health insurance which were sufficient to win acceptance from union leaders and their members. These had the potential to become a basis on which union members could later be persuaded to oppose the more generalised provision of health insurance under a "single-payer" system.

The history of the US is one of a succession of missed moments and collapsing coalitions that might have offered the possibilities of advancing to a cheaper, more effective and more inclusive system: however, each missed moment has seen the "medical industrial complex" gain in wealth and political influence. The current system delivers extravagant profits to shareholders and enormous salaries to well-placed executives and specialist doctors – all of whom have a vested interest in keeping the system the way it has developed.

Indeed, the current set-up works to the detriment of sections of manufacturing employers. Despite this, their tacit (even occasionally explicit) support for some form of single-payer system to escape the rising costs of health coverage for their staff and retirees is insufficient to force a change. General Motors, for example, is now the largest single purchaser of health care in the USA, spending more on health insurance packages for current and retired members of staff than it spends on steel to make its vehicles (Lister 2005a). But the health care industry itself has outstripped almost every other industry and now amounts to more than a seventh of the US economy, consuming over 16 per cent of GDP. It is clearly better placed to influence Congress and key decision-makers than the diminished manufacturing industry.

Marmor and other commentators (Ranade 1998) have in recent years raised doubts over the possibility of piecing together a sufficiently powerful coalition to turn the tide against such well-entrenched opposition when so many influential people and such major corporations are making so much money from the system the way it is. There are political, ideological and economic factors which underpin the eccentric status of the US on health care. In other words, it has not always been within the grasp of the US administration of the day to impose a change.

Other countries that have lagged behind the general movement towards some form of collective, social protection against prohibitive costs for health care can also point to objective, material obstacles in the way of progressive reform. Many countries have been in this situation because they were denied democratic rule; and many African, Asian and Latin American countries have also remained very much subordinate to the dominant northern financial centres, or even directly under colonial rule beyond 1945, only achieving the political space for progressive health reform much later on.

Developing countries and new industrial powers such as South Korea and Brazil also demonstrate that the implementation of social health insurance is by no means the exclusive prerogative of political regimes and parties of the left. South Korea emerged as a regime strongly influenced by the USA from a devastating civil war which in 1953 left the country in ruins. It was not until 1963 that a system of voluntary medical insurance was established, and the transition from voluntary health insurance to a Bismarck-style workplace insurance system began under the authoritarian President Park Chung-Hee in 1977, breaking from the US model to embrace a system much closer to that in Japan: within 12 years, government-mandated universal coverage had been established (Matthews and Jung 2006; Lee 2003).

Brazil

Brazil's brutally authoritarian military government, installed with CIA support in the 1960s, attempted in the 1970s to secure a degree of legitimacy in the wider population by extending social security coverage to workers previously excluded, and by offering a new entitlement to emergency health care to the whole population, regardless of social security status. The Institute of Medical Care and Social Security (INAMPS) contracted with the private sector to buy in the expanded volume of services required: by 1976, 73 per cent of all hospital beds were in the private sector. The government further encouraged this development by offering subsidies for the building of new hospitals, with guarantees of future contracts to provide care. Existing private hospitals were encouraged to provide services to INAMPS on a fee-for-service basis, which resulted in widespread fraud. Companies were also offered generous subsidies if they took responsibility for the health care of employees (Lobato and Burlandy 2000).

As the power of Brazil's military government began to unravel in the 1980s, a powerful lobby group, the Health Movement – including Communists inspired by the health reforms being carried out by their comrades in Italy in the 1970s – began to press for a democratisation and decentralisation of health care, funded and provided by the state – clashing as they did so with the power of the medical profession and the private-sector providers.

In the event, the campaigners won most of their demands. The centralised power of INAMPS was abolished, and in the early 1990s responsibility for planning and providing health care was decentralised to states and municipalities, enabling a number of progressive reforms. These included the introduction of family doctors and investment in primary care and health centres (Lobato and Burlandy 2000: 8–14).

Serious problems remain, not least in the fight for sufficient resources to run local services, and in the fee-for-service model for agreements, which gives providers the incentive to provide (or bill for) maximum services rather than support prevention and health promotion measures (Lobato and Burlandy 2000: 16). There is a serious shortage of nurses, the overall funding level is inadequate, and there are conflicts of interest between public and private sectors and between some sections of health professionals.

However, unlike many others, the Brazilian reforms appear to have delivered a more accessible and democratic structure, and positive rights to the population, sections of which had previously been cynically appeased and annexed by populist and authoritarian governments.

South Africa

South Africa is the most prosperous of the sub-Saharan Africa countries, classified by the World Bank as an "upper middle income" country, with a GNP of $113 billion in 2001 and a population of 43 million. However, more than half the population can be classified as poor, in many cases still reflecting the stark racial inequalities inherited from the apartheid regime, with poverty concentrated among black people and the rural areas (McIntyre et al. 1998).

Despite high comparative and absolute levels of health spending in South Africa,[25] life expectancy fell from 62 to just 48 years during the 1990s. This was largely a result of the raging HIV/AIDS epidemic, which had infected almost 5

---

25 Equivalent to around half the entire health budget for all the sub-Saharan Africa countries (Lister 2005a).

million adults by 2005 (almost 20 per cent of the adult population): 84,000 infants were born with HIV in 2001 (World Bank HNPstats[26] 2003).

Apartheid South Africa's health policies were regressive in every way, with more than 75 per cent of public health spending allocated to hospitals, most of which are in urban areas. Academic and specialist hospitals took 44 per cent. Just 11 per cent was allocated to primary care. A burgeoning private sector employed the majority of health staff, and controlled 61 per cent of the country's health spending.

The allocation of hospital beds and every other aspect of health care resourcing was consistently focused on the richest districts (and therefore the white minority of the population) which enjoyed almost double the allocation of hospital beds, almost seven times as many doctors, double the number of nurses and nearly four times the health budget per head compared with the poorest (Gilson et al. 1999).

However, the political and economic policies of the ANC in government have also meant that the much-promised National Health Bill (NHB), which first appeared as a draft in 1995, only passed through Parliament in 2004. It was held up by years of debate and delay, and then spent time awaiting the Presidential signature that would make it law.

The ANC has established itself as a keen proponent of public–private partnerships, and the Bill itself stresses from the very outset its objective of "establishing a national health system which encompasses the public and private providers of health services" (Pillay Y 2004). Indeed the NHB does not, as its name might suggest, focus on funding a health care system to allow the elimination of user fees, but on seeking to regulate the private sector and establish a more equitable allocation of resources and more decentralised structure – while retaining full powers at government level in the hands of the minister. Its supporters argue that the Bill does represent a real step forward for some of South Africa's most vulnerable people (Pillay K 2002).

The Bill seeks to ensure that all South Africans have access to a package of free primary health care – although even where such services are provided free of charge, many people face physical and financial problems travelling to and accessing them (Connolly 2002). There is no specific health insurance system for the whole population, although South Africa's main trade union confederation COSATU, in its initial response to the Bill, strongly urged that further measures should be brought forward to establish a system of National Health Insurance, to ensure universal access to comprehensive health care, and allow all health services to be incorporated into the public sector (COSATU 2002).

The health minister has been quoted describing the public sector provision as "in a shambles". Chronic shortages of resources in the more isolated rural areas

---

26 World Bank Health Nutrition and Population statistics can be accessed at
    http://go.worldbank.org/N2N84RDV00

have contributed to an exodus of doctors, dentists and other trained professionals – to the cities, to the private sector, or often overseas to work in developed countries for higher salaries – creating an atmosphere of growing crisis in public sector health care (Cullinan 2003).

Other African countries

We have a good idea what many countries of sub-Saharan Africa would have aspired to in the way of health services, since a number of them took the opportunity immediately after achieving independence to establish publicly funded health care, free at point of use, and supported by substantial economic expansion in the 1960s and early 1970s. Most of these – such as Kenya, Uganda and Zimbabwe – registered substantial gains in life expectancy and reductions in child mortality[27] (Colgan 2002; Gatheru and Shaw 1998).

Kenya is an especially clear example: in the period immediately after independence in 1964, its economy grew rapidly – averaging just over six per cent a year for the first decade, a rate exceeding Malaysia and Indonesia. The government began to implement its promise to develop a health care system offering free basic treatment, introducing free outpatient care in 1965. With these measures in place, Kenya achieved reductions of almost 50 per cent in mortality among the under-fives in the years to 1993. Life expectancy increased from 40 to 60 years. Rural health centres were set up, and there was an expansion of the renamed Kenyatta National Hospital which began to train more Kenyan doctors (Colgan 2002; Gatheru and Shaw 1998).

But during the 1970s, the emerging system was swamped by the demands of a rising population while the economic growth faltered, stretching resources. Bed numbers have grown more than fourfold since 1963, but have not kept pace with the rapid growth of the population. The service was never able to grow on sufficient scale to confront the major endemic threats to health. Diseases like malaria, respiratory tract disease, skin diseases, diarrhoea, and intestinal worms could all be tackled through improved primary care, preventive health policies, clean water supplies and enhanced nutrition (Gatheru and Shaw 1998).

The 1980s brought the end of economic growth and, with it, pressure from the IMF and World Bank to implement "structural adjustment" programmes, including cuts in public spending (Amrith 2001). Government health spending fell sharply in the 1990s, from $10 per capita in 1990 to just $2.90 in 2000 (Heaton 2001; Achieng 2001). User fees were imposed for health services at World Bank insistence from 1989, and this triggered a sharp reduction in numbers accessing key services: there was an especially sharp reduction in coverage for immunization, falling from 79 per cent in 1993 to just 65 per cent in 1998 (Kimalu 2001: 11).

---

27 The same was also true for post-1979 Nicaragua until the Sandinista government was destabilised by a protracted US-backed terror campaign and ousted (Birn et al. 2000).

India

India missed out on the post-war drive towards socialised systems of health care, being embroiled in the late 1940s with the pressures towards independence from British rule, the partition with Pakistan and the subsequent massive social upheavals. It remains a prime example of the failure of a largely privatised health care system.

Sixty years later, the world's second most populous country still has chronic low levels of government health spending, static for several years at around one per cent of GDP – well below the WHO's recommended minimum of five per cent. About 80 per cent of this spending is absorbed by the private sector, while 75 per cent is paid directly by households, and only 10 per cent of Indians have some form of health insurance.

User fees apply even for poor people treated in public hospitals, with upwards of 15 per cent of those hospitalised falling into poverty as a result of the costs incurred:

> Hospitalised Indians spent 58% of their total annual expenditures on health care. More than 40% of hospitalised people borrow money or sell assets to cover expenses.
>
> (Peters et al. 2002: 5)

Spending is also highly unequal, with the wealthiest 20 per cent receiving three times more government health spending than the poorest – though the pattern varies in different states (Peters et al. 2002).

The central government, with a Central Ministry of Health employing no fewer than 30,000 administrators, exerts direct and heavy-handed control over its network of under-funded and pressurised public hospitals – but little if any regulatory control over private sector providers, many of which are not formally registered.

Curative services in the rural areas have been largely left to the private sector, which as World Bank-commissioned research has concluded, is at best of uneven quality (Naylor et al. 1999; Peters et al. 2002). The neglect of rural services is also reflected in the lack of hospital provision: in 1991 just 32 per cent of hospitals and 20 per cent of beds were in the rural areas where 70 per cent of the population lives – giving just one-twelfth of the beds per head available in urban areas (Nandraj 1997).

Overt and covert government subsidies for the private sector include the training of at least 15,000 doctors every year, two-thirds of whom go to work in the private sector. Public hospitals also offer a "safety net" for under-insured Indians who cannot obtain private treatment, while the public sector also handles almost all treatment of the poorest citizens, allowing the private hospitals to 'cream-skim' those best able to pay.

Most accident victims and more serious cases are also passed on to public hospitals from the private sector: a survey in Karnatka found that just three per cent of small private hospitals had a blood bank (Naylor et al. 1999). Many of the generic problems of private medical provision are exhibited in the context of the unregulated Indian system: perverse incentives for private practitioners to give superfluous, costly "tests" and treatment, widely fluctuating levels of fees; payments flowing back to referring doctors when patients are sent for specialist treatment; and private hospitals refusing treatment without a cash payment in advance (Nandraj 1997). Small wonder a household survey in 2002 found that health care is seen as the most corrupt service in India (Kumar 2004).

Nandraj (1997) blames the lack of government investment in health care on Structural Adjustment Programmes promoted by the World Bank and IMF, and in particular India's New Economic Policy. However, it is also clear that some of the chronic lack of public sector infrastructure, the bureaucratism in the public sector and the unequal distribution of health care services have been inherited from the worst aspects of the British Raj.

CHAPTER TWELVE

Into a seventh decade: what have we got left? Alternatives and conclusions

As EARLIER CHAPTERS HAVE SHOWN, the NHS has been more "reformed" and restructured in the last seven years than in the previous 53. But this must not distract us from the progress that has been made since 1948, most of it as a result of the new possibilities that were opened up by the launch of Bevan's NHS – the national system that has developed for training doctors, nurses and professionals, the linking up of hospitals into a modern system to deliver a comprehensive range of services, and the efforts that have been made to facilitate more equal access to health care for groups who have historically been failed by market-based systems.

The NHS at 60 has 1.3 million staff, including a significant increase since 2000 in numbers of nurses, hospital doctors, GPs, health professionals, and many more skilled clinical and non-clinical support staff whose effort and dedication make the system tick. The NHS has established a national network of hospitals, health centres, clinics and community-based services, with resources allocated on the basis of maximising accessibility and meeting health needs, not on targeting the wealthy and maximising profit. NHS primary care services – involving GPs, community, district and practice nurses and midwives, health visitors, occupational, speech and physiotherapists – have improved and provide tens of millions of consultations and treatment, free of charge. For non-emergency health issues, primary care is the principal gateway for referral to specialist hospital treatment.

But there are more important strengths. The NHS is the only source of 24-hour emergency services – ambulances and A&E departments – offering a comprehensive mix of care including specialist services that the private sector does not even pretend to provide. In 2005–6, almost 18 million people attended A&E units in England. In 2006–7, NHS hospitals admitted over 4.7 million people as emergencies for hospital treatment; no such treatment is available from the private sector. Waiting times in A&E have been reduced: ambulance services have begun to improve.

Overall, NHS hospitals in England delivered 14.8 million episodes of treatment in 2006–7, 4.4 million of which were day cases, and 5.27 million (36%) of the hospital treatment was for older people (aged over 65).

In 2006–7, 7.8 million NHS patients had surgery in England. Against this, the few tens of thousands treated – at inflated expense – in independent sector treatment centres can be seen as a statistical irrelevance to the overall capacity of the system. The expansion of the NHS in the last ten years has also been dramatic. In 2006–7, the NHS delivered 289,500 cataract operations – a 44% increase on its performance in 1998–9. Numbers of heart operations have more than doubled in the same period, from 41,000 to over 81,000, with the main expansion being in the use of angioplasty by balloon or laser to free up blocked arteries. The NHS is performing 31% more hip operations now than in 1998–9, and 36% more kidney transplants; 22% more people are being diagnosed with cancer, and 18% more with ischaemic heart disease.

Another service not available from private sector health insurance or private hospitals is maternity. In 2005–6, hospitals and NHS midwife-led units gave expert help in 593,400 deliveries in England, up 1.6% on 2004–5. A further 15,900 took place at home (2.6% of all NHS deliveries) compared to 13,700 (2.3%) in 2004–5. NHS hospitals also lead the field in the care of premature and new-born babies and in specialist care for children.

Swifter access to life-saving treatment for cancer and heart problems has helped deliver improved results in the form of falling death rates; 99.9% of people with suspected cancer are now seen by a specialist within two weeks of being referred by their GP, compared with 63% in 1997. Over 99% of people with suspected cancer now receive their first treatment within a maximum of 31 days of diagnosis. An estimated 60,000 lives have been saved from cancer and 175,000 from coronary heart disease since 1997. All of these key services are delivered by the NHS.

The NHS has also trained and educated nurses and midwives, health professionals and therapists, and doctors – with large NHS district general and teaching hospitals offering the basis for the development of specialist skills, and a career structure for nurses and medical staff. Private sector hospitals do not train medical staff, but recruit from the pool of NHS-trained doctors and nurses, or poach skilled staff from overseas. Because they accept only the most minor and least complex cases, private hospitals don't offer a broad enough caseload to allow them to train specialists, or conduct research.

The last 60 years have also seen very important improvements in the treatment even of those patients often seen to be on the margins of the NHS – the elderly, and people with mental illness. Old, poorly resourced workhouse-style wards for the elderly have increasingly been superseded, and community-based services have shown a glimpse of the possibilities if adequate resources are made available and the gulf between health and social care can be bridged. Mental health services, too, are predominantly provided by the NHS, but again significant strides have been taken to break down the model of institutionalised care, and develop new and creative methods of treatment and support for service users in smaller units and in the community. Again, the glimpses of what should be possible highlight the unresolved problem of securing adequate resources for mental health against the shroud-waving pressures of the media-friendly acute hospital sector. Some of the services that have been hit first in recent cash saving measures have been among the most innovative and progressive in the possibilities they offer for service users.

As in mental health, the NHS and public sector have also led virtually all of the ground-breaking research into new techniques, new anaesthetics, drugs and surgical methods in the UK. It was the NHS which pioneered the notion of separating emergency care from non-emergencies and streaming the less complex routine operations through dedicated treatment centres – an area of care subsequently hijacked by private sector providers and now increasingly monopolised by profit-seeking multinational corporations.

NHS district and teaching hospitals are all much larger and offer a much more comprehensive range of services than the generally small-scale network of private hospitals which average just 40 beds each, and concentrate only on the least complex and most profitable types of treatment. Unlike private hospitals, NHS hospitals are staffed 24-hours a day by consultants and doctors as well as specialist nurses and experienced support staff. Furthermore, NHS hospitals maintain a network of almost 3,500 critical care beds – high dependency and intensive care – for patients suffering potentially life-threatening conditions. That's why when private hospitals face any emergency situation in which an operation goes wrong, or a patient faces complications... they rush them to the nearest NHS hospital.

It is important to keep hold of these very strong pluses in the development of the NHS as a basis for any serious critique of the inroads of market-style "reforms" and the private sector. There is still plenty worth defending in the NHS, and still large areas of NHS services which the private sector has no intention of taking over. That's why the Keep Our NHS Public campaign that took shape over the summer of 2005, and has consistently monitored the impact of New Labour reforms and offered support to local campaigns, was not a pious gesture or a desperate attempt to resist progressive change. It recognised that the public sector, public service core of the NHS has been vital to its development and remains vital to its future.

Why the market reforms matter

Opposition to the Blair and Brown government reforms has had to be carefully targeted – welcoming the overall increase that has taken place in NHS spending and resources, while deeply critical of the market-style changes and the growing involvement of the private sector, which costs more and delivers less than an expansion of the NHS to deliver the same services. Campaigners are in favour of new hospitals – but opposed to the inflated costs of PFI, and the consequent squeeze on bed numbers, pressure on Trust budgets, and the raiding of resources for mental health, services for the elderly, community and primary care to pay for new buildings which serve as a guaranteed profit stream for private-sector shareholders.

The fundamental problem is that New Labour's reforms have begun to fragment what once was a centralised national service with a degree of local control, and which attempted to address health inequalities and match resources to health needs. Instead, increasingly, we have the rules of the market, which have brought a range of conundrums and contradictions, among which:

- Foundation Trusts now sit on £1 billion of surpluses drawn from their local health economies, but are now accountable only to an independent regulator, who will monitor them as businesses, but has no responsibility to ensure generalised access to health services

- NHS budgets have been opened up through Payment by Results to fund high-cost and inflexible contracts for private sector treatment and diagnostics for low-risk patients, leaving correspondingly reduced resources available to deal with the most complex and chronic cases

- NHS Trusts have now been excluded from all of the decision-making processes, but are required to meet stiff targets and balance their books each year with virtually no guaranteed basic level of income as a result of Payment by Results

- Trusts with new PFI-funded hospitals face all of these pressures, plus the inflated overhead costs of unitary charge payments for 30 or more years to come, including early deals which would never have been signed under 2006 Department of Health rules limiting the share of Trust revenue to 12.5%

- Specialist services and specialist Trusts face a tariff payment system that understates the costs of their services and therefore puts them at risk

- PCTs remain under pressure to divest themselves of directly provided services… and to bring in high-cost management consultants from a list of 14 major private sector corporations to help them spend a total of £75 billion in commissioning budgets

- GPs, seeking to respond to patient choice by referring them for treatment to a specific hospital find referral management teams intervening to alter their proposals and override any choices that may have been made.

In addition to these new problems arising from New Labour's market-style "reforms", the ongoing problems arising from the effective privatisation of long-term care of the elderly, the loss of NHS specialist capacity for long-term care and the continued yawning gulf between health and social care budgets have run alongside tightened eligibility criteria in cash-strapped social services departments, making the quest for a seamless service into mission impossible.

While these flaws have undermined the possibility for the NHS and its local organisations to plan services and allocate resources according to social and health needs, the constant churn of reorganisation has also taken its toll – in the demoralisation of staff, the disorientation of management and the squandering of resources. To make matters worse, it is increasingly obvious to NHS staff, to some journalists, and to a confused and unconvinced general public, that the reorganisations are taking the NHS around in circles.

In 1997 the Tories lost power having reorganised the NHS in England to consist of 100 District Health Authorities, 3,500 fundholding GPs and eight regional offices on the purchasing side, and NHS Trusts as providers.

In 1998 New Labour slimmed down the fundholders to 480 Primary Care Groups, working alongside the health authorities. In 2002 these were slimmed down to 303 Primary Care Trusts; then the health authorities were abolished; and in 2006 the number of PCTs was cut back again to 152.

But GPs, reorganised into PCTs in 1998, dispersed in the establishment of PCTs in 2002, have been urged since 2006 to take on practice-based commissioning, which could push the numbers of distinct groups well above the 3,500 fundholders.

At regional level, the eight regional offices were replaced by 28 Strategic Health Authorities in 2002, only for the number to be slimmed back down to ten in 2006, covering essentially the same areas as the regional offices (Halligan 2007).

The chaos on patient representation is possibly even worse. Well-established Community Health Councils were eventually dissolved in 2003, to be replaced by a complex and confusing mess involving Patient and Public Involvement Forums, Trust-level Patient Advocacy Liaison Services and council Oversight and Scrutiny Committees. Now the PPIFs are to be abolished in April 2008, and replaced by even more toothless and pointless Local Involvement Networks. The one consistent message is that however much they may talk about patient choice, ministers do not want a well-entrenched, knowledgeable and forceful voice for patients because they are too likely to disagree with the enforced "reconfiguration" of hospital care and to ask awkward questions about resources for promised alternatives.

None of these reforms appears to have made any positive contribution to the task of improving and expanding the NHS to meet the challenges of the 21st century; but nearly all of them carry a fearful cost. With the exception of scrapping the wasteful and divisive system of GP fundholding (which is now making a reappearance in the guise of practice-based commissioning), most of the reorganisations, coupled with the complex and costly system of Payment by Results, and the use of private-sector providers, have served to force up costs and increase the numbers of senior managers and administrative staff required.

Then add the constantly rising and still not finalised £12 billion costs of the computerisation required for Blair's "choose and book" system and for the Electronic Patient Record – which in the light of a succession of catastrophic losses of sensitive data by government departments, may never lift off as a completed national scheme (Brooks 2007).

An international market?

The extent of marketisation that has already taken place within the NHS also has the danger that it could lead to further inroads as a result of pressure through the World Trade Organisation or the European Union. The WTO, of which Britain is a member, has for many years been trying to open up markets in the highly lucrative health care market, estimated to be worth a global total of $3.5 trillion per year, around half of that underwritten by public funds or social insurance systems in the wealthiest countries. The WTO objective is to pressurise governments to allow private providers from anywhere in the world to bid to provide any public services they wish to, including health services: the larger the share of the NHS budget that is spent with private providers, the stronger the case US and other expansionist multinationals may have to force other work to be put out to tender.

A powerful lobby, inside the EU, which instigated the abortive Bolkestein directive, is pushing in the same direction. Interestingly, the final few days of 2007 saw an unlikely coalition of New Labour ministers with leaders of European Public Sector Unions, Europe's hospital managers, the governments of Germany and Spain, and the European Parliament's socialist group – to oppose a new directive which was due to be issued on cross-border health care (EPSU 2007). In the event, the promised European Commission directive was abruptly withdrawn at the last minute on 19 December. The new directive would not only open up the possibility of patients who could afford to pay up front seeking treatment in another EU country and sending the bill back to their own health service, it would also permit companies to provide health services from one member state to another, or to set up a health service in another member state, and also covers the right of health professionals to move between EU member states with minimal regulation.

Critics of the new proposal argue that it is transparently designed to benefit private health care providers rather than help patients, and that it raises all kinds of issues in relation to quality control, safety monitoring and adherence to standards of training and qualifications. The requirement for patients to pay for their own treatment before reclaiming the money would exclude poor people with severe health needs accessing care, but allow the wealthy to jump queues or opt for treatment elsewhere in the EU. Opinion polls show only a tiny minority of EU citizens want the right to seek treatment abroad: most prefer to get treatment close to home (EPSU 2007).

New Labour ministers who have invested such faith in market-style changes within the NHS appear to fear a wider EU market in health services, and are understood to oppose the scheme because it would mean local health commissioners would effectively lose control of budgets, although it is clear that with waiting lists and waiting times much reduced the level of interest is marginal.

There was a flurry of activity back in 2001, when the government bowed to the European court and announced that patients facing 'undue delay' [undefined] could, with the agreement of local health authorities, seek treatment abroad. Some were even sent from south coast Primary Care Trusts for treatment in French and German hospitals. But at the high point of interest figures show only 1,000 people took advantage; last year, the figure stood at just over 350.

However, last year Bedford pensioner Yvonne Watts won her long-running appeal for reimbursement of £3,900 she had paid in 2003 to get a hip operation in France two months earlier than she would have done under the NHS. Her case seems to have been a catalyst for the latest EU plan. But some patients from overseas are coming to Britain to seek operations from the NHS. Last year, an estimated 750 patients from EU countries came to the UK for non-emergency treatment, paid for by their own home country, many of them for specialist care, such as liver transplants.

What is clear is that these transactions are once more restoring the cash nexus and tending to recommodify health, with some private-sector providers in Eastern Europe looking to compete on price and speed of treatment with other health services.[28] The creation of an enlarged market in health care spanning the whole of Europe is no more progressive than transforming the NHS in England or across the UK into a market. However, it appears that the pace of privatisation of health, education and many other public services is set to increase across the EU with the imposition of the controversial Lisbon Treaty. This effectively reinstates many of the centralising and neoliberal policies of the abandoned constitution.

The door to privatisation is being opened up by political leaders willing to concede that health care can be a service to be traded commercially, like hairdressing. The contradiction of the British government's stance will undermine its opposition to the revised EU directive on cross-border health when it is published in the spring, while the rapid pace towards privatisation of primary care services give us a glimpse of the brave new world to be ushered in by the Lisbon Treaty. This has now been forced through the Commons without the referendum that had been promised on the constitution.

BMA offers a "rational way forward"

One interesting aspect of the government's drive towards market-style reforms is that it has forced the BMA into the role of defender of the core values of the NHS. The BMA whose GP members in 1946 and 1948 forced it into opposition to the very establishment of the NHS, and which clung so tenaciously to pay beds, part-time consultant contracts and GP status as independent contractors now argues that it has "consistently championed the founding principles of the NHS" (BMA 2007: 49).

It is now the BMA, pressing its alternative as *A Rational Way Forward*, which argues against Gordon Brown's Labour Party that the core values of the NHS are "less of a financial arrangement and more of a social agreement", and that:

> Commercial motives have the potential to undermine this social contract. For this reason NHS clinical services should be publicly provided as far as capacity allows.

---

2 On a global level the notion of "health tourism" is being taken to an altogether higher level in countries like Thailand and India, which is projecting a $1 billion dollar annual turnover from health tourism in the next few years.

(BMA 2007: 49)

The BMA, with reference to the danger of "patchwork privatisation" that has been identified by the Keep Our NHS Public campaign (Nunns 2007), also offers a hard-edged critique of the corrosive effect of private-sector involvement:

> Doctors do not want to see English healthcare shaped according to the financial interests of profit making entities and are opposed to privatisation, defined as the 'clear transfer of crucial decision making responsibilities from the public to the private sector and an effective transfer of power over assets.' ...Opportunities for conflicts of interest are much too prominent for currently proposed structures to be something that any society could accept.

> We are concerned by evidence of a trend towards a 'commodification' of healthcare, drawing out and isolating some services from others, ostensibly to improve their management, but with the effect of packaging services for competitive award. This managerial reductionism has a corrosive influence on the operation of a health system. It ignores the economic benefits, and quality of service, gained from service integration that make an overwhelming case against disaggregating care from integrated systems.

(BMA 2007: 54)

Unfortunately the BMA does not consistently follow through the logic of these statements, or take on the full implications of the political problems that would arise from its proposal for a constitution for the NHS – a recommendation which appears to have received a distorted echo in Gordon Brown's 2008 New Year message.

The difficulty is that any constitution would inevitably reflect the political ideology and prejudices of the government of the day; and right now, the government of today is the one undermining the core values that the BMA wants enshrined in a binding document. The BMA goes on to concede that the constitution should include a version of the Brown/Blair/New Labour mantra of "rights and responsibilities" ("what the NHS expects from them") – which offers the opportunity to exclude people from care and restrict rights and entitlements.

Nor is there any mechanism to get around the total control that the government would inevitably have over the process of drafting, debating and "consulting" on any "constitution". We have already seen a first round of Lord Darzi's stage-managed so-called consultations, in which critics and opponents are excluded, and hand-picked groups of largely uninformed people are fed one-sided information and then "consulted". Neither this, nor the more conventional NHS-style consultation in which public views are invited and ignored, and difficult questions swept aside, would offer any hope of securing a constitution along the lines the BMA, the health unions and many more would find acceptable.

If a constitution is a utopian vision, the notion that it could be upheld and the organisational integrity of the NHS defended by an independent board of governors is equally fanciful. We should note the immense political pressure which ministers are able to bring to bear on the BBC and its governors, both politically – as during the Andrew Gilligan affair – and financially through control over the licence fee. Even now the BBC is planning drastic cuts in news budgets as a result of the squeeze on funding imposed by ministers – and there is every reason to believe an NHS Board of Governors would be treated with as little respect in the event of any disagreements with the government of the day.

There are other problems with the BMA's recommendations. It rashly concedes in point 2 that "rationing is inevitable" – a point immediately seized upon by the right-wing press and Doctors for Reform as a means to buttress their call for the NHS budget to be bolstered by user fees and private medical insurance.

And while many of the BMA recommendations seek to integrate services and ensure collaboration between primary and secondary care, it would seem more appropriate for them to look to the Scottish model of health boards rather than their strange hybrid proposal of a "Health Economy Foundation Trust" which again seems to concede too much value to the New Labour concept of Foundations:

> A health economy foundation trust (HEFT) model could be created to overlay the purchaser–provider divide. The board of the HEFT would include provider and commissioner representation from hospitals, general practice, community providers and public health representatives. They would plan and deliver healthcare across a local health economy.
>
> (BMA 2007: 17)

There is no doubt that the HEFT model would offer more possibilities of collaboration and cooperation between the different sections of the NHS than PCTs, and would also potentially break down the isolationism of Foundation Trusts. Another positive BMA proposal is for the formation of new local health councils as a fully elected and independent forum that would link local communities and the health professionals shaping their services (BMA 2007: 19).

In general the BMA's proposals are more consistently social democratic than anything on offer from New Labour ministers since the NHS Plan. The organisation has embraced the need for extra resources and powers for public health as well as systems and structures that bridge the gaps between primary and secondary care, and between health and social care.

But its "rational way forward" does not emphasise the need to scrap the purchaser–provider split which lay at the centre of Thatcher's market-style reforms and continues to underpin New Labour's drive towards a more developed market. There is no evidence to demonstrate that the market mechanism – rather than the massive injection of additional staff, the increase in beds and the increase in funding – was responsible for the reduction in NHS waiting times. But there is growing evidence that the new market, with cream-skimming contracts for private-sector providers, surplus-hunting Foundation Trusts, and a hefty bill for overpaid management consultants, is an obstacle to cooperation, collaboration and the most effective use of NHS resources.

Another NHS is possible

A solid basis for a new NHS that can win the confidence and engagement of its staff and service users would be the abolition of the purchaser–provider split, and the establishment of joint health boards on the Scottish model – or as outlined in the BMA proposal. This would establish a management structure capable of linking primary and secondary care with public health, mental health and continuing care for the elderly, and would plan and provide services in each locality.

Practice-based commissioning should be scrapped in favour of arrangements to incorporate representatives from Local Medical Committees, including GPs and staff from practices in socially deprived areas, in the decision-making process of health boards. Health service provider units should work to three- or five-year service agreements guaranteeing funding in return for meeting service targets, with the possibility of additional funding if targets are exceeded while maintaining service quality.

Foundation Trusts must be reintegrated with the local NHS, and any expanded private wings and deals with private for profit companies must be wound up to focus management time and resources on NHS services for NHS patients. The short-term pain of sharing their pool of unspent resources with the local health economy will be compensated by the long-term gain of cooperative working relations and greater long-term financial security for services.

The terms of reference of NICE should be widened to enable it, together with the Healthcare Commission, to draw up a basic charter identifying the core services that must be provided to a specified standard in every area of the country, in proportion to local population. This must include a minimum requirement for resourcing the improvement of mental health, care for elderly patients, palliative care and preventive care. On this basis, a new system of democratic local control needs to be introduced, with the establishment of a system of elected health boards or health authorities to take the place of Primary Care Trusts and to take over the social care elements of social services.

While the track record of local councils in stewarding and providing social care is seriously discouraging, in the NHS 60 years of control by non-elected quangos – all of them controlled from the top downwards and therefore responding to ministers and NHS bureaucrats rather than the needs and wishes of local people – have failed to deliver equity or even the most rudimentary degree of accountability. The health boards in Scotland and Northern Ireland aim to deliver both health and social care (with Scotland now planning the first fresh approach to public health in over a century). Scotland, Wales and Northern Ireland all have a far greater degree of democratic control over health services, through their elected assemblies and Parliament, than England, where there is no democratic voice. Popular models for successful tax-funded health care systems similar to the NHS can be found in Norway, Sweden and Denmark, where elected county councils control services (Lister 2005a). However, the long-standing antipathy between the medical profession and local government in Britain may well indicate that a parallel system of elections to local health boards in England would be less instantly controversial. Either way the elected body should be required to work to NICE and Healthcare Commission guidelines.

There is also a democratic deficit in the involvement (or lack of it) of NHS professional and support staff in the planning and development of services. Over 24 years of research on NHS policies and issues, talking with health workers, campaigners and the wider public have brought this author copious anecdotal evidence that the existing systems generate frighteningly large numbers of avoidable errors at every level. These include delays and errors in diagnosis and treatment, deficiencies in nursing care, lack of adequate help in eating, nutritional problems, poor coordination of discharge procedures, sloppy notification of appointments, and many other errors which may put patients' lives or the quality of their care at risk. However, the accumulation of problems – especially those attributable to short staffing and excessive pressures on those in post – can result either in total demoralisation and the loss of highly trained and experienced staff. Alternately, it produceds a variant form of demoralisation, in which staff distance themselves from problems and failings which they feel unable to remedy, and become reconciled to delivering a sub-standard service, effectively operating as conventional "wage slaves" delivering commercial services.

In the 1970s there was a flurry of discussion in the trade unions on the concept of "workers' control", although little of this was followed through to build new systems to make it work. The NHS, dependent as it is upon the commitment and dedication of workers required to demonstrate caring skills as well as professional competence, is a good example of the consequences of excluding workers from any genuine control over the quality of the work they do. It is vital that the workforce is recognised to be a key resource in improving the quality of care, and that nursing and other staff themselves recognise that they must stand up for their right to deliver care of an adequate standard – and to the resources they need if they are to do so.

One obvious starting point should be for health unions to begin to invoke the Nursing and Midwifery Council's Code of Conduct as a challenge to managers who attempt to run down staffing levels and skill mix to dangerous levels. Complaints should be laid, backed up by the union, and managers with nursing qualifications must be required to respect the code of conduct and ensure that their staff members are enabled to comply with it in their work. Unions should also be pressing for the vague words about "partnership working" that have littered NHS management documents since 1997 to be transformed into genuine mechanisms that allow NHS staff to challenge and force changes in systems that deliver poor care for patients. Weak and marginalised unions, leaving workers without a voice, lead to a loss of professional pride and a decline in workplace morale – with the consequence being a reduced quality of service in the midst of incessant marketising reforms.

These changes are needed across the board in the NHS. One of the areas where morale has fallen among nursing staff has been mental health, where ministers and management constantly talk about "partnership" that includes service users and even sometimes their carers, but ignores the frontline staff and their organisations.

There must be an immediate audit of mental health services and services for older people to identify areas where the National Service Framework targets still have not been met. Any cutbacks must be halted, and resources made available to meet these basic requirements. Where serious gaps are identified in nursing and residential home provision, the NHS and social services in each area should be empowered and required to investigate the viability of public sector investment in new purpose-built accommodation, to be staffed to specified standards.

Many younger GPs are reported to be reluctant to make the commitment involved in becoming practice partners, and are expressing a preference to work on a salaried basis which does not carry the financial liability or bureaucratic and managerial responsibility. In "under-doctored areas" the NHS and local government need to pool resources to build NHS health centres (or even polyclinics) combining a range of health care and therapeutic services, and recruit salaried GPs, nurses and therapists on the basis that the management and administration will be run by the joint health board. If necessary, recruitment premium payments could be used to fill vacancies, keeping the service under the control of the NHS.

The droves of private-sector management consultants should be released into the community, and an intensive programme of training NHS managers, doctors, and nurses on quality issues and effective management techniques should be launched, with the involvement of professional organisations and trade unions. The career structure of senior NHS management should be reviewed to bring an end to the constant insecurity and lack of local commitment that flows from short-term contracts.

Hospital support services, especially cleaning, catering, portering and laundry that have been contracted out to private firms should be brought back in house, with resources made available to improve staffing levels and raise standards of hygiene and patient care.

Contracts for independent sector treatment centres should be terminated as soon as possible without incurring punitive costs, and no further deals should be signed. Instead, the model of NHS treatment centres, pioneered in Central Middlesex, SW London and elsewhere, should be rolled out as a cost-effective way to separate elective from emergency treatment and hold down waiting lists.

PFI, too, must be brought to a halt, and serious debate begun on how to stem the flow of NHS revenues into private consortia on deals already signed and operational. In the short run, the law should be changed as necessary to ensure that the public sector recoups the lion's share of any future windfall profits from refinancing PFI deals. In place of PFI, a process of "smart procurement" developed in the public sector should be applied, with specified new building projects put out to competitive tender and strict scrutiny of the building process and the standard of materials used. In the longer run there seems little alternative but some form of enabling act to force the sale of existing PFI schemes back to the Treasury or the NHS. If the government can wheel out £100 billion to back the crisis-ridden Northern Rock bank, it can find a much smaller sum to buy out its own ill-considered contracts and stem the haemorrhage of cash to PFI consortium shareholders.

The historic debts that in many cases have rolled over on Trust books for a decade or more, together with the heavy borrowing that has taken place in other Trusts to cover the scale of the shortfall, must be also written off, to allow the new local health boards to begin with a clean sheet and on a basis of mutual trust and collaboration. In most cases this will carry no real cost, since the debts cannot be paid without ruinous local cutbacks in services, and the accountancy and other managerial time involved in dealing with the deficits could be better devoted to developing patient care.

With the financial pressure removed, existing plans to reconfigure services, downgrade A&E units and close popular local hospitals should be halted for a moratorium, reviewed and revisited in a joint process involving the new health boards, the trade unions, the local authorities and other representatives of service users. Hospitals and existing services should be permitted to close only when and if a full-scale and properly resourced alternative community-based service has already been put in place, and begun to win the confidence and change the behaviour pattern of the local community.

These few points do not pretend to answer every question that would necessarily arise from a change of regime in the NHS in England – which unfortunately is such a hypothetical scenario at the beginning of 2008 that it seems superfluous at this point to go any further. We could discuss the joyous prospect of a bonfire of quangos, the scrapping of costly and useless computer systems, even policies to force down the exorbitant prices charged to the NHS for drugs, equipment and other supplies.

Indeed, while the historic demand of socialists for the nationalisation of the drug industry appears overly simplistic and unrealistic in an era of global capital and vast multinational pharmaceutical corporations, few of which are British-owned – systems to stimulate public sector-funded research and development, coupled with the use of the NHS's status and power as a monopoly purchaser and new and tighter regulation of drug companies operating here, could yield useful results.

These proposals do offer broad lines of approach that would lay the basis for a consistent alternative based on the values of public service, the spirit of collaboration in place of competition, of planning in place of the market, of integration of primary, secondary and public health functions in place of the competition and fragmentation that has flowed from New Labour's reforms. They are consistent with the approach of Keep Our NHS Public, and with the core values of the joint NHS trade unions, NHS Together, which have tried to challenge New Labour's marketisation and privatisation without confronting

Gordon Brown or breaking from the political link with the Labour Party.

This book has studiously avoided drawing party political conclusions from the various issues that have been discussed. After 24 years as a campaigner working for London Health Emergency (LHE), and working with people from a wide range of political persuasions I have come to the conclusion that drawing hard political lines and hard conclusions can put people off the content of the debate. Suffice it to say that while New Labour has driven through the most far-reaching and objectionable reforms, I and many others would not turn for relief to David Cameron's Conservatives, the party which vigorously opposed the NHS at the outset, and which began the whole drive towards market-style policies. Nor am I persuaded that the as yet largely anonymous Nick Clegg and the Lib Dems have anything of great value to contribute as an alternative – indeed they appear to be sliding in a pro-market direction themselves.

LHE and Keep Our NHS Public have both made a point of reaching out to people of any party, or none, who value the NHS, regard it as a historic gain worth saving, and who are prepared to stand up and campaign for it, along with health workers, service users and the wider public. I hope this book has provided more ammunition to all those wanting to pursue this fight. There is still plenty of the NHS to defend, and plenty to be lost if our most popular public service is further carved up for the benefit of private profit.

REFERENCES

Abel-Smith B (1978) *National Health Service: The First Thirty Years.* London & New York: HMSO

Academy of Medical Royal Colleges (2007) *Acute health care services.* September, available at: http://www.aomrc.org.uk/documents/Acutehealthcareservicesreportofaworkingparty2.pdf

ACCA (2002) *Do PFI schemes provide value for money? ACCA member's survey.* September, available at: http://www.accaglobal.com/doc/publicsector/ps_ms_aw1.pdf

Achieng J (2001) Kenya: NGOs seek to import generic drugs from India. *Third World Network*, 22 February, available at: http://www.twnside.org.sg/title/generic.htm (accessed 6 October 2002)

Adam Smith Institute (1984) *The Omega Health Papers.* London: Adam Smith Institute

Albreht T, Cesen M, Hindle D, Jakubowski E, Kramberger B, Petric VK, Premik M and Martin Toth M (2002) *Slovenia: Health Care Systems in Transition.* Denmark: WHO European Observatory

Allsop J (1984) *Health Policy and the National Health Service.* London: Longman

Alvarez-Rosete A, Bevan G, Mays M and Dixon J (2005) The Effect of Diverging Policy Across the NHS. *British Medical Journal*, 331: 946–50

Alzheimer's Disease Society (1993) *NHS Psychogeriatric Continuing Care Beds.* London: ADS

Amicus the union (2007) *Briefing on Social Enterprises and the NHS.* London: Amicus, available at: http://www.amicustheunion.org/PDF/AmicusInformationSocialEnterprisesandtheNHS.pdf (accessed 3 February 2008)

Amrith S (2001) Democracy globalisation and health: the African dilemma. December, Centre for History and Economics, Cambridge, available at: http://www.kings.cam.ac.uk/histecon/papers.htm (accessed 7 July 2003)

Appleby J (2005) *Independent Review of Health and Social Care Services in Northern Ireland.* Department of Finance and Personnel, available at: http://www.dfpni.gov.uk/appleby_review_final_report.pdf

_____ (2006) Where's the money going? *King's Fund Briefing*, February, available at: http://www.kingsfund.org.uk/publications/briefings/wheres_the.html

Appleby J, Smith P, Ranade W, Little V and Robinson R (1994) Monitoring managed competition. In Robinson R and LeGrand J (eds) *Evaluating the NHS Reforms.* London: King's Fund Institute

Appleby L (2007) *Mental Health Ten Years On: Progress on Mental Health Care Reform.* Department of Health, available at: http://www.dh.gov.uk/en/Publicationsandstatistics/Publications/PublicationsPolicyAndGuidance/DH_074241 (accessed 29 April 2007)

Ashton J and Seymour H (1993) *The New Public Health.* Buckingham: Open University Press

Aubrey ME (2001) Canada's fatal error – health care as a right (part 1). *Medical Sentinel*, 6(1): 26–8, Ass of American Physicians and Surgeons, Macon Georgia

Audit Commission (1986) *Making a Reality of Community Care.* London: HMSO

_____ (1996) *By Accident or Design: Improving A&E Services in England and Wales.* London: HMSO

_____ (2005) *Queen Elizabeth Hospital NHS Trust: Public Interest report Government and Public Sector.* PwC, December, available at: http://www.audit-commission.gov.uk/pir/downloads/QEHPIR.pdf

_____ (2006) *Report in the Public Interest Good Hope Hospital NHS Trust.* Audit Commission, June, available at: http://www.audit-commission.gov.uk/pir/downloads/GoodHopeHospitalNHSTrustPIR.pdf

Audit Scotland (2002) *Taking the initiative – Using PFI contracts to renew council schools.* Available at: http://www.audit-scotland.gov.uk/utilities/search_report.php?id=342, (accessed 17 December 2007)

Barnet Health Authority (1997) *Progress Report on Wellhouse Trust Phase Ib Project.* London: BHA

Barrett E (2006) *Privatising primary care: a personal account.* Keep Our NHS Public, available at: http://www.keepournhspublic.com/pdf/Barrattletter.pdf (accessed 3 February 2008)

Barros PP and de Almeida Simões J (2007) *Portugal: Health Care Systems in Transition.* Denmark: WHO European Observatory

BBC News (2003a) Clinics could "poach" NHS staff. 12 September, available at: http://news.bbc.co.uk/go/pr/fr/-/1/hi/halth/3096126.stm (accessed 12 September 2003)

_____ (2003b) Hip op ruling: Freedom to travel? 1 October, available at: http://news.bbc.co.uk/1/hi/health/3156386.stm

_____ (2006) Patients rejecting hospital food. Monday, 16 October, available at: http://news.bbc.co.uk/1/hi/health/6054408.stm

_____ (2007a) Food in hospitals "unacceptable". 17 December, available at: http://news.bbc.co.uk/1/hi/health/7144557.stm

_____ (2007b) Ambulances queue at full hospital. 21 November, available at: http://news.bbc.co.uk/1/hi/england/norfolk/7106402.stm

_____ (2007c) Bed crisis sparks hospitals alert. 22 November, available at: http://news.bbc.co.uk/1/hi/england/7106938.stm

_____ (2007d) Caution as health plans "on hold". 7 June, available at: http://news.bbc.co.uk/go/pr/fr/-/1/hi/wales/6728827.stm

_____ (2007e) Hospital campaigners say it big. 21 July, available at: http://news.bbc.co.uk/go/pr/fr/-/2/hi/uk_news/wales/mid_/6908949.stm

_____ (2007f) Powys health board chief to quit. 19 June, available at: http://news.bbc.co.uk/1/hi/wales/mid/6766601.stm

_____ (2007g) EU "health tourism" plan delayed. 19 December, available at: http://news.bbc.co.uk/1/hi/health/7151339.stm

_____ (2007h) Health care across Europe's borders. 19 December, available at: http://news.bbc.co.uk/1/hi/uk/7147971.stm

BBC News Online (2006a) Thousands march over health cuts. 22 July, available at: http://news.bbc.co.uk/1/hi/england/gloucestershire/5205804.stm

_____ (2006b) Lanarkshire loses A&E department. 22 August, available at: http://news.bbc.co.uk/1/hi/scotland/glasgow_and_west/5270736.stm

_____ (2007) Plans to end private cash for the NHS. 22 June, available at: http://news.bbc.co.uk/1/hi/scotland/6225328.stm

Belfast Telegraph (2007) Shocking state of our waiting lists. 20 February, available at: http://www.belfasttelegraph.co.uk/news/local-national/article2287528.ece

Bell D and Bowes A (2006) *Financial care models in Scotland and the UK.* Joseph Rowntree Foundation, available at: http://www.jrf.org.uk/bookshop/eBooks/1859354408.pdf

Bennett E (2006) DoH scraps £167m Colchester hospital. *Building Design online*, 23 June, available at: http://bdonline.co.uk/story.asp?storyCode=3069372 (accessed 3 February 2008)

Benson M (1994) Doctors forced into rationing care. *The Observer*, 13 November: 24

Bevan A (1952) *In Place of Fear: A free health service.* Available at: http://www.sochealth.co.uk/history/placeofear.htm (accessed 28 February 2008)

Bevan G and Hood C (2006) Have targets improved performance in the English NHS? *British Medical Journal*, 332: 419–22, doi:10.1136/bmj.332.7538.419

Birn AE, Zimmerman S and Garfield R (2000) To Decentralize or not to Decentralize; is that the Question? Nicaraguan Health Policy under Structural Adjustment in the 1990s. *International Journal of Health Services*, December 30(1): 111–28

Black D et al. (1980) *Inequalities in Health.* London: DHSS

Black N (1992) Jennifer's ear: airing the issues. *Quality and Safety in Health Care*, December, 1(4): 213–4

Blake J (2007) Are GPs exploiting NHS markets? *Channel 4 News*. Available at: http://www.channel4.com/news/articles/society/health/are+gps+exploiting+nhs+markets/7 58447 (accessed 29 December 2007)

Blears H, Mills C and Hunt P (2002) *Making Healthcare Mutual*. London: Mutuo

Bloom G and Tang S (eds) (2004) *Reforming Health Services in Urban China*. London: Ashgate

Bloor K, Maynard A and Street A (1999) *The cornerstone of Labour's "New NHS": reforming primary care*. Discussion paper 168, University of York Discussion Paper, available at: http://www.york.ac.uk/inst/che/pdf/DP168.pdf (accessed 2 March 2008)

BMA (2005) "Cleaner hospitals" – more important to patients than choice. *Press release*, 26 June, available at: http://www.bma.org.uk/ap.nsf/Content/PressconfARM05?OpenDocument&Highlight=2, YouGov

_____ (2007) *A rational way forward for the NHS in England, A BMA discussion paper outlining an alternative approach to health reform*. May, BMA London, available at: http://www.bma.org.uk/ap.nsf/Content/rationalwayforward

BMA Health Policy and Economic Research Unit (1997) *Leaner and Fitter What Future Model of Delivery for Acute Hospital Services*. London: BMA

Boardman J and Parsonage M (2007) *Delivering the Government's Mental Health Policies: Services, staffing and costs*. Sainsbury Centre for Mental Health, 12 January

Bower P, Roland M, Campbell J and Mead N (2003) Setting standards based on patients' views on access and continuity: secondary analysis of data from the general practice assessment survey. *British Medical Journal*, 326: 258

Braine B (1967) quote from *International Medical Tribune*, 26 October, cited in Lister (1988: 36)

Brent and Harrow Health Authority and Barnet Health Authority (1994) *Changes in Service Provision in the Edgware Area*. London: B&HHA & BHA

Brindle D (1993) Bottomley steps into NHS market to aid hospital caught in cash trap. *Guardian*, 27 May: 11

_____ (1994) Trusts first NHS chief condemned. *Guardian*, 14 November: 2

_____ (1995) Spending up to £1 bn on NHS bureaucrats. *Guardian*, 28 February: 3

Brittan L (1988) *A New Deal for Health Care*. London: Conservative Political Centre

Bromley Hospitals Trust (1998) FBC *section 13*. London: BHT, pp.97–8

Brooks R (2007) System failure: How this government is blowing £12.4 billion on useless IT for the NHS. *Private Eye*, 2–15 March

California Nurses Association (1997) *Kaiser Watch: Report on Kaiser Permanente*. 1 December, CAN, available at: http://www.califnurses.org/cna/press

Cambridge and Huntingdon Health Authority (1996) *Draft Annual Plan* 1997–98. Cambridge: CHHA

Cambridge and Huntingdon Health Commission (1995) *Local Policies and Eligibility Criteria for Formal Consultation*. Cambridge: CHHC

Campbell J (1987) *Nye Bevan and the Mirage of British Socialism*. London: Weidenfield & Nicholson

Carlisle D (2007a) A different Kind of revolution. *Health Service Journal*, 3 May: 22–4

_____ (2007b) Controversial and divisive: Whitehall's own Big Brother. *Health Service Journal*, 28 June: 14–15

_____ (2007c) £35m ISTC deal scrapped. *Health Service Journal*, 28 June

Carlton Club Political Committee (1988) *The NHS & the Private Sector (confidential)*. London: Carlton Club

Carvel J (2004) Chaos ahead for foundation hospitals. *Guardian*, 21 January, available at: http://www.guardian.co.uk/medicine/story/0,1127474,00.html (accessed 26 December 2007)

_____ (2006a) Time to make the figures add up. *Guardian*, 12 April, available at: http://www.guardian.co.uk/money/2006/apr/12/publicfinances.politics1

_____ (2006b) Cut more beds, says NHS official. *Guardian*, 22 May, available at: http://www.guardian.co.uk/society/2006/may/22/health.politics

_____ (2006c) Plan for wave of closures of NHS services. *Guardian*, 13 September, available at: http://www.guardian.co.uk/society/2006/sep/13/health.politics

_____ (2006d) Blair says shake-up of health service crucial to its survival. *Guardian*, 6 December, available at: http://www.guardian.co.uk/guardianpolitics/story/0,1964913,00.html

_____ (2006e) £64bn NHS privatisation plan revealed. *Guardian*, 30 June

Carvel J and Mostrous A (2006) Where the government is feeling the heat. *Guardian*, 26 October

Carvel J and White M (2004) Reid seeks to rekindle the Nightingale philosophy. *Guardian*, 20 October

Central Health Services Council (1969) *The Functions of the District General Hospital (The Bonham-Carter Report)*. London: HMSO

Charter D (2004) Ministers snub MPs' hospital questions. *The Times*, 18 October, available at: http://www.timesonline.co.uk/tol/news/uk/article495644.ece

Chief Medical Officer (2002) *Getting ahead of the curve*. Department of Health

CIPFA (1988) *Health Service Trends* 1987. London: CIPFA

Coates K and Topham T (1974) *The New Unionism: Case for Workers' Control*. London: Pelican

Coates P (2001) *Soft Services in PFI Projects: the Retention of Employment Model*. DoH Circular from PFIC, 21 June, London

COHSE (1992a) *Under Pressure. COHSEs evidence to the Tomlinson Inquiry into London's health services*. London: COHSE

_____ (1992b) *Privatising the Elderly: Why COHSE Says No*. Reading: COHSE

Colgan AL (2002) Hazardous to Health: the World Bank and IMF in Africa. *Africa Action Position Paper*, April, available at: http://www.africaaction.org/action/sap0204.htm (accessed 29 June 2002)

Committee on the Future of Emergency Care in the United States (2006) *Health System. Hospital-based emergency care: at the breaking point*. Washington, DC: National Academies Press

Commons Health Committee (2006) *UK Health spending as a percentage of GDP*. Available at: http://www.publications.parliament.uk/pa/cm200506/cmselect/cmhealth/1692-i/169202.htm (accessed 15 December 2007)

Connolly G (2002) South African Health Care a system in transition. *Background paper for Asian Social Forum Hyderabad,* January 2003, available at: http://www.cehat.org/rthc/paper6.htm

Cook R (1988) *Life Begins at Forty: In Defence of the NHS*. London: Fabian Society

Corens D (2007) *Belgium: Health Care Systems in Transition*. Denmark: WHO European Observatory

COSATU (Congress of South African Trade Unions) (2002) *Initial submission on the Draft National Health Bill*. COSATU, 8 March, available at: http://www.cosatu.org.za/docs/2002/initial.htm (accessed 11 June 2004)

Counsel and Care (2007) Care Home Fees: paying them in Scotland. Information from *Counsel and Care,* 52: October, available at: http://www.counselandcare.org.uk/assets/library/documents/52_Care_Home_Fees_paying_them_in_Scotland.pdf

Courtney M and Walker M (1996) *Stand and Deliver: Making Pensioners Pay for Care*. London: NHS Support Federation

Coyle A (1986) *Dirty Business*. Birmingham: West Midlands Low Pay Unit

Craig F (1990) *British General Election Manifestos* 1959–87. Aldershot: Dartmouth Publishing

Cressey D (2006) Millions wasted in oxygen fiasco. *Pulse*, 22 December, available at: http://www.pulsetiday.co.uk/story.asp?sectioncode=23&storycode=4011530 (accessed 27 December 2007)

Crisp N (2005) *Commissioning a Patient Led NHS*. Department of Health, 28 July, available at: http://www.dh.gov.uk/en/Publicationsandstatistics/Publications/PublicationsPolicyAndGui dance/DH_4116716

Crook A (2007) Nurse suspended for "speaking out". *Manchester Evening News*, 19 June

Cullinan K (2003) Legal vacuum hampers health for all. *HIVAN* (Centre for HIV/AIDS Networking), 31 March, available at: http://www.hivan.org.za (accessed 11 June 2004)

Darzi A (2007a) *Healthcare for London: A Framework for Action*. NHS London, July
_____ (2007b) *Our NHS Our future: NHS next stage review – interim report*. Department of Health, 4 October, available at: http://www.dh.gov.uk/en/Publicationsandstatistics/Publications/PublicationsPolicyAndGui dance/dh_079077
_____ (2007c) *A Framework for London – Technical Paper*. NHS London, available at: http://www.healthcareforlondon.nhs.uk/pdf/FFA-Technical-Paper.pdf (accessed 18 March 2008)

Davies M and Elwyn G (2006) Referral management centres: promising innovations or Trojan horses? *British Medical Journal*, 332: 844–6, doi:10.1136/bmj.332.7545.844

Dawe V (1996) More trust mergers on the cards. *British Medical Journal*, 313: 773 (News, 28 September)

Deber R (2000) Getting what we pay for: myths and realities about financing Canada's health care system. *Background papers for the Dialogue on Health Care reform*, available at: http://www.utoronto.ca/hpme/dhr/4.html (accessed 11 May 2003)

Democratic Health Network (2003) *A briefing for non-experts*. London: UNISON, available at: http://www.unison.org.uk/acrobat/13620.pdf (accessed 15 December 2007)

Den Exter A, Hermans H, Dosljak M and Busse R (2004) *Netherlands: Health Care Systems in Transition*. Denmark: WHO European Observatory

Denham J (2000) Commons written answer, *Hansard*, 2 February

Department of Health (DoH) (1989a) *Working for Patients*. London: HMSO
_____ (1989b) *Caring for People*. London: HMSO
_____ (1989c) *Self Governing Hospitals: Briefing for Managers*. London: HMSO
_____ (1991) *The Patients' Charter*. London: HMSO
_____ (1993a) *Health and Personal Social Services Statistics for England*. London: HMSO
_____ (1993b) *Making London Better*. Lancashire Health Publications Unit
_____ (1994) *Guidance on Discharge of Mentally Disordered People and Their Continuing Care in the Community*. London: DoH
_____ (1995a) *NHS Responsibilities for Meeting Continuing Health Care Needs*. London: DoH
_____ (1995b) *NHS's 1.6 per cent budget boost*. Press Release, 28 November
_____ (1996) *Personal Services Key Indicators*. London: HMSO
_____ (1997a) *The New NHS: Modern, Dependable*. London: HMSO
_____ (1997b) *Personal Social Services Key Indicators 1997*. London: DoH
_____ (1998a) *The Future of London's Health Services*. London: HMSO
_____ (1998b) *Health Services in London: A Strategic Overview*. London: HMSO
_____ (1998c) *The Government's Expenditure Plans 1998–1999*. Fig 2.7, available at: http://www.archive.official-documents.co.uk/document/cm39/3912/3912.htm (accessed 15 December 2007)
_____ (2000a) *Shaping the Future NHS: Long Term Planning for Hospitals and Related Services. Consultation Document on the Findings of The National Beds Inquiry*. February, available at: http://www.dh.gov.uk/en/Publicationsandstatistics/Publications/PublicationsPolicyAndGui dance/DH_4009640
_____ (2000b) *The NHS Plan: a plan for investment, a plan for reform. July,*

available at:
http://www.dh.gov.uk/en/Publicationsandstatistics/Publications/PublicationsPolicyAndGui
dance/DH_4002960

_____ (2000c) *Departmental Investment Strategy*. November. London: DoH

_____ (2001) *The NHS Plan: investment and reform for NHS Hospitals. Taking forward the NHS Plan*. Stationery Office, February

_____ (2002a) *Delivering the NHS* Plan. Stationery Office, April

_____ (2002b) *The Government's Expenditure Plans 2000–01. Chapter 4, Fig 4.1.*
Available at:
http://www.dh.gov.uk/en/Publicationsandstatistics/Publications/AnnualReports/Browsable
/DH_4097428

_____ (2002c) *Growing Capacity. Independent Sector Diagnosis and Treatment Centres*. December, available at:
http://www.dh.gov.uk/en/Publicationsandstatistics/Publications/PublicationsPolicyAndGui
dance/DH_4005842

_____ (2002d) *Growing Capacity. A new role for external healthcare providers in England*. June, available at:
http://www.dh.gov.uk/en/Publicationsandstatistics/Publications/PublicationsPolicyAndGui
dance/DH_4009238

_____ (2005) *Independent Sector Procurement Programme Phase 2 Electives CPD0083: Phase 2 – Elective Care Services PQQ (Parts 1 and 2 and Rev A Annex)*.
Department of Health, 8 September

_____ (2006a) *No excuses. Embrace partnership now. Step towards change!* Report of the third sector commissioning task force, July, available at:
http://www.dh.gov.uk/en/Publicationsandstatistics/Publications/PublicationsPolicyAndGui
dance/DH_4137144

_____ (2006b) *Billion pound boost for new NHS hospitals*. Press Release, 12 April,
available at:
http://www.dh.gov.uk/en/Publicationsandstatistics/Pressreleases/DH_4133762

_____ (2006c) *Alternative Provider Medical Services (APMS) Q&A*. DoH website,
12 September, available at:
http://www.dh.gov.uk/en/Policyandguidance/Organisationpolicy/Primarycare/Primarycare
contracting/APMS/DH_4125919 (accessed 14 December 2007)

_____ (2006d) *The Mental Capacity Act and the Independent Mental Capacity Advocate (Imca) Service*. Local Authority Circular LAC 2006 (15), available at:
http://www.dh.gov.uk/en/Publicationsandstatistics/Lettersandcirculars/LocalAuthorityCirc
ulars/AllLocalAuthority/DH_4140232

_____ (2007a) *Departmental Report 2007*. London: The Stationery Office, May

_____ (2007b) *Have your say. Consultation on the regulations for Local Involvement Networks (LINks)*. Available at:
http://www.dh.gov.uk/en/Consultations/Liveconsultations/DH_078794

_____ (2007c) *Payment by results*. Available at:
http://www.dh.gov.uk/en/Managingyourorganisation/Financeandplanning/NHSFinancialR
eforms/index.htm

_____ (2007d) *Sharing the learning: Payment by results*. Available at:
http://www.dh.gov.uk/en/Healthcare/Secondarycare/NHSfoundationtrust/DH_4088993

_____ (2007e) *NHS financial performance: quarter four 2006–07*. 6 June, available at:
http://www.dh.gov.uk/en/Publicationsandstatistics/Publications/PublicationsPolicyAndGui
dance/DH_075230

_____ (2007f) *Making Decisions; the Independent Mental Capacity Advocate (IMCA) service*. Available at:
http://www.dh.gov.uk/en/Publicationsandstatistics/Publications/PublicationsPolicyAndGui
dance/DH_073932

Department of Health and Home Office (1991) *The Reed Report: Review of Health and Social Services for Mentally Disordered Offenders and Others Requiring Similar*

Services. London: DoH

Department of Health and Social Security (DHSS) (1975) *Better Services for the Mentally Ill*. London: HMSO

_____ (1976) *Sharing Resources for Health in England: Report of the Resource Allocation Working Party*. London: HMSO

_____ (1977) *The Way Forward: Priorities in the Health and Social Services*. London: DHSS

_____ (1979a) *Royal Commission on the NHS*. London: HMSO

_____ (1979b) *Patients First: The Reorganisation of the NHS*. London: HMSO

_____ (1981a) *Care in Action*. London: HMSO

_____ (1981b) *Growing Older*. London: HMSO

_____ (1981c) *Care in the Community*. London: HMSO

_____ (1983) *NHS Support Services: Contracting Out*. London: DHSS

_____ (1987) *Determination of Private Patient Charges*. London: DHSS

_____ (1988) *London Study Acute Health Services in London*. Unpublished Paper

Department of Health Commercial Directorate (2004) IS-TC *Market Sustainability Analysis*. July, available at: http://www.dh.gov.uk/en/Publicationsandstatistics/Freedomofinformationpublicationsche mefeedback/FOIreleases/DH_4102647 (accessed 28 December 2007)

Department of Health DTC Programme (2002) *Independent sector Diagnosis & Treatment Centre programme Independent sector Ophthalmology chains Project Memorandum of Information*. December

Department of Health Information Centre (2007) *NHS staff numbers*. April, available at: http://www.ic.nhs.uk/statistics-and-data-collections/workforce/nhs-staff-numbers (accessed 24 December 2007)

Department of Health Press Release (2003) *250,000 NHS patients to receive quicker treatment in new treatment centres*. Department of Health, 23 September, available at: http://www.dh.gov.uk/en/Publicationsandstatistics/Pressreleases/DH_4054251 (accessed 28 December 2007)

Department of Health Statistics (1993) *Bed Availability for England 1991–2*. Fylde: DoH Statistics Division

_____ (1997) *Bed Availability and Occupancy for England 1996–97*. Wetherby: DoH Statistics Division

Derby Royal Infirmary and Derby City General Hospital NHS Trusts (1997) *Working Together for the People of Derbyshire*. Derby: DRI & DCGH

Dixon C (1994) Health reforms close 88 casualty units. *Independent on Sunday*, 14 August

Dixon A and Mossialos E (eds) (2002) *Health care systems in eight countries: trends and challenges*. European Observatory on Health Care Systems and London School of Economics

Donatini A, Rico A, D'Ambrosio MG, Lo Scalzo A, Orzella L, Cicchetti A and Profili S (2001) *Italy: Health Care Systems in Transition*. Denmark: WHO European Observatory

Donnelly L (2007) Plan would give UK patients free care in EU. *Daily Telegraph*, 25 November, available at: http://www.telegraph.co.uk/news/main.jhtml?xml=/news/2007/11/25/nhealth125.xml

Doughty S (2007) Care homes fleecing middle-class residents. *Daily Mail*, 17 October

Doyal L (1985) *The Political Economy of Health*. London: Pluto Press

Dunlop DW and Martins JM (eds) (1996) *An International Assessment of Health Care Financing: Lessons for Developing Countries*. Washington, DC: World Bank

Dunnigan MG and Pollock AM (2003) Downsizing of acute inpatient beds associated with private finance initiative: Scotland's case study. *British Medical Journal*, 326: 905

Durán A, Lara JL and van Waveren M (2006) *Spain: Health Care Systems in Transition*. Denmark: WHO European Observatory

Dyer O (1994) London scientists blame NHS reforms for brain drain. *British Medical Journal*, 309: 291

Eaglesham J (2003) Blair finds words to explain core belief. *Financial Times*, October 2001

Ebrey G and Revel P (2005) In need of treatment. *Newshopper*, 4 May, available at: http://www.newsshopper.co.uk/search/display.var.593322.0.in_need_of_treatment.php

Eckstein H (1970) *The English Health Service (Third reprint).* Cambridge, MA: Harvard University Press

Economist (1997) Dobson's choice. The internal market is dead. Long live the internal market. 11 December

Edinburgh Evening News (2006) Consort vows to clean up its act at the ERI. 26 September, available at: http://news.scotsman.com/edinburgh.cfm?id=1422792006

Edwards N (2007) RAB axed as Hewitt defends year of pain. *Health Service Journal*, 29 March: 12–13

eGov Monitor (2007) 500m pound annual PFI bill for Scottish Health Service. *eGov Monitor*, 24 October, available at: http://www.egovmonitor.com/node/15393

Elliott L (2003) Third Way addicts need a fix. *Guardian*, 14 July

Elwell H (1986) *NHS; The Road to Recovery.* London: Centre for Policy Studies

Engels F (1977) *The Condition of the Working Class in England.* London: Lawrence & Wishart

Ennals D (1977) Speech to the Socialist Medical Association. 27 March, available at: http://www.sochealth.co.uk/history/ennalspeech.htm (accessed 18 September 2007)

Enthoven AC (1985) National Health Service: some reforms that might be politically feasible. *The Economist*, 22 June: 9

_____ (1997) Market-based reform of US health care financing and delivery: managed care and managed competition. In Schieber (1997) *Innovations in Health Care Financing.* World Bank Discussion Paper 365 March. Washington, DC: World Bank

_____ (2003) Employment-based health insurance is failing: now what? *Health Affairs web exclusive*, available at: http://www.healthaffairs.org/WebExclusives/Enthoven_Web_Excl_052803.htm (May 280) (accessed 19 June 2003)

EPSU (European Public Sector Unions) (2007) EPSU BRIEFING on draft EU directive on Cross-Border Healthcare. December, available at: http://www.akeuropa.eu/documents/daseinsvorsorge/EPSU_briefing_for_Health_Trade_U nions.pdf

Evans CM (2007) No cuts say Morriston protesters. *Wales on Sunday*, 29 April

Evans JR (2007) *The Scottish Regional Treatment Centre Pilot Project at Stracatho Hospital.* 31 March, available at: http://www.keepournhspublic.com/pdf/ShortSRTCfinal.pdf

Evans O (2007) Diagnostics firm found inadequate. *Health Service Journal*, 11 October: 9

Eversley J and Shepherd C (1988) *Changes in Primary Care Draft final report to Health Rights.* Unpublished

Fleming N (2006) Ministers "are trying to privatise NHS by stealth". *Daily Telegraph*, 1 July

Foot M (1982) *Aneurin Bevan: A Biography (Vol.2) 1945–1960.* London: Granada

Frankel S, Ebrahim S and Davey Smith G (2000) The limits to demand for health care. *British Medical Journal*, 321: 42–5, 1 July

Freeman R (2000) *The Politics of Health in Europe.* Manchester: Manchester University Press

Gaál P (2004) *Hungary: Health Care Systems in Transition.* Denmark: WHO European Observatory

Gadelrab R (2006) £175m windfall may be spent on "super hospital". *Camden New Journal*, available at: http://www.thecnj.co.uk/camden/081006/news081006_21.htm

_____ (2007) Mentally-ill patients to be released early. Fears £8m savings target will squeeze NHS services. *Camden New Journal*, 22 March, available at: http://www.thecnj.com/camden/032207/news032207_02.html

Gaffney D and Pollock AM (1997) *Can the NHS Afford the Private Finance Initiative?* London: BMA Health Policy and Economic Research Unit

Gaffney D, Pollock AM, Price D and Shaoul J (1999a) PFI in the NHS – is there an economic case? *British Medical Journal*, 319, 10 July

_____ (1999b) NHS capital expenditure and the Private Finance Initiative – expansion or contraction? *British Medical Journal*, 319, 48–51 (3 July)

Gainsbury S (2007a) Fresh row erupts over plans for private GP practices. *Public Finance*, 13–19 April: 7

_____ (2007b) Bitter inheritance. *Public Finance*, 27 April, available at: http://www.publicfinance.co.uk/search_details.cfm?News_id=30450&keysearch=Gainsbury

_____ (2007c) PFI debt fears as district general hospitals feel the squeeze. *Health Service Journal*, 15 November

_____ (2007d) PFI hospitals costing NHS extra £480m a year. *Public Finance*, 23–9 March

_____ (2007e) Seven new PFI hospitals given the green light. *Public Finance*, 2–8 March: 8

_____ (2007f) NAO cast doubt on value of PFI schemes. *Public Finance*, 8–14 June: 12

_____ (2007g) District general hospitals face heavy specialist service losses. *Health Service Journal*, 8 November, available at: http://www.hsj.co.uk/news/district_general_hospitals_face_heavy_specialist_service_losses.htm

Garcia A (2001) *Healthcare reform in Germany: the search for efficiency and cost control.* 30 November, available at: http://www.frost.com/prod/news.nsf

Gatheru W and Shaw R (eds) (1998) *Our problems our solutions*. Nairobi: Institute of Economic Affairs

Gilson L, Doherty J, McIntyre D, Thomas S, Briljal V and Bowa C (1999) The Dynamics of Policy Change: health care financing in South Africa 1994–1999, Major Applied Research 1, *Technical Paper*, 1 November. Bethesda, MD: Partnerships for Health Reform

Gordon P (1999) Primary care in context. In Sims J (ed.) (1999) *Primary Health Care Sciences*. London: Whurr Publishers

Gorsky (2006) Hospital governance and community involvement in Britain: evidence from before the National Health Service. *History and Policy*, February, available at: http://www.historyandpolicy.org/archive/pol-paper-print-40.html (accessed 28 August 2007)

Gosling P (2007) End of the line for the PFI? *Public Finance*, 27 July–2 August: 18–21.

Grabham Sir A (1989) *The End of the Dream*. London: BMA News Review

Green B (1997) *Deputy PFI Director Report to Barnet Health Authority*. 23 July, London: BHA

Green D (1986) *Challenge to the NHS*. London: IEA

_____ (ed.) (1988) *Acceptable Inequalities?: Essays on the Pursuit of Equality in Health Care*. London: IEA Health Unit paper

Greener I and Mannion R (2006) Does practice based commissioning avoid the problems of fundholding? *British Medical Journal*, 333: 1,168–70, doi:10.1136/bmj.39022.486921.94

Grey-Turner E and Sutherland F (1982) *History of the British Medical Association 1932–1982*. London: BMA

Griffiths R (1983) *NHS Management Enquiry*. London: DHSS

_____ (1988) *Community Care: An Agenda for Action*. London: HMSO

Guy's and Lewisham Mental Health Trust (1997) *Chief Executive's Report September.* London: G&LMHT

Hall C (2006) Doctors to slow down treatment to save money. *Daily Telegraph*, 23 November, available at: http://www.telegraph.co.uk/news/main.jhtml?xml=/news/2006/11/23/ndoctor23.xml (accessed 3 February 2008)

Hall C and Rozenberg J (2006) NHS may have to pay for surgery abroad. *Daily Telegraph*, 17 May, available at: http://www.telegraph.co.uk/news/main.jhtml?xml=/news/2006/05/17/nhs17.xml

Hall S (2007) Will Life After Blair be Different? *British Politics*, 2, 118–22, doi:10.1057/palgrave.bp.4200045

Halligan L (2007) Ten years of going round in circles. *Sunday Telegraph*, 25 February, available at:
http://www.telegraph.co.uk/news/main.jhtml?xml=/news/2007/02/25/nrhewitt125.xml

Ham C (1994) *Health Policy in Britain (3rd edn)*. London: Macmillan

_____ (1996) *Public, Private or Community: What Next for the NHS?* London: Demos

_____ (1997) Why rationing is inevitable in the NHS. In New B (ed.) (1997) *Rationing: talk and action in health care*. London: BMJ Publishing Group/King's Fund

_____ (1999) *Health Policy in Britain (4th edn)*. London: Macmillan

_____ (2006) Creative destruction in the NHS. *British Medical Journal*, Editorial 332: 984–5, 29 April, doi:10.1136/bmj.332.7548.984

Ham C and Honigsbaum F (1998) Priority setting and rationing health services. In Saltman R, Figueras J and Sakellarides C (eds) (2000) *Critical Challenges for Health Care Reform in Europe*. Buckingham: Open University Press

Hands Off Our Hospitals (1989) *A Response to the White Paper*. London: HOOH

Hanna J (2006) Memorandum submitted by Jane Hanna, Former Non-Executive Director of South-West Oxfordshire Primary Care Trust. Keep Our NHS Public, available at:
http://www.keepournhspublic.com/pdf/JaneHannaOxonEyes.pdf

Hansard (1946) *House of Commons Debates April 30th*. London: HMSO

_____ (1948) *House of Commons Debates February 9th*. London: HMSO

_____ (1985) *House of Commons Written Answers October 30th*. London: HMSO

_____ (1988) *Written Answers March 10th*. London: HMSO

_____ (1997) *Written Answers December 11th*. London: HMSO

Hart E (2007) *News: Neurosurgery Services 2007*. Press Release, Welsh Assembly Government, 4 July, available at: http://www.wales.nhs.uk/newsitem.cfm?contentid=7028

Hart J (1971) The Inverse Care Law. *The Lancet*, 1: 405–12

_____ (1994) *Feasible Socialism: The National Health Service, Past, Present and Future*. London: Socialist Health Association

_____ (2006) *The political economy of health care: a clinical perspective*. Bristol: Policy Press

Hawkes N (2006a) Secret NHS plan to ration patient care. *The Times*, 7 April

_____ (2006b) American firm is hired to do all NHS shopping. *The Times*, 26 July, available at: http://www.timesonline.co.uk/article/0,11069-2285857,00.html (accessed 3 February 2008)

_____ (2006c) PFI hospital deal was unacceptable face of capitalism. *The Times*, 3 May

_____ (2007) Hospitals project abandoned after cost increased by £200m. *The Times*, 21 July

Hayek F (1976) *The Road to Serfdom*. London: Routledge & Kegan Paul

HDA (Health Development Agency) (2004) Lessons from health action zones (Choosing Health? briefing). June, available at:
http://www.nice.org.uk/niceMedia/documents/CHB9-haz-14-7.pdf (accessed 2 March 2008)

Health Service Journal (1999) Profits for Industry. 13 May

_____ (2006) Trusts' admin bills on the rise. 20 July: 9

_____ (2007) Hewitt vows to end mental health "bail-outs". 11 April, available at:
http://www.hsj.co.uk/news/hewitt_vows_to_end_mental_health_bailouts.html (accessed 10 February 2008)

Health Service Journal reporters (2007) Flagship ISTC comes back into the NHS fold. 24 May: 5

Heart of England NHS Foundation Trust (2006) *Overview of the three Independent Reports into the Financial Position of Good Hope Hospital*. Birmingham: Heart of England NHS Foundation Trust

Heaton A (2001) *Joint public-private initiatives: meeting children's right to health?* Save the Children Fund UK, May

Hellowell M (2006) Alive and kicking. *Public Finance*, 21 November, available at: http://www.cipfa.org.uk/publicfinance/features_details.cfm?news_id=29388

Hellowell M and Pollock AM (2007a) New Development: The PFI: Scotland's Plan for Expansion and its Implications. *Public Money & Management*, Vol. 27, Issue 5, pp.351–4, November

_____ (2007b) The big payback. *Guardian*, 12 September

Helm T and Hall C (2006) NHS chief quits and carries can for record deficit. *Daily Telegraph*, 8 March, available at: http://www.telegraph.co.uk/news/main.jhtml?xml=/news/2006/03/08/nhs08.xml (accessed 27 December 2007)

Hemmings J (2007) "Free" care for elderly to cause a few more headaches in long term. *The Scotsman*, 15 December, available at: http://news.scotsman.com/carefortheelderly/39Free39-care-for--elderly.3593583.jp

Hencke D (2007a) Health trust chief and MPs attack maternity unit closures. *Guardian*, 25 August, available at: http://www.guardian.co.uk/guardianpolitics/story/0,2155906,00.html

_____ (2007b) Taxpayer may have to pay £170bn for PFI schemes, says Treasury. *Guardian*, 27 November, available at: http://www.guardian.co.uk/uk_news/story/0,2217576,00.html

Henwood M (1992) *Through a Glass Darkly: Community Care and Older People*. London: King's Fund Institute

Hertfordshire Councils (1995) *Acute Concern*. Welwyn Garden City: Welwyn Hatfield Council

Hertfordshire Health Agency (1994) *A&E Review*. Hertfordshire: HHA

_____ (1995) *Where do we want to be?*. Hertfordshire: HHA.

Hertfordshire PCTs (2007) *Delivering Quality Health Care for Hertfordshire*. East and North Herts and West Herts Primary Care Trusts, June 2007

Hewitt P (2005) *Speech to NHS Confederation Conference*. Department of Health, 17 June, available at: http://www.dh.gov.uk/en/RemovedSections/Speecheslist/DH_4113723 (accessed 10 February 2008)

Hinchcliffe D (1992) *Towards a Policy Programme for Community Care (Confidential draft for consultation and comment by SHA members)*. London: Unpublished

Hindle D and McAuley I (2004) The effects of increased private health insurance: a review of the evidence. *Aust Health Review*, 28(1): 119–38

Hines N (and agencies) (2007) NHS back in the black, but 17 trusts in dire straits. *Times Online*, 6 June, available at: http://www.timesonline.co.uk/tol/news/uk/health/article1893988.ece

Hinkov H, Koulaksuzov S, Semerdjiev I and Healy J (2005) *Bulgaria: Health Care Systems in Transition*. Denmark: WHO European Observatory

HM Treasury (1986) *Using Private Enterprise in Government*. London: Treasury

_____ (2000) *Pre-budget report 2000*. Available at: http://archive.treasury.gov.uk/pbr2000/leaflets/pbrl3.htm (accessed 31 December 2007)

_____ (2001) *Budget, Chapter C*, Table C24. London: Treasury

Hofmarcher MM and Rack HM (2006) *Austria: Health Care Systems in Transition*. Denmark: WHO European Observatory

Holland W (1992) *Letter to Virginia Bottomley*. London

Hornagold and Hills (2003) *Post project evaluation report*. Prepared for East London Community & Mental Health Trust, 4 November

House of Commons Expenditure Committee (1974) *Expenditure Cuts in Health and Personal Social Services*. Social Services sub-committee, Fourth Report. London: HMSO

House of Commons Health Committee (2002) First report The Role of the Private Sector in the NHS (1 May), available at: http://www.publications.parliament.uk/pa/cm200102/cmselect/cmhealth/308/30807.htm#a 17

_____ (2006) *NHS deficits: First report of Session 2006–7.* The Stationery Office, December

House of Commons Social Services Committee (1985) *Session 1984–85 Community Care.* Vol.1, London: HMSO

_____ (1988) *First Report: Resourcing the NHS, Short Term Issues.* London: HMSO

_____ (1990) Eleventh Report: *Community Care: Services for People with Mental Handicap and People with Mental Illness.* London: HMSO

Hughes D (1993) *Health policy: letting the market work.* In Page R and Baldock J (eds) *Social Policy Review 5, The Evolving State of Welfare.* Canterbury: Social Policy Association

Hunt L (1993) Parents to sue Guy's over £8,500 operation. *The Independent,* 5 July: 7

Hutton J (2004) *Practice Based Commissioning. Speech given at Health Service Journal Conference,* 7 December 2004, available at: http://www.dh.gov.uk/en/News/Speeches/Speecheslist/DH_4099631 (accessed 14 December 2007)

_____ (2007) *The Future of Public Service Reform.* Speech to CBI Public Services Forum, 17 May, available at: http://www.publictechnology.net/modules.php?op=modload&name=News&file=article&s id=9285

Iggulden A (2007) Wards and staff cut at bankrupt hospital. *Evening Standard,* 9 November

Iliffe S (1983) *The NHS: A Picture of Health?* London: Lawrence & Wishart

Imai Y (2002) Health Care Reform in Japan. *Economics Department Working Paper,* No. 321, February, Paris: OECD

Institute of Medicine (National Academy of Sciences) (2006) The future of emergency care in the United States health system. Washington, DC: National Academies Press, available at: http://www.nap.edu

IPPR (Institute for Public Policy Research) (2006) *Hospital reconfiguration: IPPR briefing.* September, available at: http://www.ippr.org.uk/uploadedFiles/research/projects/Health_and_Social_Care/hospital _reconfiguration_QA.pdf

James Paget Hospital NHS Trust (1994) *Strategic Direction and Business Plan.* Lowestoft: JPH

Jarman B (1993) Is London over-bedded? *British Medical Journal,* 306: 979–82

_____ (1994) *The Crisis in London Medicine How many hospital beds does the capital need?* London: University of London

Jervis P (2008) *Devolution and Health.* London: Nuffield Trust

Johnston C (2005) £3 billion for NHS patients to have private treatment. *Times Online,* 13 May, available at: http://www.timesonline.co.uk/article/0,2-1610957,00.html

Joint NHS Privatisation Research Unit (1987) *Contractor's Failures: The Whole Story.* London: JNHSPRU

_____ (1990) *The NHS Privatisation Experience.* London: JNHSPRU

Jones K (1972) *A History of the Mental Health Services.* London: Routledge and Kegan Paul

Keep Our NHS Public (2006) *News Briefing.* Available at: http://www.keepournhspublic.com/newsroundup.php?allrecs=ALL

Kelly S (2005) Letter. *Hospital Doctor,* 6 October

Kensington Chelsea and Westminster Health Authority (2001) *Report HA(01)30.2.* 13 June, London: KCWHA

Kerr D (2005) *Building a health service Fit for the future.* NHS Scotland, May, available at: http://www.scotland.gov.uk/Resource/Doc/924/0012113.pdf

Kettle M (2005) Pollsters taxed. *Guardian,* 4 April

Kimalu PK (2001) Debt relief and health care in Kenya. 24 July, Nairobi: Kenya Institute for Public Policy Research and Analysis (KIPPRA)

King's Fund (1983) *Health Finance: Assessing the Options.* London: King's Fund

_____ (1992) *London Health Care 2010.* London: King's Fund

_____ (1995) *London Monitor,* No.2. London: King's Fund

Kirby D (2007) Health in 2007 under the microscope. *BBC News*, 25 December, available at: http://news.bbc.co.uk/1/hi/northern_ireland/7140949.stm

Klein R (2006) *The new politics of the NHS, from creation to reinvention* (fifth edn). Abingdon: Radcliffe Publishing

Knight R (2004) Consumer group attacks "illusion of choice" in public services. *Financial Times*, December, available at: http://search.ft.com/nonFtArticle?id=041201001729

Kumar S (2004) India's treatment programme for AIDS is premature. *British Medical Journal*, 328: 70

Kuszewski K and Gericke C (2005) *Poland: Health Care Systems in Transition*. Denmark: WHO European Observatory

Labour Research Department (1987) *Privatisation: Paying the Price*. London: LRD

Laing and Buisson Healthcare Consultants (1997) *Care of Elderly People Market Survey* (10th edn). London: L&BHCC

_____ (2007) *Ten year decline in care homes set to reverse*. Press release, 27 April, available at: http://www.laingbuisson.co.uk/portals/1/MarketReports/CareofElderly2007_PR.pdf

Lancashire Evening Post (2008) Lack of patients forces firm to pull out. *Lancashire Evening Post*, 17 January, available at: http://www.lep.co.uk/news/Lack-of-patients-forces-firm.3683151.jp

Lancashire PCTs (2008) *Development of clinical assessment, treatment and support services*. Report to Lancashire Overview and Scrutiny Committee. 22nd January, available at: http://www3.lancashire.gov.uk/council/meetings/displayFile.asp?FTYPE=A&FILEID=27530

Lancet Editorial (1961) Everybody's business: Report of the Annual Conference of the National Association for Mental Health. *The Lancet*, 1: 608–9

Laurance J (2006) Millions for NHS pay, but little for beds and operations. *The Independent*, 18 January

Lawrence F (2001) Crisis-hit hospital finds that private finance for NHS comes at a price. *Guardian*, 23 July, available at: http://www.guardian.co.uk/society/2001/jul/23/hospitals.ppp

Lawrence H (2007) Everything to gain. *Public Finance*, 31 August–6 September: 17

Lea R and Mayo E (2002) *The Mutual Health Service*. London: New Economics Foundation

Lee J-C (2003) Health Care Reform in South Korea: Success or Failure? *American Journal of Public Health*, January, 93(1): 48–51

Lee P (2004) *Public Service Productivity: Health. Estimating the change in productivity of public expenditure on health*. October, London: National Statistics

Leftly M (2007) Who owns this place? *Building*, Issue 19, 11 May, available at: http://www.building.co.uk/story.asp?sectioncode=667&storycode=3086637&c=1

Leicester Mercury (2007a) Mental health care cutbacks debated. Tuesday 23 January

_____ (2007b) Mental health wards are to remain closed to save money. Friday 23 March

Lenaghan J (1997) *Hard Choices in Health Care*. London: BMJ Publishing Group

Lewis RQ, Mays N, Curry N and Robertson R (2007) Implementing practice based commissioning. *British Medical Journal*, (Editorial) 335: 1,168

Light D (1997) The real ethics of rationing. *British Medical Journal*, 315: 112–15 (12 July)

Lister J (ed.) (1988) *Cutting the Lifeline, the Fight for the NHS*. London: Journeyman

_____ (1989a) Cheap and Cheerless: a response to Kenneth Clarke's proposals for community care. July, London: London Health Emergency

_____ (1989b) Passing the Buck. *Community Care*, 774: 21–2 (3 August)

_____ (1990) *Acute Agony A Survey of Opt Out Bids*. London: LHE

_____ (1991) *Where's the Care? An Investigation into London's Mental Health Services*. London: COHSE

_____ (1992a) *Prescription for disaster, A detailed reply to the Tomlinson report*. London: COHSE

_____ (1992b) *Countdown to Crisis: The Government's Hidden Agenda for London's*

Health Services. London: LHE

_____ (1992c) *Under Pressure, COHSE's evidence to the Tomlinson Inquiry.* Banstead: COHSE

_____ (1995) *Passing the Buck: A UNISON Response to Cambridge & Huntingdon Health Commission*. Cambridge: UNISON

_____ (1996a) *The Two-Way Squeeze: How Cambridge NHS Cuts Would Hit the Frail Elderly.* Cambridge: UNISON

_____ (1996b) *Passing the Buck: A Survey of Eligibility Criteria for Continuing Care in the East Midlands*. Nottingham: UNISON

_____ (1996c) *Passing the Buck (Cambridge)*. April, Chelmsford: UNISON Eastern Region

_____ (1997a) *Squeezing out the elderly: the impact of NHS eligibility criteria on services for the elderly in Cambridge and Suffolk*. April, Chelmsford: UNISON Eastern Region

_____ (1997b) *Checking out Community Care: a UNISON campaign kit for health and social services staff*. June, Chelmsford: UNISON Eastern Region

_____ (1997c) *The Credibility Gap: Rhetoric Versus Reality in London's Mental Health Services*. London: UNISON

_____ (1998a) *Taking Liberties, a response to the North Essex Health Authority consultation document Taking the Initiative*. January, Chelmsford: UNISON Eastern Region

_____ (1998b) *Into the Wilderness: a response of West Hertfordshire Health Authority's document Choosing the right direction*. September, UNISON Eastern Region, available at: http://www.healthemergency.org.uk (accessed 1 November 2003)

_____ (1998c) *Casting Care Aside, a response for Wyre Forest District Council to plans by Worcestershire Health Authority*. Available at: http://www.healthconcern.org.uk/carereport2.htm (accessed 17 December 2007)

_____ (1999) *The Care Gap*. 27 May, London: UNISON

_____ (2001) *PFI in the NHS: A dossier, GMB, London*. Available at: http://www.epolitix.com/NR/rdonlyres/3F394786-780B-4D4E-ABCE-B8A7EC087250/0/pfiinthenhsadossier.pdf (accessed 17 December 2007)

_____ (2002) *Penny Pinchers*. An analysis of the privatisation of home care services by London Borough of Wandsworth, Battersea & Wandwworth TUC

_____ (2003a) *The PFI Experience, Voices from the frontline*. London: UNISON

_____ (2003b) *Not So Great: voices from the frontline at Swindon's Great Western Hospital*. London: UNISON

_____ (2003c) *SW London Hospitals Under Pressure*. London: Battersea & Wandsworth TUC

_____ (2003d) *The Central Manchester PFI Scheme: Reinventing the flat tyre?* Central Manchester Community Health Council, available at: http://www.healthemergency.org.uk/pdf/ManchesterPFI.pdf (accessed 18 December 2007)

_____ (2005a) *Health Policy Reform: Driving the wrong way?* London: Middlesex University Press

_____ (2005b) *Cleaners' Voices: interviews with hospital cleaning staff*. January, London: UNISON

_____ (2006a) *System Failure, North Staffordshire's health care services stuck in a downward spiral*. UNISON North Staffs and West Midlands

_____ (2006b) Mergers and markets: a magical mystery tour – A response drafted for UNISON East Midlands Region to the 2006 proposals for a single East Midlands Strategic Health Authority. East Midlands UNISON

_____ (2006c) A blank cheque for privatisation – A response drafted for UNISON West Midlands Region to the 2006 proposals for a single West Midlands Strategic Health Authority

_____ (2006d) *Castles in the air – Response to Public Consultation Document Gwent Clinical Futures*. December, UNISON Gwent Healthcare Branch, available at: http://www.healthemergency.org.uk/workingwu/Castlesintheair.pdf

_____ (2007a) *Too high a price to pay. The case against closing the Felix Post Unit*. UNISON South London & Maudsley Branch.

_____ (2007b) *The Darzi Report: the critical gaps*. London Health Emergency, available at: http://www.healthemergency.org.uk/pdf/Darziresponsecriticalgaps.pdf

_____ (2007c) *Hertfordshire's health services: Back To The Future?* Chelmsford: Eastern Region UNISON

_____ (2007d) *Under the Knife: a response to A Picture of Health*. Staff side unions, Queen Mary's Hospital, Sidcup, available at: http://www.healthemergency.org.uk/workingwu/Undertheknife.pdf

_____ (2007e) *Carving up the NHS: Dangers to staff, services and patients from "social enterprises"*. UNISON Oxfordshire Health Branch

_____ (2007f) Mental health care under the axe – A response by UNISON to the consultation document "Mental Health Services in North Essex". Chelmsford: UNISON Eastern Region.

_____ (2007g) *Markets versus mental health: the inappropriateness of the mainstream health reform agenda*. In Benos A, Deppe HU and Lister J (eds) (2007) *Health Policy in Europe: Contemporary dilemmas and challenges*. IAHPE, available at: http://www.healthp.org

_____ (2007h) Caught in the Crossfire – The plight of Hinchingbrooke Health Care Trust. February, Chelmsford: Eastern Region UNISON

_____ (2007i) Hiving off Peterborough – A response to a consultation document "The Next Steps". Peterborough: UNISON

Lister J and Martin G (1988) *Community Care: Agenda for Disaster*. A reply to the Griffiths Report. London: London Health Emergency

_____ (1996) *Accidents Waiting to Happen: A Survey of Acute Hospital Services in London*. London Region UNISON

Lister S (2006) Stealth plan to "privatise" NHS care. *The Times*, 30 June

Lloyd I and Donnelly L (2005) DoH allows commissioning to be outsourced in Oxfordshire. *Health Service Journal*, 20 October: 7

Lobato L and Burlandy L (2000) The context and process of health care reform in Brazil. In Fleury et al. (2000)

London Health Economics Consortium (1992) *Beds for Londoners. The current state of London's acute care*. London: Inner London Chief Executives Group

London Health Planning Consortium (1979) *Acute Health Services in London*. London: HMSO

Lords Hansard (2004) Lord Warner response to Baroness Noakes. Available at: http://www.parliament.the-stationery-office.com/pa/ld200304/ldhansrd/vo040419/text/40419w03.htm (accessed 26 December 2007)

McCartney I (2002) NHS Foundation Trusts aren't elitism, but localised public ownership. *Guardian*, 2 December

Macdonell H and Robertson J (2007) 9,000 elderly fear axe for free care after ruling. *The Scotsman*, 18 October, available at: http://news.scotsman.com/carefortheelderly/9000-elderly-fear-axe-for.3471672.jp

McGimpsey, M (2007a) McGimpsey dismisses hospitals closure proposals. Northern Ireland Executive Press Release, 06 December, available at: http://www.northernireland.gov.uk/news/news-dhssps-061207-mcgimpsy-dismisses-hospitals

_____ (2007b) McGimpsey opens "state of the art" nursing home accommodation in Cookstown. Northern Ireland Executive Press Release, 5 December, available at: http://www.northernireland.gov.uk/news/news-dhssps/news-dhssps-051207-mcgimpsey-opens-state.htm

McIntrye D, Gilson L, Valentine N and Soderlund N (1998) Equity of health sector revenue generation and allocation: a South African Case Study. *Major Applied Research 3, Working Paper,* 3 August, Bethesda, MD: Partnerships for Health Reform

Mandelstam M (2007) *Betraying the NHS. Health abandoned.* London: Jessica Kingsley

Marchildon GP (2005) *Canada: Health Care Systems in Transition.* Denmark: WHO European Observatory

Marsh B (2006) Rush to take GPs into private sector. *Daily Telegraph,* 18 June

Martin G (1997) *Into the Red A Survey of Trusts in UNISON Eastern Region.* Chelmsford: UNISON

Matthews B and Jung Y (2006) The Future of Health Care in South Korea and the UK. *Social Policy and Society,* 5: 375–85

Maxwell R (1988) *Reshaping the National Health Service.* London: Policy Journals

Maynard A (1998) Happy days are here again. *Health Service Journal*

Maynard A and Bosanquet N (1986) *Public Expenditure on the NHS: Recent Trends and Future Problems.* London: IHSM

MCMHT (Manchester Community and Mental Health Trust) (2004) *Visioning mental health services for Manchester.* 20 September, Manchester

Meads G (1999) The organisational development of primary care. In Sims J (ed.) (1999) *Primary Health Care Sciences.* London: Whurr Publishers

MEN (2007a) Mental health nurses out on strike. *Manchester Evening News,* 31 January, available at:
http://www.manchestereveningnews.co.uk/news/health/s/234/234799_mental_health_nurses_out_on_strike.html

_____ (2007b) Reissmann strike to continue. *Manchester Evening News,* 11 December

Mental Health Forum (2007) Modernising mental health to embrace business challenges and achieve service transformation. *Health Service Journal,* available at: http://www.hsj-mentalhealthforum.co.uk/homepage.asp

Mental Health Foundation (1990) *Mental Illness: The Fundamental Facts.* London: MHF

Merton, Sutton and Wandsworth Health Authority (1998) Service and Financial Framework. London: MSWHA

Mid Ulster Mail (2007) New extension for Fairfields. 13 December, available at:
http://www.midulstermail.co.uk/news/New-extension-for-Fairfields.3580163.jp

Milburn A (2002) Power and resources shift to NHS frontline. *Department of Health Press Release,* 11 December, available at:
http://www.dh.gov.uk/en/Publicationsandstatistics/Pressreleases/DH_4026008 (accessed 26 December 2007)

Milne S (2007) Only dogma and corporate capture can explain this. *Guardian,* 18 October, available at: http://www.guardian.co.uk/comment/story/0,2193282,00.html

MIND (1986) *When the Talking has to Stop.* London: MIND

Ministry of Health (1920) *Interim Report on the Future provision of Medical and Allied Services.* London: HMSO

_____ (1956) *Report of the Committee of Enquiry into the Cost of the National Health Service.* London: HMSO

_____ (1957) *Royal Commission on the Law relating to Mental Illness 1954–57.* London: HMSO

_____ (1959) *Report of the Maternity Services Committee.* London: HMSO

_____ (1962) *A Hospital Plan for England and Wales.* London: HMSO

Mohan J (1995) *A National Health Service?* London: Macmillan

_____ (2003a) The past and future of the NHS: New Labour and foundation hospitals. *History and Policy,* June, available at:
http://www.historyandpolicy.org/archive/pol-paper-print-14.html (accessed 28 August 2007)

_____ (2003b) *Reconciling Equity and Choice? Foundation hospitals and the future of the NHS.* London: Catalyst

Monbiot G (2007) This great free-market experiment is more like a corporate welfare scheme. *Guardian*, 4 September

Monitor (2006) Annual Report 2005–6. *Monitor*, July, The Stationery Office, available at: http://www.regulator-nhsft.gov.uk/documents/Monitor_2005_06_annual_report_final.pdf

Mooney H (2007a) Trusts hail £178m windfall as "unfair" finance system is axed. *Health Service Journal*, 29 March: 5

_____ (2007b) Acute trust set to privatise all elective ops. *Health Service Journal*, 9 August: 8

_____ (2007c) DoH may pull private scanning schemes. *Health Service Journal*, 11 October: 9

_____ (2007d) Trusts face monitoring on take-up of private services. *Health Service Journal*, 14 June: 7

_____ (2007e) DoH to get the measure of PCTs working with the private sector. *Health Service Journal*, 26 April: 5

_____ (2007f) BUPA to plug skills gap in Hillingdon. *Health Service Journal*, 27 September: 13

_____ (2007g) PCT denies new director has conflict of interest. *Health Service Journal*, 11 October: 8

Moore A (2006a) Are paid-up ITC millions being consigned to the scrapheap? *Health Service Journal*, 21 September: 12–15

_____ (2006b) Trust faces bill for dropped PFI deal. *Health Service Journal*, 6 July: 13

_____ (2006c) Herts and minds: £100m hole that could defeat protestors. *Health Service Journal*, 6 July: 14–15

_____ (2007a) Costly ITC plans scrapped. *Health Service Journal*, 8 June: 21

_____ (2007b) Money for nothing in the ISTC labour crisis. *Health Service Journal*, 4 October: 16–17

_____ (2007c) Shelved report exposes PFI management problems. *Health Service Journal*, 28 June: 8

_____ (2007d) Trusts shell bed space to keep grip on PFI approval. *Health Service Journal*, 1 November: 15

Moore W (2002) Public bodies should take more care in managing PFI contracts. *British Medical Journal*, 325: 66

MORI (1998) *Poll conducted for BBC State of the Region*. London: MORI/BBC

MSI Healthcare (2000) *MSI healthcare: Germany*. October, MSI, Devon, UK

Mudur G (2004) Hospitals in India woo foreign patients. *British Medical Journal*, 328: 1,338

Mulholland H (2005) Hewitt apologises to nurses over NHS reforms. *Society Guardian*, Thursday 10 November

_____ (2006) Blair welcomes private firms into NHS. *Guardian Unlimited*, Thursday 16 February, available at: http://www.guardian.co.uk/society/2006/feb/16/health.politics

Nandraj S (1997) Unhealthy prescriptions: the need for health sector reform in India. *Informing and Reforming*, 2: 7–11, April–June

National Assembly for Wales (2001) *Improving Health in Wales: a plan for the NHS with its partners*. February, Cardiff: NAW

National Audit Office (1999) *The PFI contract for the new Dartford & Gravesham Hospital*. 1 May, London: NAO

_____ (2000) *The Management and Control of Hospital Acquired Infection in Acute NHS Trusts in England*. February, National Audit Office

_____ (2006) *The Paddington Health Campus scheme*. HC 1045 Session 2005–2006, The Stationery Office, May

National Coalition on Health Care (2004) *Building a Better Health Care System: Specifications For Reform*. Washington, DC: National Coalition on Health Care

National Union of Public Employees (1978) *Under the Axe*. London: NUPE

Navarro V (1983) Radicalism, Marxism and Medicine. *International Journal of Health Services*, 13(2): 179–202

_____ (ed.) (1992) Why the United States does not have a national health program. Amityville, NY: Baywood Publishing

Naylor DC, Jha P, Woods J and Shariff A (1999) A fine balance. Some options for private and public health care in urban India. *Human Development Network*, May, Washington, DC: World Bank

Newbigging R and Lister J (1988) *Privatising health care: the record of private companies in NHS support services*. Association of London Authorities

NHS Confederation (2004) *Practice based commissioning guidance*. Wednesday 15 December

_____ (2005) *Money in the NHS: the facts*. September, available at: http://www.nhsconfed.org/membersarea/downloads/listings1.asp?pid=392 (accessed 27 December 2007)

NHS Emergency Action Committee (1985) *Occupy and Win: A Manual for Fighting Hospital Closures*. London: Emergency Action Committee

NHS Estates (2004) *Revised Guidance on Contracting for Cleaning December*. London: Department of Health

NHS Executive (1994a) *Introduction of Supervisory Registers for Mentally Ill People from 1 April 1994*. London: HMSO

_____ (1994b) *Developing NHS Purchasing and General Practice Fundholding: Towards a Primary-care Led NHS*. EL(94)79, London: NHSE

_____ (1996) *The Spectrum of Care – a Summary of Comprehensive Local Services for People with Mental Health Problems*. London: HMSO

_____ (1998) *The new NHS Modern and Dependable, Developing Primary Care Groups*. HSC 1998/139, 13 August

NHS Health and Social Care Information Centre (2006) *Personal Social Services expenditure and unit costs: England: 2004–2005,* available at: http://www.ic.nhs.uk/statistics-and-data-collections/social-care/adult-social-care-information/personal-social-services-expenditure-and-unit-costs:-england:-2004-2005

NHS London (2007a) *Healthcare for London, consulting the capital*. November, available at: http://www.healthcareforlondon.nhs.uk/pdf/consultingTheCapital.pdf

_____ (2007b) *Better healthcare for London – a capital idea*. Press release, 30 November, available at: http://www.healthcareforlondon.nhs.uk/pressRelease-betterHealthcare.asp (accessed 14 December 2007)

NHS National Leadership Network (2006) *Strengthening Local Services: The Future of the Acute Hospital*

NHS Trust Federation (1996a) *Inner City Mental Health*. London: NHS Trust Federation

_____ (1996b) *Health Trusts Spending £1m a Year Each on GP Paperwork*. London: NHS Trust Federation

NHS Wales (2001) *Improving Health in Wales, a plan for the NHS and its partners*. January, available at: http://www.wales.nhs.uk/Publications/NHSStrategydoc.pdf

_____ (2005) *Designed for Life*. Available at: http://www.wales.nhs.uk/documents/designed-for-life-e.pdf

Nicholl J, Turner J and Dixon S (1995) *The Cost Effectiveness of the Regional Trauma System in the North West Midlands*. University of Sheffield: Medical Care Research Unit

Nicholson D (2007) *The Year*. NHS Chief Executive's annual report. June, London: Department of Health

No Turning Back Group (1988) *The NHS: A Suitable Case for Treatment*. London: Conservative Political Centre

Norfolk A and Lister S (2006) Thousands threatened by oxygen shortage. Woman dies as chaos follows privatisation of vital NHS supplies. *The Times*, 17 February, available at: http://www.timesonline.co.uk/tol/news/uk/health/article731872.ece

North East Thames RHA Consultation Unit (1993) *The St Bartholomews, Royal London and London Chest Hospitals Application for Trust Status*. London: NETRHA

North Essex Health Authority (1997) *Taking the Initiative*. Chelmsford: NEHA

North Thames RHA (1995) *Performance Management report* (9). Mental Health Task Force,

London: NTRHA

Northern Ireland Assembly (2007) *Committee for Health, Social Services and Public Safety Minutes of Proceedings*. 4 June 2007, available at: http://www.niassembly.gov.uk/health/2007mandate/minutes/070614.htm

Northern Ireland Executive (2007) *Building a Better Future Draft Budget 2008–2011*. October, available at: http://www.pfgbudgetni.gov.uk/draftbudget1007new2.pdf

Nowottny S (2007) Practices offered to high-street stores in franchise plan. *Pulse*, 13 November, available at: http://www.pulsetoday.co.uk/story.asp?sectioncode=23&storycode=4115856&c=5 (accessed 10 February 2008)

Nunns A (2006) Derbyshire goes private. *Red Pepper*, March
_____ (2007) *The "Patchwork Privatisation" of our health service: a User's Guide*. Available at: http://www.keepournhspublic.com/pdf/Patchworkprivatisation.pdf

O'Grady S (2007) The Big Question: what is the PFI, and why is it in such trouble on the London Underground? *Independent on Sunday*, 17 July

O'Sullivan E and medical directors (1995) South West Thames Area Provider Advisory Committee Letter to William Wells, Regional Chair, 5 December, London

OECD (2001) *Health At A Glance*. Paris: OECD

OHE (Office of Health Economics) (1981) *Compendium of Statistics*. London: OHE
_____ (1989) *Mental Health in the 1990s: From Custody to Care*. London: OHE

OJEU (Official Journal of the European Union) (2006) Contract Notice: UK-London: management related services. *OJEU* (Supplement), 17 June, S114 121806-2006-EN, ted.europa.eu

OPCS (1991) *Health Survey for England 1991*. London: HMSO
_____ (1995) *Social Trends No 25*. London: HMSO
_____ (1997) *Social Trends No 27*. London: HMSO

Osborne D and Gaebler T (1992) *Reinventing government*. Massachusetts: Addison Wesley

Paige V (1985) *Competitive Tendering. Note to RHAs in improving procedures by DMAs*. London: DHSS

Palmer K (2007) The reconfiguration challenge in SE London: implications for NHS reform policies (Powerpoint presentation). Unpublished, 19 July, London: King's Fund

Parliamentary Labour Party (2006) *Brief from Labour's Health Team*. November

Pater JE (1981) *The making of the National Health Service*. King Edward's Fund for London

Paterson R and Walker M (1997) *A Very Peculiar Practice: The Case Against GP Fundholding*. London: UNISON

Pattanaik S (2007) French election debate dodges healthcare reform. Reuters, Thursday 19 April, available at: http://uk.reuters.com/article/worldNews/idUKL1921092020070419?pageNumber=2&virtualBrandChannel=0&sp=true

Pelling H (1973) *A History of British Trade Unionism*. London: Penguin

Peters DH, Yazbeck AS, Sharma RR, Ramana G, Pritchett LH and Wagstaff A (2002) *Better health systems for India's poor*. Human Developmen Network, Washington, DC: World Bank

Phillips L (2007) Cost of long-term care really hits home. *Daily Mail*, 28 September

Picture of Health (2007) *Project Team perspective on the implications of fixed costs and PFI schemes for service redesign in SE London*. 14 April, available at: http://www.apictureofhealth.nhs.uk/documents/view.aspx?id=38 (accessed 15 December 2007)

Pierson C (1998) *Beyond the Welfare State?* Cambridge: Polity Press

Pillay K (2002) The National Health Bill: a step in the right direction? *ESR Review*, (3)2 September, available at: http://communitylawcentre.org.za/ser/esr2002/2002sept_national.php (accessed 11 June 2004)

Pillay Y (2004) The National Health Bill: Key Issues That Impact On The Public & Private Health Sectors. Paper delivered at Public Health 2004 Conference, 8 June, Durban, available at: http://www.mrc.ac.za/conference

Player S and Leys C (2008) *Confuse & Conceal, The NHS and Independent Sector Treatment Centres*. London: Merlin Press

Plumridge N (2007) Healthy Differences. *Public Finance*, 1–7 June: 18–21

_____ (2008) Better than cure? *Public Finance*, 18–24 January: 20–3

Politics of Health Group (1979) *Cuts and the NHS*. London: BSSRS

Pollitt C (2000) Is the Emperor in his underwear? An analysis of the impacts of public management reform. *Public Management*, Vol.2, No.2 pp.181–99

Pollock AM (1997) *The Private Finance Initiative and the Future of NHS Hospital Development*. London: UNISON

_____ (2001) Will primary care trusts lead to US-style health care? *British Medical Journal*, 322, 21 April.

_____ (2002) *PFI versus democracy*. Lecture to the Regeneration Institute, Cardiff University, available at: http://www.cardiff.ac.uk/news/02-03/021114/lecture.html (accessed 20 October 2003)

_____ (2004) *NHS plc The privatisation of our health care*. London: Verso

Pollock AM and Dunnigan MG (2000) Beds in the NHS: the National Beds Inquiry exposes contradictions in government policy. *British Medical Journal*, 320: 461–2

Pollock AM, Dunnigan M, Gaffney D, Macfarlane A and Majeed FA (1997) What happens when the private sector plans hospital services for the NHS: three case studies under the private finance initiative. *British Medical Journal*, 314: 1,266

Pollock AM, Price D, Viebrock E, Miller E and Watt G (2007) The market in primary care. *British Medical Journal*, Vol.335, pp.475–7, 8 September

Price D (1997) Profiting from closure: the private finance initiative and the NHS. *British Medical Journal*, 315, 6

Price D, Gaffney D and Pollock AM (1999) *The only game in town? A report on the Cumberland Infirmary*. December, London: UNISON

PricewaterhouseCoopers (2005) *Surrey and Sussex Healthcare NHS Trust Public Interest Report*. March, available at: http://www.surreyandsussex.nhs.uk/about_us/documents/public-interest-report.pdf

Project Finance (2006) *Birmingham Hospital*. July/August, available at: http://www.projectfinancemagazine.com/default.asp?page=7&PubID=4&ISS=22232&SID=642152

Public Accounts Committee (2000) *The PFI Contract for the new Dartford and Gravesham Hospital*. Twelfth Report, March

_____ (2007) *Update on PFI Debt Refinancing and the PFI Equity Market*. May

Public Finance (anon) (2007a) News analysis – Data doubts leave social care in the cold. 5 January, available at: http://www.publicfinance.co.uk/search_details.cfm?News_id=29692&keysearch=social%20care

_____ (2007b) *Urgent debate needed on state's role in social care*. 12 January, available at: http://www.publicfinance.co.uk/search_details.cfm?News_id=29748&keysearch=social%20care#email#

Pulse (2006a) PCTs rush to bring in private providers to run GP services. *Pulse*, 8 June, available at: http://www.pulse–i.co.uk/articles/fulldetails.asp?aid=9778 (accessed 14 December 2007)

_____ (2006b) PCTs too poor to bring in GP private providers. Pulse, exclusive, 8 December

Puttick H (2007a) *Protesters plan rally opposing hospital closures*. 8 September, available at: http://www.theherald.co.uk/news/news/display.var.1674596.0.0.php

_____ (2007b) Controversial PFI contracts on hospitals to be detailed. *The Herald*, November 2007, available at: http://www.theherald.co.uk/news/news/display.var.1813994.0.0.php

_____ (2007c) Radical shake-up of health services revealed. *The Herald*, 13

December, available at:
http://www.theherald.co.uk/news/news/display.var.1901223.0.Radical_shakeup_of_health
_services_revealed.php
Radical Statistics Health Group (1976) *Whose Priorities?* London: RSHG
_____ (1987) *Facing the Figures*. London: RSHG
Ranade W (ed.) (1998) *Markets and health care a comparative analysis*. London: Longman
Redwood J and Letwin O (1988) *Britain's Biggest Enterprise: Ideas for Radical Reform of the NHS*. London: Centre for Policy Studies
Reed K (2006) NHS becomes fourth largest consulting market. *Accountancy Age*, 29 September
Relman AS (1980) The new medical-industrial complex. *New England Journal of Medicine*, Vol.303: 17, 963–97, 23 October
Rethink, SANE and Zito Trust (2004) *Behind closed doors*. Available at:
http://www.rethink.org/applications/site_search/search.rm?term=behind+closed+doors&se
archreferer_id=3940 (accessed 26 December 2007)
Revill J (2005) Flagship hospital pays heavy price for independence. *The Observer*, 16 January
_____ (2006) Doctors back mass hospital closures. *The Observer*, 17 September
_____ (2007) He was the architect of Labour's health service reforms. Now he is at the centre of a storm over NHS "privatisation". *The Observer*, 11 November 2007, available at: http://www.guardian.co.uk/politics/2007/nov/11/uk.publicservices
Richardson A and Mmata C (2007) *NHS Maternity Statistics. England: 2005–06*. London: National Statistics Information Centre
Ritchie J, Dick D and Lingham R (1994) *The Report of the Inquiry into the Care and Treatment of Christopher Clunis*. London: HMSO
Rivett G (1986) *Development of the London Hospital System 1823–1982*. London: King's Fund
_____ (1998) *From Cradle to Grave: Fifty Years of the NHS*. London: King's Fund
Robinson R (2002) Who's got the master card? *Health Service Journal*, 26 September, 22–4
Robson J (1973) The Social Consequence of the Professional Dominance in the National Health Service. *International Journal of Health Services*, Vol.3, No.3
Roehr B (2007) US has highest dissatisfaction with health care. *British Medical Journal*, 335: 956 (10 November), doi:10.1136/British Medical Journal.39388.639028.DB
Rokosová M and Háva P (2005) *Czech Republic: Health Care Systems in Transition*. Denmark: WHO European Observatory
Royal College of General Practitioners (1993) *Response to the Tomlinson Report*. London: RCGP
_____ (2004) *The Future of Access to General Practice-based Primary Medical Care – Informing the Debate*. RCGP, June, available at:
http://cms.rcgp.org.uk/staging/pdf/publicationsDatabase/FutureAccess.pdf (accessed 26 December 2007)
Royal College of Psychiatrists (1996) *Report of the Confidential Inquiry into Homicides and Suicides by Mentally Ill People*. London: RCP
_____ (2007) *Briefing for House of Lords debate on the NHS in London*. Royal College of Psychiatrists Press release, available at:
http://www.rcpsych.ac.uk/pdf/RCPSYCH%20HOL%20NHS%20LONDON%20DEBAT
E%2010.10.07.pdf
Royal College of Surgeons of England (1988) *The Management of Patients with Major Injuries*. London: RCS
Royal College of Surgeons (1997) *The provision of Emergency Surgical Services, An organisational Framework*. London: RCS
Royal Commission on Long Term Care (1999) *With Respect to Old Age: Long Term Care – Rights and Responsibilities*. Stationery Office, March, available at:
http://www.archive.official-documents.co.uk/document/cm41/4192/4192.htm

RPA (Review of Public Administration) (2006) *Summary of decisions*. 21 March, available at: http://www.rpani.gov.uk/summary-of-decsions.htm (accessed 1 August 2007)

Russell V (2004) Hospitals need to spend more on cleaning. *Public Finance*, 10–16 December

Sandier S, Paris V and Polton D (2004) *France: Health Care Systems in Transition*. Denmark: WHO European Observatory

Schieber G and Maeda A (1997) A curmudgeon's guide to financing health care in developing countries. In Schieber (1997) *Innovations in Health Care Financing*. World Bank Discussion Paper 365 March, Washington, DC: World Bank

Schofield K (2007) Welcome for rejection of A&E closures proposals. *The Herald*, 13 November, available at: http://www.theherald.co.uk/politics/news/display.var.1828003.0.0.php

Scott F (2007) Superhospitals shock deficit: £40 million. *Coventry Telegraph*, 15 October

Secretary of State for Health (2006) *The government's response to the Health Committee's report on Independent Sector Treatment Centres*. CM 6930, October

Sheldon J (1994) Public service ethos under attack. *Guardian*, 31 January, Section 1: 9

Shifrin T (2004) Pain but no gain. *Guardian*, 25 August

Sikora K (2006) Sorry, Ms Hewitt, the NHS can't go on like this. *Daily Mail*, 25 April

Smith D (2001) Who picks up the bill? *Sunday Times*, 15 July

Smith R (1993) Doctors and markets. *British Medical Journal*, 307: 216–7

_____ (1996a) Being creative about rationing. *British Medical Journal*, 312: 391–92 (17 February)

_____ (1996b) Rationing health care: moving the debate forward. *British Medical Journal*, 312: 1,553–4 (22 June)

_____ (1999) PFI: Perfidious Financial Idiocy. *British Medical Journal*, 318 (3 July)

Social Policy on Ageing Information Network (SPAIN) (2001) *The Underfunding of Social Care and its Consequences for Older People*. London: SPAIN

South Essex Health Authority (1997) 1998/9 *Contracting Round: Chief Executive Paper to Health Authority*. 20 November, Brentwood: SEHA

South West Thames Medical Directors (1996) *Letter to Stephen Dorrell, Health Secretary*. 26 February, London

Stanton T (1992) *Press Statement London Medical Committees*. 7 December, London

Stark Murray D (1971) *Why a National Health Service?: the part played by the Socialist Medical Association*. Pemberton

Stevens S (2004) Reform strategies for the English NHS. *Health Affairs*, 23, 3: 37–44

Stewart J (1999) *The battle for health: a political history of the Socialist Medical Association*. Ashgate

Stone P (ed.) (1980) *British Hospital and Health Care Buildings*. London: Architectural Press

Sussex J (2001) T*he Economics of the Private Finance Initiative in the NHS*. April. London: Office of Health Economics

Swansea Hospitals Trust (2007) *Swansea Infection Control good practice highlighted in WAO report*. 8 November, available at: http://www.wales.nhs.uk/sites3/news.cfm?orgid=100&contentid=7922

Talbot Smith A and Pollock AM (2006) *The New NHS: A Guide*. London: Routledge

Taylor D (1984) *Understanding the NHS in the 1980s*. London: Office of Health Economics

The Information Centre (2007) *General and Personal Medical Services; Medical and Dental Workforce Census; Non-medical Workforce Census*. London: National Statistics Information Centre

Thunhurst (1982) *It makes you sick: the politics of the NHS*. London: Pluto Press

Timmins N (1995) *The Five Giants: A Biography of the Welfare State*. London: Harper Collins

_____ (2002) Warning of spurious figures on value of PFI. *Financial Times*, 5 June

_____ (2005a) Hewitt warns that failing hospitals will be closed. *Financial Times*, 14

May, available at: http://search.ft.com/nonFtArticle?id=050514001329
_____ (2005b) Election 2005: from millions to billions in eight years. *Financial Times*, 19 April
_____ (2006a) How the mighty came to fall. *British Medical Journal*, 332: 628, doi:10.1136/bmj.332.7542.628
_____ (2006b) Hewitt admits need for hospital closures. *Financial Times*, 26 January, available at: http://search.ft.com/ftArticle?queryText=Patricia+Hewitt+AND+reconfiguring&y=4&aje=false&x=9&id=060126001093&ct=0
_____ (2006c) Five named on shortlist for £1bn NHS deals. *Financial Times*, 31 July
_____ (2006d) Watchdog brands profits on PFI scheme unacceptable. *Financial Times*, 3 May, available at: http://www.ft.com/cms/s/0/eb886818-da40-11da-b7de-0000779e2340.html
_____ (2007a) Trust takeover of failed hospital shows way forward. *Financial Times*, 2 April, available at: http://www.ft.com/cms/s/0/253bf6d4-e0b6-11db-8b48-000b5df10621.html (accessed 26 December 2007)
_____ (2007b) Hospitals told to focus on profit centres. *Financial Times*, 12 March, available at: http://www.ft.com/cms/s/0/21f089aa-d03e-11db-94cb-000b5df10621.html
_____ (2007c) Health trusts sitting on £995m in cash. *Financial Times*, 22 August, available at: http://www.ft.com/cms/s/0/1874edba-5047-11dc-a6b0-0000779fd2ac.html
_____ (2007d) No U-turn on reforms of public services, says Hutton. *Financial Times*, 17 May
_____ (2007e) Healthy predictions fall short. *Financial Times*, 30 April: 3
_____ (2007f) PM backs health job offer for US executive. *Financial Times*, 1 May, available at: http://search.ft.com/ftArticle?queryText=Channing+Wheeler&y=8&aje=true&x=15&id=070501000504&ct=0
_____ (2007g) Backing for private sector's NHS role. *Financial Times*, 5 October
_____ (2007h) Hospital building scheme cut by £4bn. *Financial Times*, 1 June
Timmins N, Masters B and Knight R (2007) US health executive offered top NHS role. *Financial Times*, 30 April, available at: http://www.ft.com/cms/s/0/19942f56-f6b7-11db-9812-000b5df10621.html
Titmuss R (1968) *Commitment to Welfare*. London: Allen & Unwin
Tomlinson B (1992) *Report of the Inquiry into London's Health Service, medical Education and Research*. London: HMSO
Toynbee P (2006) This brutal surgery is a godsend for those who wish to kill off the NHS. *Guardian*, 22 September
Tragakes E and Lessof S (2003) *Russian Federation: Health Care Systems in Transition*. Denmark: WHO European Observatory
Trueland J (2007) Scotland health spending flatlining for three years. *Health Service Journal*, 22 November: 12
Turnberg, Sir L (1997) *Health Services in London – A strategic review*. London: Department of Health
UHBFT (2005) *University Hospital Birmingham NHS Foundation Trust Full Business Case Executive Summary*. March, Birmingham
UNISON (1996) PFI in the NHS. *Survey of NHS Trust Chief Executives*. London: UNISON Health Care
_____ (1997) *PFI: Dangers, Realities, Alternatives*. London: UNISON
_____ (2000) *Evidence to the IPPR Commission on Public Private Partnerships*. Section III, August, available at: http://www. unison.org.uk
_____ (2007) *In the interest of patients?* UNISON, January 2007
UNISON Manchester Community and Mental Health (2007) Karen Reissmann: *Overview of the Case*. Available at: http://www.labournet.net/ukunion/0711/karen13.html (accessed 26 December 2007)
United Kingdom Central Council (1997) *The Continuing Care of Older People*. London:

UKCC

United Steel Workers of America (2007) *Labour History Timeline*. Available at: http://uswalocal752l.com/labor_history.htm (accessed 4 November 2007)

University Hospitals Coventry and Warwickshire (2007) *Tomorrow's Healthcare Today, Annual report 2006–7*. Available at: http://www.uhcw.nhs.uk/about/annualreport

Valentine R (1996) *Asylum, Hospital, Haven: A History of Horton Hospital*. London: Riverside Mental Health Trust

Vize R (2007) Payment by results: top-up scheme clears the way for back-door reconfiguration. *Health Service Journal*, 8 November, available at: http://www.hsj.co.uk/opinion/payment_by_results_topup_scheme_clears_the_way_for_ba ckdoor_reconfiguration.html

Vladescu C, Radulescu S and Olsavsky V (2000) *Romania: Health Care Systems in Transition*. Denmark: WHO European Observatory

Walshe K, Smith J, Dixon J, Edwards N, Hunter DJ, Mays N, Normand C and Robinson R (2004) Primary care trusts. *British Medical Journal*, Oct 2004, 329: 871–2, doi:10.1136/bmj.329.7471.871

Wanless D (2001) *Securing our Future Health: Taking a Long-Term View An Interim Report*. HM Treasury, November, available at: http://www.hm-treasury.gov.uk/consultations_and_legislation/wanless/consult_wanless_interimrep.cfm

_____ (2002) *Securing our Future Health: Taking a Long-Term View Final Report*. HM Treasury, April

_____ (2003) *The Review of Health and Social Care in Wales The Report of the Project Team advised by Derek Wanless*. June, available at: http://www.hsmc.bham.ac.uk/torfaen/Wanless%20Welsh%20Review.pdf

Ward J (1995) Reality gap in the health service. *Guardian*, 28 January: 24

Ward S (2005) Questions over PFI follow Paddington failure. *Public Finance*, 1–7 July: 12

WCMH (Wales Collaboration for Mental Health) (2005) *Under Pressure*. NHS Wales, August, available at: http://www.wales.nhs.uk/documents/EnglishUnderPressureReportAug05.pdf

Webster C (1988) *The Health Services Since the War*, Vol.1. London: HMSO

_____ (1991) *Bevan on the National Health Service*. Oxford: Wellcome

_____ (ed.) (1993) *Caring for Health: History and Diversity*. Buckingham: Open University Press

_____ (1996) *The Health Services since the war*. London: Stationery Office, Vol.2: 99

_____ (2002) *The National Health Service: A Political History*. Oxford: Oxford University Press

West Berkshire Health Authority (1997) *New Services for the Elderly, Elderly Mentally Infirm and Ill*. Reading: WBHA

West Hertfordshire Health Authority (1997) *Moving Forward: Choosing the Right Direction for Health and Health Services*. St. Albans: WHHA

West Midlands Health Service Monitoring Unit (1987) *Birmingham's Health Needs and Resources*. Birmingham: WMHSMU

White M (2005) Hewitt challenge to £1bn Bart's plan raises NHS finance fears. *Guardian*, 28 December

Whitehead M (1992) *The Health Divide*. London & New York: Penguin

_____ (1994) Is it fair? Evaluating the equity effects of the NHS Reforms. In Robinson R and LeGrand J (eds) *Evaluating the NHS Reforms*. London: King's Fund Institute

Whitfield L (2005) Not such a swell party. *Public Finance*, 22–5, 29 July–4 August

Whittington Hospital (1992) *Application for Trust Status*. London: Whittington Hospital

WHO (2006) *Working Together for Health (World Health Report 2006)*. Geneva: WHO

Willetts D and Goldsmith M (1988) *A Mixed Economy for Health Care: More Spending Same Taxes*. London: Centre for Policy Studies

Williams J and Ham C (2006) Cut and thrust: how Wales went its own way. *Health Service*

Journal, 3 August, 18–19

Wintour P and Carvel J (2006) Leaked paper reveals Labour fears on NHS. *Guardian*, 5 December

Wise J (1996) Sick doctors need special treatment. *British Medical Journal*, 313: 771 (28 September)

Worcestershire Health Authority (1998) *Investing in Excellence*. Worcester: WHA

Yates D, Woodford M and Hollis S (1990) Preliminary analysis of the care of injured patients in 33 British hospitals: first report of the UK major trauma outcome study. *British Medical Journal*, 305: 737–40

INDEX

A

Academy of Medical Royal
  Colleges 316
Accenture 239
accountability 7, 24, 27, 40,
  53–4, 60, 117, 127, 152–4,
  188, 215, 254, 276, 312
Adam Smith Institute 61, 154
Addenbrookes Hospital 57, 105,
  203
additionality 226
administrative staff 41, 53, 59,
  79, 83, 90, 96, 122, 141, 172,
  230, 238, 249, 251, 286, 307
Aetna 201
Age Concern 116
Agenda for Change 56, 174
AIDS 94, 316
Alternative Provider Medical
  Services (APMS) 279
Alzheimer's Disease Society
  102
American (USA) 76, 97, 146,
  184, 238, 296
ancillary 55, 56, 58–9, 82, 223,
  224, 245, 259
Anglian Harbours Trust 118
Appointments Commission 152
Area Health Authorities (AHA)
  40–1, 44, 46, 53–4
Asda 202, 239, 288
assertive outreach 143
Association of London
  Authorities (ALA) 102
Association of Metropolitan
  Authorities 105
AT Kearney 239
Atos Healthcare 234
Audit Commission 67, 71–2, 98,
  142, 237, 240, 270
Australia 294
Austria 292, 294

B

Bacon, John 183, 281
bad debt 65
Banstead Hospital 39, 70, 106
Barber, Anthony 39–40
Barking and Havering 93, 96,
  262–3
Barking Hospital
  strike 56
Barnet 58, 91, 98, 113, 247, 250
Bart's Hospital 129
Beckett, Margaret 125
beds
  Beds Inquiry 136–7, 248

blocking 46, 102, 105, 109,
  116, 150
Belfast 207
Belgium 292–3
benchmark 103, 126, 146, 150,
  255
Better Services for the Mentally
  Ill 70
Bevan, Aneurin 2, 15
Beveridge 2, 4, 28, 293
Bexley Care Trust 149
Birmingham 73, 79, 96, 99, 100,
  156–7, 170, 186, 202, 233,
  237, 239, 257, 261, 264, 288
Black Report 49–52
Blackpool 65
Blair, Tony 1, 7, 89, 112, 125,
  133, 135, 137, 145, 159, 167,
  168, 175, 177, 181–2, 187,
  189, 190, 194–5, 202, 205,
  216, 218, 223–4, 227, 233,
  239, 260, 273, 280, 305, 307,
  310
Bloomsbury 65, 90
Blue Arrow 57
Blunkett, David 86
Bogle, Ian 109, 272
Bolkestein directive 308
Bonham Carter Report 100
Bottomley, Virginia 95–6, 97,
  107, 123, 129, 130, 187, 271,
  277
Bradford Hospitals 158
Braine, Bernard 3
Brazil 297–8
Brent and Harrow 98, 191, 249,
  283
Bristol 165, 257, 263
British Medical Association 14
  BMA 19–20, 33, 64, 75, 78,
  84–5, 101, 102, 105, 109,
  110, 115, 125, 131, 154, 161,
  171, 187, 198, 230, 231, 234,
  268–9, 272, 273, 284, 309–12
Brittan, Leon 63, 76
Bro Morgannwg 215
Bromley 58, 196, 199, 203, 240,
  248, 249, 256
Brown, Gordon 1, 7, 89,
  114–15, 120, 122, 125, 133,
  137, 159, 162, 164, 167, 173,
  180, 189, 190, 192, 194–5,
  197, 200, 224, 227, 282, 305,
  309, 310, 316
Bulgaria 292, 295
BUPA 60, 62, 66, 128, 183, 185,
  188, 229, 238
Bureaucracy 4, 59, 82–3, 110,

  113, 117, 122, 139, 152, 179,
  231, 271
Burnley 73, 79
By Accident or Design 98

C

Calman Report 100
Camden 192, 283
Cameron 4, 186, 316
Canada 229, 301
cancer 16, 33, 34, 49, 69, 73,
  111, 174, 216, 223, 304
Capio 156
capital
  charges 84, 124, 244, 245
  investment 21, 24, 39, 47,
    194, 239, 244, 245, 250
  shortage 21–2, 78
  stock 16, 21, 34, 35, 242
capitation funding 44, 115
Cardiff 95, 209, 212, 213, 215
Care First 128
Care in the Community 66, 70,
  91, 189
Care Programme Approach 107
Caring for People 80
Carlisle 206, 236, 239, 248, 251,
  256
Carlton Club 63
cash-limit 45, 54, 67, 81, 102,
  103, 113, 121, 123, 126, 146,
  273, 274, 275, 279
catchment 27, 35, 41, 97, 99,
  100, 101–2, 149, 187, 243, 274
catering 39, 56, 57, 95, 124,
  142, 250, 257, 314
Central Manchester 73, 260
Central Middlesex Hospital 314
Centre for Policy Studies 62, 76,
  77
Charing Cross Hospital 92,
  95,111, 36
charities 34, 83, 144, 188, 258
Chase Farm Hospital 99
Cheltenham 186, 187
Chessells, Tim 95
Chichester 186
Child B (Jaymee Bowen) 112
Chinese Revolution 295
Churchill, Sir Winston 31, 269
Cinderella service 106
City and East London 58, 90,
  93, 94, 96, 98, 110, 149, 157,
  164, 191, 196, 218, 240–1,
  251, 261, 263, 281
Clarke , Kenneth 21, 58, 59, 60,
  79, 80, 85, 87, 89, 105–6,
  114, 120, 223, 239

class 2, 11, 13, 19, 26, 30, 43, 49–51, 57, 64, 87, 291, 295
Clean Hospitals Programme 140
Clinicenta 236
Clunis, Christopher 107
Code of Conduct 313
COHSE 39, 77, 79, 89, 91, 93
Colchester 116, 185, 262
commercial secrecy 23
commissioning
    Patient-Led NHS 171, 177, 280
Community Care
    Agenda for Action 85
Community Health Councils (CHCs) 27, 40, 46, 53, 81, 91, 110, 152, 171
competition 4, 77, 82–3, 120, 139, 141, 160, 168, 182, 200, 205, 207, 216, 217, 232, 234, 274, 315
competitive tendering 55, 56, 82, 139, 141, 214, 223
computerisation 307
concessions 2, 17, 18, 20, 32, 80, 85, 154, 224, 296
Concordat 151, 228–9
consensus 2, 4, 7, 23, 41–2, 49, 53, 59, 61, 140, 153, 206, 208, 243, 271, 293
constitution for the NHS 1, 3, 295, 309, 310
consultation 12, 32, 49, 74, 103–4, 131, 157, 172, 177, 179, 193, 201, 212–13, 215, 220, 254, 263, 267, 271, 274, 281, 282, 283, 286, 303, 310
contestability 135, 195, 200, 207, 226, 232, 234
continuing care 66, 85–6, 91, 102–5, 109, 115–16, 126–8, 145, 151, 190, 312
contracting out 56, 57, 77, 223
contracts 56
Cook, Robin 78, 86
cooperation 23, 120, 123, 150, 274, 311
cooperatives 5, 278
Cornwall 165, 187
cost improvement programme 61, 250
Coventry 73, 241, 248
Cox, Alfred 19
creative destruction 161, 182
Crisp, Sir Nigel 171–2, 177–9, 280–1
cross-border health care 308
Crossman, Richard 39, 44, 100
Crothalls 56, 58
Currie, Edwina 78, 86
Czechoslovakia 295

D

Dartford 247–8, 251–6
Darzi, Lord Ara 2, 197–203, 216, 220, 236, 239, 243, 282–9, 310
Dawson, Lord 13, 268, 282
day centre 71, 105, 283
decommodified 6
Delivering the NHS Plan 135, 138, 150
Deloitte 239
democratic deficit 313
Denmark 292, 312
dentistry 8–9, 20, 26, 29–31, 39, 52, 75, 267, 268, 276, 300
Derby City General 118
Designed for Life 209–11, 215
Diagnostic & Treatment Centres 151
District Health Authorities (DHAs) 53, 66, 117, 270, 273, 275, 307
divest 177, 178, 306
Dobson, Frank 113–15, 117, 126, 128–30, 136, 154, 260, 273
Doctors for Reform 3, 4, 311
domestic 5, 56–9, 115, 139, 214, 283
domiciliary services 87, 148
Doncaster 73
Dorrell, Stephen 108, 110–11, 127, 128
Downe Hospital 208
downsize 46
drugs 31–3, 37, 42, 95, 121, 122, 131, 144, 165, 174, 220, 305, 315
Dudley 249

E

Eastbourne 186
Edgware Hospital 58, 95, 99, 112, 113–14
Edinburgh 95, 218, 252, 253, 257, 259, 264
Edinburgh Royal Infirmary 218, 252, 253, 259
elective operations 151–2, 161, 196, 224–6, 228, 234, 280
Electronic Patient Record 307
eligibility criteria 103, 105, 116, 146, 148, 189, 283, 306
Elizabeth Garrett Anderson Hospital 46
Elliott, Larry 125
Elwell, Hugh 62
Emergency Medical Service 14, 217
emergency services 76, 97, 181, 187, 199, 217, 303

enabling act 315
Ennals, David 49–50
Enniskillen and Omagh Hospital 208–9
Enthoven, Alain 80–1
Epsom 99, 186, 235, 263
Epsom and St Helier hospitals 99, 186, 235, 263
Essex Rivers 116, 185, 262
estate 42, 245–6
European Observatory on Health Care Systems 162
European Union 133, 307
European Working Time Directive 174
eye tests 52, 75

F

Falkirk and Stirling Royal Infirmaries 218, 257
Fallon, Michael 77
Family Health Services Authority (FHSA) 96
Family Practitioner Services (FPS) 44, 72
flag-days 15
Foley, Sheila 149
for-profit 179, 185, 188, 190, 226, 231, 279, 281
Forth, Eric 77
Foundation Trusts 54, 154–76, 193–4, 196, 197, 205, 207, 216, 227, 235, 236, 238–9, 264, 306, 311, 312
Fowler, Norman 60, 67
Fox, Liam 231
Fox, Marcus 58
frail elderly 46, 66, 67, 85, 102–4, 115, 277
Framework for Procuring External Support for Commissioners (FESC) 238
France 4, 292, 293, 309
franchising 75, 153, 156, 228, 236–7
free personal care 206, 215, 220–1
Froggatt, Clive 76

G

Gaitskell, Hugh 29
geriatric beds 66–7, 91, 117, 127, 141, 147, 190
Germany 4, 19, 30, 292, 308
Giddens, Anthony 145
gift economy 23
Glasgow 58, 95, 217–18, 257
Gloucestershire 102, 106, 116
Godber, Sir George 24
Goldsmith, Michael 76
Good Hope Hospital 79, 156, 237

Goodenough Report 14
GP fundholders 81, 123
Greece 32, 113, 115
Green, David 77
Griffiths, Peter 88, 110
Griffiths, Roy 59, 67, 76, 80,
    85–7, 104, 106, 147, 190
Griffiths Now! 104
    Report 85–6, 106, 147, 190
Grossman, Lloyd 142
Guillebaud Committee 28, 30–1,
    34–5, 41, 242
Guy's Hospital 45, 83, 88, 90,
    92, 95, 99, 110, 128–9, 157
Gwent 211–13, 215

H

Hairmyres Hospital 218
Hamilton, Neil 77
Hammersmith Hospital 57, 165,
    235
Harman, Harriet 191
Harris, Nigel 73
Hart, Edwina 213, 215
Hastings 186
Health Action Zones (HAZs)
    120–1
health care closer to home 136,
    182
health centres 6, 21, 268–9, 303,
    314
Health Dialog Services 201
Health Economy Foundation
    Trust (HEFT) 311
health insurance 3, 11–12, 14,
    20, 60–4, 76, 133, 293–7,
    299, 301
Health Maintenance
    Organisation (HMO) 76, 80
Health Services Act 1980 55, 64
Healthcare Financial
    Management Association
    (HFMA) 113, 132
Heart of Birmingham PCT 202,
    239, 288
Heartland Institute 4
Heath, Edward 39
Help the Aged 116
Hemel Hempstead 46, 196, 236
Hertfordshire 46, 99–100, 132,
    196, 236, 262–3
Hewitt, Patricia 166–92, 196,
    224, 232–4, 260–1
Hillingdon Hospital 112, 238,
    263
Hinchingbrooke Hospital 194,
    227
Hoffenberg, Sir Raymond 73
Homerton Hospital 157
Horton General Hospital
    (Banbury) 118

Horton Hospital Surrey 37–8, 70
Hospital Acquired Infection
    (HAI) 140
Hospital Alert 73
Hospital Hygiene Services 58
Hospital Management
    Committees 21, 23, 26, 40
Hospital Plan for England &
    Wales 1962 35, 43, 242–3
Howe, Sir Geoffrey 53
Humana 201, 238
Hungary 32, 294
Hutton, John 195, 227, 279

I

ICATS 207, 236
Independent Reconfiguration
    Panel 152
Independent Sector Treatment
    Centres (ISTCs, ITCs) 151,
    160, 175, 183, 196, 201–2,
    224–30, 236
India 301–2
Institute of Directors 154
Institute of Economic Affairs 77
Institute of Health Services
    Management 102
International Monetary Fund
    (IMF) 44
inverse care law 11–12, 21, 44,
    49, 51, 200, 226
IPPR 187
Ipswich 118
Italy 32, 291–3, 298

J

Japan 294, 297
Jarman, Brian 93, 114
Jenkin, Patrick 49–55
Jennifer's Ear 91
Joffe, Joel 145
John Radcliffe Hospital, Oxford
    59
Johnson, Alan 1, 199, 220,
    237–8
Joseph, Sir Keith 40, 53, 62
Jowell, Tessa 96, 191

K

Keep Our NHS Public 9, 187,
    281, 305, 312, 315–16
Kenya 300
Kerr, David 216–17
Kidderminster 235, 248, 253,
    261
King George's Hospital 99, 263
King's College Hospital 87, 98,
    157
King's Fund 45, 72, 76, 93–8,
    136, 138, 175, 198, 206, 271
Kingston Hospital 119, 202

Klein, Rudolf 23, 29–32, 42, 44,
    54, 89, 92, 118–121, 137,
    153, 268–9
Korean War 29

L

Langlands, Alan 109, 272
Largactil 33, 37
Lawson, Nigel 72, 75
Leadership Centre for Health
    152
learning disabilities 8
Leeds 73, 79, 103, 118, 165
Leigh, Edward 62, 77, 195, 258
Lelliott, Paul 144
Letwin, Oliver 77
Lewisham and North Southwark
    54, 65, 128, 164–5, 169, 196,
    199, 240, 264, 283
LIFT 15, 60, 75, 186, 224, 228,
    240, 287, 307
Lipsey, David 145
Lisbon Treaty 309
Liverpool 95–6, 263
lobby of Parliament 188
Local Government Act 15
Local Involvement Networks
    153, 307
London
    Health Economics
        Consortium 93
    Health Planning Consortium
        92
    Implementation Group (LIG)
        95, 98, 130
    Initiative Zone 96
    London Study 93
London Bridge train crash 95
long-term care 2, 69, 90, 96,
    128, 145

M

Maidstone and Tunbridge Wells
    58, 141–2, 263
Major, John 7, 75, 92, 118, 124,
    224
Making it Happen 188
malaria 37, 292, 300
managed care 80, 81
management consultants 6, 61,
    141, 159, 180, 228, 238–9,
    248, 253–4, 306, 311, 314
Manchester 73–5, 79, 96, 149,
    165, 186, 191, 199, 207, 245,
    247, 260
Maudsley Hospital 79, 191
Maxwell, Robert (King's Fund)
    76–7
Maynard, A 113, 123
McKinsey's 185, 238–9
McNalty, Sir Arthur 22

Meacher, Michael 66
means-test 2, 16, 62, 67, 83–7, 128, 144, 146, 150, 190, 220
Mediclean
ISS 57, 214
Mental Capacity Act 151
mental health
    asylums 16, 36–7, 39, 42
    community-based care 36, 243
    Mental Health Forum 2007 192
    specific grant 107
merit payments 18
Merton and Sutton 65, 131–2, 283
    and Wandsworth 131–2
Metronet 264
Middlesex Hospital 155, 235, 258
Milburn, Alan 103, 114, 125, 135–40, 148–57, 216, 228, 248–50, 254–5, 261, 273
Mind 8, 36–7, 70, 192
Minor Accident Treatment Services 99
Minor Injury Units 99, 285
Modern Matrons 140
Modernisation Agency 152
Monitor 42, 103, 154, 156, 159, 169, 193, 218, 238, 264, 306
Monklands 217–18
Moore, John 74–5
Morgan, Rhodri 205, 213–14
Morrison, Herbert 17
Mount Vernon Hospital 99, 112
Moyes, Bill 169–70, 193
MRSA 140–2
Murphy, Elaine 88
mutuals 5, 154

N

National Audit Office 140, 174, 254, 263
National Health Insurance Act 1911 11
National Institute for Clinical Excellence (NICE) 121, 165
National Service Frameworks 121
nationalisation 3, 6, 13, 42, 242, 294–5
Netcare 196, 219, 231
Netherlands 294
New Public Management 61, 121, 135
New Zealand 292
Newcastle 73, 154
Newham General Hospital 129
Newton, Tony 73, 75, 78

NHS
    and Community Care Bill 80, 85
    Confederation 170, 172–4, 181, 218
    Institution for Innovation and Improvement 152
    Logistics 186
    Support Federation 110, 273
    Together 21, 80, 85, 106, 135, 141, 148, 186, 285, 315
    Trust Federation 108, 110
Nichol, Sir Duncan 112
Nightingale, Florence 59
No Turning Back group 77
Norfolk and Norwich Hospital 118, 166, 175, 203, 252, 254, 256, 259
Normansfield 39
North Derbyshire
    Langwith 281
North Durham 247, 248, 251, 254, 256, 258
North Essex 132, 193
Northern Ireland
    Stormont 7, 206
    Unionist 7
Northern Rock 136, 315
Northwick Park Hospital 87
Nuffield Orthopaedic Centre 90

O

O'Brien, Mike 118
O'Donnell, Gus 195, 220
occupational health 9, 25, 47
OCS 57
Octagon 252–3
OECD 6, 113, 115, 137, 293
Omega Report 61–2
One Wales 214–15
Ophthalmic services 5, 31, 232
opticians 26, 267
opting out 54, 81, 83, 90, 270
Oxfordshire 115–16, 153, 170–3, 191, 230–1, 278
    Eye Hospital 153, 230, 278
Oxford 116, 153, 170, 230, 278

P

Paddington Health Campus 259, 261
Paige Victor 58, 60
Panorama 74
Patel, Chai 145
paternalism 26
Patient
    Advocacy and Liaison Services 152
    and Public Involvement Forums 142, 152, 307

Environment Action Teams 14–1
Patients Awaiting Appropriate Facilities Elsewhere (PAAFE) 126
Patients Charter 77
payment by results
    PBR 159, 168, 194, 225, 241
Peach, Len 60
pharmacists 26, 276, 295
Pinker, George 73–4
PMS contract 273
poaching 111, 156, 181, 231
Poland 295
Pollock, Allyson 4, 116, 121, 135, 145, 218, 240, 245, 256, 264, 268–9, 273–4, 277–9, 282, 288
polyclinic 199, 284–8
poor law 11, 19, 291
Portugal 32, 113, 115, 154, 294
Powell, Enoch
    Hospital Plan 35, 242
    prescription charge 35
    water tower speech 36–7, 106
Powys 214
Practice-based commissioning 172, 189, 279, 288, 307, 312
Prescott, John 115
prescription
    charges 5, 29, 31–2, 35, 39, 41, 51–2, 67, 209, 215
Primary Care Groups (PCGs) 120, 122–3, 153, 273–7, 307
Primary Care Trusts (PCTs) 27, 122, 143, 146, 153, 155, 161–2, 167–71, 173, 178, 180, 184–90, 196, 201–2, 231, 234, 274–80, 307–8, 312
private beds
    in NHS hospitals 18
Private Finance Initiative (PFI) 7, 35, 124–5, 136, 151, 164, 180, 186, 194–7, 203, 214, 224, 228, 239, 244, 260–1, 305
psychiatric beds 38, 69, 71, 121
purchaser–provider split 7, 120, 122, 172, 207, 215, 274–5, 311–12

Q

quangos 54, 88, 95, 120, 130, 152, 276
Queen Elizabeth Hospital, Woolwich 240
Queen Mary's Hospital, Roehampton 95, 99, 112, 119
Queen Mary's Sidcup 199
Queen's Hospital Romford 73, 125, 262

R

Rational Way Forward 309
rationing
  debate 112
  materials 34
  treatment 28, 112
Reckitts 57
Redbridge 78, 96, 263, 283
  and Waltham Forest 96
Redhill 229
Redwood, John 77
Reed Report 107
Reeves, Colin 72, 132
referral management centres 183
Regional Health Authorities
  (RHAs) 41, 43, 53–4, 97,
  117, 123, 153, 171
Regional Hospital Boards 21
Regional Offices 123, 153, 307
regional trauma centres 97
Regulator 22, 154, 156, 158–9,
  169, 172, 238, 264, 306
Reid, John 140, 159, 161, 167,
  224
Reissmann, Karen 149, 191
Renton, Timothy 62
residential care 71, 86, 106,
  146–8
Resource Allocation Budgeting
  (RAB) 159, 166
Resources Allocation Working
  Party (RAWP) 43
Retention of Employment 249
Rethink 144
Revised Guidance on
  Contracting for Cleaning 139,
  141
Romania 295
Romford 112, 129, 262–4
Royal College of Psychiatrists
  108, 143
Royal College of Surgeons
  (RCS) 73, 97, 101, 187, 200
Royal Commission
  1926 14
  1979 41, 53–4
  and 1959 Mental Health Act
  37
  on Long Term Care 1999 144
  on Lunacy and Mental
  Disorder 37
Royal Free Hospital 36, 244
Russia 32, 291

S

Sainsbury Centre for mental
  health 144, 191
salaried GPs 268, 285, 314
Scarsdale Hospital 57
Scotland 7, 13, 27, 47, 73, 205,
  215–21, 257–9, 312

Secta 237
Sefton 106
Selbie, Duncan 177
self-governing hospitals 83–4
Semashko 292, 295
Shropshire 73
Sikora, Karel 3–4
Silcock, Ben 107
Skanska Innisfree 260–1
Smee, Clive 117, 136–7
social care waiters 126
Social Security Act 67, 293
Socialist Health Association 2,
  17, 268–9
Socialist Medical Association 2,
  17, 25, 49, 268
Solihull 73
South Africa 183, 196, 219, 229,
  231, 298–9
South Essex 132
Spain 113, 115, 154, 294, 308
St Goran's 156
St Mary's Hospital, Paddington
  73, 90
St Thomas Hospital 45, 92, 95,
  157
stakeholders 157
Standardised Mortality Ratios
  (SMRs) 44, 215
steady state 88–9, 111
Stevens, Simon 135, 202
Stobhill and Victoria hospitals
  218
Stracathro Hospital 219
Strategic Health Authorities
  (SHA) 27, 153, 171, 177,
  183, 307
Sturgeon, Nicola 217–21
Sunlight 57
Surrey and Sussex 39, 166, 170,
  229
Sutherland Commission 145
SW London Elective
  Orthopaedic Centre
  (SWLEOC) 199, 235
Swansea 212–15
Sweden 32, 150, 154, 156,
  291–2, 294, 312
Swindon 246, 259

T

targets
  bed quota 46
  contradictory 180, 231
  performance 60, 138, 173,
  192
tariff 52, 161, 177, 194, 216,
  225, 231, 241, 306
Tebbit, Norman 3
Tesco 202, 239, 288
Thames Regions 92–3

Thatcher, Margaret 3, 7, 40, 47,
  49–53, 61, 63, 72, 74–6,
  80–1, 85, 87, 92, 120, 154,
  156, 160, 163, 190, 198, 223,
  311
third sector 5, 22, 121, 188–9
Todd, Ian 73
Tomlinson, Sir Bernard
  (Tomlinson Report) 89, 92–5,
  98, 114, 130, 198, 271–2
trade unions 5–6, 11, 125, 149,
  186, 198, 292, 296, 313–15
transitional funding 89
Trauma Centres 97, 198
Treasury 63, 75–6, 122, 124–5,
  159, 162, 174, 203, 208,
  244–5, 255, 264, 315
trolleys crisis 1995–6, 111
Trust Boards 27, 84, 119
tuberculosis (TB) 49, 292
TUC
  day of action on NHS pay 55
Tudor Hart, Julian 12, 30, 44,
  49, 51, 267, 268
Turnberg, Sir Leslie 114, 129,
  130

U

Uganda 300
Under Pressure 28–9, 87, 97,
  114, 127, 211, 213, 271, 281,
  306
under-doctored areas 12, 273,
  279, 314
unitary charge 124, 218, 240–2,
  252, 254, 261, 264, 306
United Health 176, 179, 183–5
United Kingdom Central
  Council
  UKCC (now Nursing and
  Midwifery Council) 126
University College Hospital
  Trust 155, 157, 235, 248
University Hospital for
  Birmingham 261
University Hospitals of North
  Staffordshire Trust 179, 262
Urgent Treatment Centres 99
user fees 31–2, 299–301, 311

V

Virgin 202, 239, 288
voluntary
  hospital 12, 14–16, 21, 26,
  37, 155, 178
  sector 5, 11–12, 14–15, 69,
  86, 127, 151, 172, 178, 188,
  279

W

Wakefield 80, 86, 204

Waldegrave,.William 82, 96
Wales
    National Assembly 32, 205,
        209, 211–12
Walsall Hospital Trust 262
Wandsworth 131–2, 283
Wanless, Sir Derek 2, 136, 147,
        162–3, 173, 209
Warner, Lord Norman 140, 156,
        182
Webster, Charles 20, 24, 27–8,
        31, 242
Wellhouse Trust 91, 113, 250
Welsh Assembly 5, 7, 205, 209,
        214
Welwyn Garden City 27
West Berkshire 91
West Midlands 73, 79, 87, 176,
        236, 288
Western Provident Association
        66
Wheeler, R. Channing 195, 202,
        228
Whittington Hospital 129, 142
Willetts, David 76
winter crisis (1987–8) 66, 78–9
Wishaw Hospital 218
Worcestershire 101, 248, 250,
        253–4, 256, 261
workers' control 313
Working for Patients 80, 270
working-to-contract 79
World Trade Organisation
        (WTO) 307
World War ll 293–6
Worthing 186

Y

Yorkshire 73, 79, 233, 254, 263

Z

Zito, Jonathan 107, 144